Death, Posthumous Harm, and Bioethics

Routledge Annals of Bioethics

Series Editors: MARK J. CHERRY, *St. Edward's University, USA*
ANA SMITH ILTIS, *Wake Forest University, USA*

Death, Posthumous Harm, and Bioethics

James Stacey Taylor

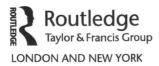
Routledge
Taylor & Francis Group

LONDON AND NEW YORK

First published 2012
by Routledge
711 Third Avenue, New York, NY 10017

Simultaneously published in the UK
by Routledge
2 Park Square, Milton Park, Abingdon, Oxfordshire OX14 4RN

First issued in paperback 2014

*Routledge is an imprint of the Taylor & Francis Group,
an informa business*

Library of Congress Cataloging-in-Publication Data
Taylor, James Stacey, 1970–
    Death, posthumous harm, and bioethics / James Stacey Taylor.
      p. cm. — (Routledtge annals of bioethics)
    Includes bibliographical references (p.) and index.
  1. Death.   2. Death—Moral and ethical aspects.   3. Respect for
persons.   4. Dead.   5. Bioethics.   I. Title.
    BD444.T39 2012
    128'.5—dc23
    2012002725

ISBN 978-0-415-51884-0 (hbk)
ISBN 978-1-138-89157-9 (pbk)
ISBN 978-0-203-10642-6 (ebk)

Typeset in Sabon
by IBT Global.

For Oliver

8th January 1976–2nd May 2011.

Contents

Acknowledgments

This volume has been several years in the making, during which time I have accumulated many intellectual and personal debts associated with its writing. The most significant of these is owed to the Social Philosophy & Policy Center at Bowling Green State University, which graciously invited me to spend the summer of 2007 in residence as a Visiting Scholar. If there actually is a Platonic Form of the ideal place to engage in academic work the Policy Center would be its closest earthly approximation. Dedicated to intellectual pursuits, its quiet broken only by the tapping of computer keys, the occasional hum of conversation on research topics, and the soft padding of research assistants bringing in requested books and articles, the Policy Center is a wonderful place to study and write. My sincere thanks go out to Fred D. Miller, Jr., Ellen Frankel Paul, and Jeffrey Paul, the Directors of the Center, as well as to its staff, Tamara Sharp, Terrie Weaver, and Mary Dilsaver. Thanks, also, to Ben Dyer and Richard McNeillie, who served as my research assistants that summer, and whose dedication and diligence (and impressive ability to secure the often obscure articles and books that I requested, frequently within mere hours of my asking!) greatly aided my writing. I hope though, that the production of this volume is itself the best way to thank the Center, for it was during my tenure there that the bulk of it was written, including drafts of Chapters 2 through 7, inclusive, and a draft of Chapter 9.

In addition to the support that I have received from the Social Philosophy & Policy Center I have also received considerable institutional support from The College of New Jersey. My first thanks here go to my colleagues in the Department of Philosophy and Religion—Joanne Cantor, Holly Haynes, Richard Kamber, Pierre Le Morven, Consuelo Preti, Melinda Roberts, and Morton Winston—for uniformly contributing to a wonderfully collegial and congenial atmosphere in which to work. My thanks, too, to the College for providing me with research leave each year through the Support of Scholarly Activities program. I have also been fortunate to have had the opportunity to discuss the issues addressed in Chapters 1–3 and 5 with my students in four Freshman Seminars at the College of New Jersey during the Fall semesters of 2006 and 2011. It is a tribute to the students in those

xii *Acknowledgments*

Seminars that there were conducted at a level that would be considered to be suitable for graduate work at some other institutions. I thank both the students of those Seminars for their invigorating discussions of these issues, and also to the College's students in general for their contribution to its rigorous and collegial intellectual climate.

I also thank the Institute for Humane Studies for support during the writing of this volume through giving me the opportunity to have stimulating and cross-disciplinary conversations on these issues that I would otherwise have missed out on. Thanks, too, are owed both to the Departments of Moral Philosophy and of Logic and Metaphysics at the University of St. Andrews and to the Department of Philosophy at Bowling Green State University, for generating and fostering my interest in well-being during both my undergraduate and postgraduate studies.

I have also benefitted from presenting aspects of my work on these issues to various audiences. Thanks to the Economics Departments at New York University and George Mason University both for indulging my discussions of posthumous organ conscription and its relationship to the postmortem ownership of organs—and for their trenchant and (very, very) helpful criticisms of my views in these areas. Thanks, too, to my audiences at Bowling Green State University, the 2010 Central Division meeting of the American Philosophical Association, and at Princeton Theological Seminary for their thoughtful and helpful comments on my work.

I have also been greatly helped in formulating my ideas on the metaphysical and bioethical issues surrounding death that I address in this volume through conversations with many people, including (but, obviously, not limited to) Paul Bentley, Paul Tudico, James Spence, Jason Grinnell, Francois Raffoul, Mary Sirridge, Greg Shrufreider, Chris Belshaw, David Benatar, Stephan Blatti, Griffin Trotter, Tom Bell, Mark Pennington, Glen Whitman, Larry White, Geoffrey Scarre, James Worth, Gordon Graham, Barbara Baum Levenbook, R. G. Frey, Michael Gill, Aaron Spital, Ben Hippen, Mark J. Cherry, Sam Zinaich, Adam Engel, Alex Sisko, Neil Tennent, Harry Silverstein, Stephen Winter, Kai Draper, Jens Johansson, Walter Glannon, Josie Fisher, Margaret P. Battin, Tom Beauchamp, Jim Childress, Mark Bernstein, Charles Griswold, Daniel Sperling, Alastair V. Campbell, Pete Boettke, Russell DiSilvestro, Marina A. L. Oshana, Stephen Rosenbaum, John Hardwig, David Friedman, Gillian Haddow, Ben Bradley, Steven Luper, Martha Nussbaum, Don Marquis, Jeff McMahan, Katariina Mustakallio, Doug Portmore, C. G. Prado, James Warren, and T. M. Wilkinson, many of whom graciously provided me with copies of their unpublished work on the issues that I address in this volume. I thank, too, Routledge's anonymous referee for this volume who kindly provided me with extensive and very helpful suggestions on how to improve it, and who saved me from several philosophical infelicities.

Since I am defending an Epicurean approach to these thanatological and bioethical issues I would be remiss were I not to thank Fred D. Miller,

Jr., for his extreme patience in teaching me Greek over the course of several years during my graduate work at Bowling Green State University. No doubt he will be worried to hear that (unless otherwise indicated) all of the translations of Greek (and Latin) texts in this volume are my own—but this worry will, I hope, be mitigated by my noting that none of my arguments in this volume turn on any exegetical issues!

I thank, too, John Martin Fischer for his exceptionally kind encouragement during the writing of this volume, as well as for the continuous encouragement and support that I received from Ana Iltis and (and especially) Mark J. Cherry from its initial conception through to its completion. Thanks, too, to both Julie Ganz and Felisa N. Salvago-Keyes at Routledge and Michael R. Watters at Integrated Book technology, Inc., for their help in preparing this volume (and their patience!)

Sections of Chapter 1 previously appeared in "The Myth of Posthumous Harm," that was published in *American Philosophical Quarterly* 42, No. 4 (2005), pp. 311–322. Sections of Chapter 8 previously appeared in "Personal Autonomy, Posthumous Harm, and Presumed Consent Policies for Organ Procurement," *Public Affairs Quarterly* 20, No. 4 (2006), pp. 381–404, and "The Unjustified Assumptions of Organ Conscripters," HEC Forum 21, no. 2 (2009), pp. 115–133. I thank both the *American Philosophical Quarterly* and *Public Affairs Quarterly* for allowing me to reprint the material which originally appeared in their pages, and acknowledge with thanks the original publication of "The Unjustified Assumptions of Organ Conscripters" in *HEC Forum*, whose copyright is Springer 2009. I also thank the anonymous referees of these papers for their very helpful comments on each.

Finally, I thank my beloved wife, Margaret, and daughter, Octavia, for their continuous support during the writing of this volume.

January 9th, 2012
Old Waterhollow Dairy
Pennington, New Jersey.

Introduction
Death Unterrible

"Death," wrote Aristotle in the *Nicomachean Ethics*, "is the most terrible of all things".[1] Worse yet, for an Aristotelian, a person contemplating her own death cannot even take comfort in the belief that once dead she will be "beyond evils and misfortunes," for Aristotle cautiously endorsed the Solonic view that persons can still be adversely affected by events that occur after their deaths.[2] Against this bleak view of the inescapability of human misfortune Epicurus famously (or notoriously) argued that "death is nothing to us," for "good and evil imply sentience, and death is the privation of all sentience," a view that leads naturally to the equally-comforting claim that posthumous harm is impossible.[3] Yet despite its comforting appeal the Epicurean position has been almost universally rejected by both philosophers and lay persons alike, almost all of whom tend to endorse the bleaker conclusion of Aristotle.[4]

This volume sides with Epicurus. This in itself is a bold move, for not only do almost all people side with Aristotle's views that death is the most terrible of all evils, and that posthumous harm is (at least) not obviously impossible, but they tend to reject the Epicurean alternative forcefully. The view that death is not a harm to the person who dies has been variously ridiculed as being "inane," "absurd," "very odd," and "freakish."[5] Kierkegaard even claimed that it was a "jest," and not something to be taken seriously,[6] while Mary Mothersill holds that Epicurus' argument "will hardly bear looking into."[7] This volume does not, however, merely support the classic (and ridiculed) Epicurean position that death is not a harm to the one who dies. Instead, it supports a much more radical, *full-blooded* Epicureanism, arguing that not only is death not a harm to the person who dies (either intrinsically, or extrinsically), but *also* that posthumous harm is impossible, *and* that persons cannot be wronged after their deaths. This volume should hence not be understood as offering either an exegesis or a defense of the views of the historical Epicurus or his followers.[8] Instead, it will offer an account and defense of views that are in the spirit of Epicurean thanatology.[9] With this initial caveat concerning the scope of this volume in place, a second should also be noted. While this volume will defend some bold anti-Aristotelian thanatological claims one should still be mindful of

Aristotle's distinction between bravery and recklessness, and so it will not be so bold as to attempt to address all of the metaphysical questions that surround the nature and value of death. In particular, this volume will not examine the nature of death itself, but will simply take as its starting point the plausible (if not uncontroversial) claim of Joel Feinberg, that an agent's death begins at the first moment of her nonexistence.[10] It will thus be assumed that agents will not exist after the deaths of their physical bodies (or those parts of them that are relevant to the ascription of death) in any state in which they can have conscious experiences,[11] whether this state be one that they enter from the moment of their deaths (e.g., as disembodied spirits),[12] or one that they enter after they have been reconstructed (e.g., by God) for this purpose.[13] Finally, this volume will not address the question of which criteria for death should be adopted in clinical practice. An engagement with the discussion of whether these clinical criteria should be cardiopulmonary or neurological, and, if the latter, whether they should be based on whole-brain, higher-brain, or brainstem criteria would take this volume too far afield from the metaphysical questions and their bioethical implications that are its primary foci.[14]

FULL-BLOODED EPICUREANISM AND CONTEMPORARY BIOETHICS

The thanatological positions that will be argued for in this volume are thus threefold: that death is not a harm to the person who dies, that posthumous harm is impossible, and that the dead cannot be wronged.[15] It is clear that these positions have important implications for various issues in applied ethics—and that they are *especially* important within bioethics. The question of whether death can be a harm to the person who dies is obviously relevant to debates over the morality of suicide, euthanasia, and abortion,[16] as well as to questions concerning how to adjudicate between the needs for resources of persons involved in palliative care and those involved in attempting to combat mortality.[17] It is also relevant to the question of whether or not there is a duty to die,[18] and to the question of whether human extinction would be a bad thing.[19] Similarly, the questions of whether the dead can either be harmed or wronged are clearly relevant to debates concerning the ethics of posthumous organ procurement,[20] the ethics of research on dead human bodies,[21] the ethics of research on the health status that historical figures enjoyed while they were alive,[22] posthumous medical confidentiality,[23] posthumous reproduction,[24] the moral status of postmortem pregnancy,[25] and the moral status of living wills.[26] That these Epicurean thanatological positions can be used to illuminate so many questions in bioethics would no doubt be pleasing to Epicurus, for he stressed the therapeutic power of philosophy, comparing its proper use to the medical arts.[27] Outside the realm of bioethics the question of whether death can be a harm to the person who dies is relevant to, for example, tort law as this pertains to killing,[28] the morality of the death penalty,[29] and (for some types of consequentialists), the moral status of killing.[30] The questions of whether the dead can be harmed or wronged are also directly relevant to debates concerning the ethics of writing biographies,[31] the ethics of musical interpretation,[32] archeological ethics,[33] and both the morality and rationality of bequeathing and inheriting property.[34] These questions are also relevant to questions of intergenerational justice,[35] to questions concerning reparations for past wrongs,[36] the efficacy of postmortem punishment or reward,[37] and to the status of religious relics.[38] More generally, the question of whether posthumous harm is possible will be of obvious interest both to utilitarians and to liberal political theorists.[39]

Yet although this volume will not shy away from making and defending bold claims in the realm of philosophical thanatology this boldness will not always directly carry over into making equally revisionary claims in the context of bioethical debate. Although certain revisionary claims will be made in the context of the debate over using policies of presumed consent to procure transplantable cadaveric organs, and the full-blooded Epicureanism developed in this volume will support the bold dismissal of prominent arguments offered in the context of the debates over assisted posthumous reproduction, research on the dead, and posthumous patient confidentiality, the thanatological views defended here will not directly support the drawing of many bold bioethical conclusions. However, it must be stressed—and stressed *strongly*—that this relative lack of secondary boldness does *not* undermine the importance of full-blooded Epicureanism for those debates in bioethics in which the questions of the possibility of posthumous harms and wrongs, and the question of whether death can be a harm to the person who dies, play a central role. The relative lack of Epicurean boldness in the bioethical sphere results from the fact that while the questions that Epicurean thanatology addresses play an important role in many areas of bioethical debate, the debates in question often do not turn exclusively upon the answers to them. Thus, while the questions of whether a person can be harmed or wronged by events that occur after her death are important to the debate over the ethics of research on the newly dead establishing that both posthumous harms and wrongs are impossible does not itself demonstrate that such research can progress with impunity. The questions of whether the person whose body is at issue could be harmed or wronged by certain ways in which it is used of after her death are only two facets of this debate. Others include, for example, the question of who owns (or should own) the body in question, what limitations such ownership should place on the ways in which it is used by those who do not own it, and whether and to what extent the interests of those who are concerned about how it is treated should be taken into account. Moreover, even if the debates in question *do* turn on the answers to the thanatological questions addressed by the Epicurean, even if full-blooded Epicureanism is true this does not entail that the best-justified practice is that which the Epicurean would hold was theoretically best supported. This is because (as will be discussed in Chapter 4) even if a practice lacks direct theoretical justification persons might have such antipathy to abandoning it *even once they cognitively acknowledge that it is unjustified* that concern for persons' well-being could *indirectly* justify its retention, even though it was not *directly* justifiable in its own right.[40]

Yet even once it is acknowledged that for these two reasons the Epicurean would not be justified in making as many bold claims in the context of bioethics as she is justified in making in the context of philosophical thanatology this does *not* mean that a defense of full-blooded Epicureanism is not of central importance to those areas of bioethics in which the questions of posthumous harms and wrongs and the putative harmfulness of death play a central role. First, to believe that a set of arguments $A_1 \ldots A_n$ that show that an argumentative position P is untenable where P is not a decider for the debate D in which it plays a role (e.g., that posthumous harm is possible, and so persons' interests concerning the disposal of their post-mortem bodies should be taken into account), are not important because they do not decide D is to commit what might be termed "the irrelevance of non-deciders fallacy". Eliminating one set of arguments for a position in a debate (indeed, even better, eliminating one set of arguments that supports a position that plays a role in *multiple* debates) is clearly important for the debate in question, even if this elimination does not lead immediately to its conclusion. Thus, that full-blooded Epicureanism does not itself decide certain debates in bioethics does not show that it is not important to them.

What, then, of the second reason mentioned above—that even if it is shown that a practice is unjustifiable this would not necessarily lead to its being altered, for persons might be so attached to it that considerations of their well-being would support its retention despite its inability to secure independent justification? Here, it should be acknowledged that accepting the truth of full-blooded Epicureanism might not lead to any radical revisions in either clinical practice or medical policy. In part, this might be because (as discussed in Chapter 4) persons are biologically hardwired to hold *anti*-Epicurean views concerning the questions of posthumous harms, posthumous wrongs, and the putative harm of death, and so even if they can be brought to see the truth of full-blooded Epicureanism there still would be hedonistic reasons for both individually behaving, and crafting policy, as if posthumous harms and wrongs *were* possible, and as if persons *could* be harmed by their own deaths. Having noted this, there is certainly no *a priori* reason for believing that persons are hardwired in the way that the brief sociobiological account offered in Chapter 4 suggests, and hence there is no *a priori* reason for believing that persons' beliefs—and hence their behavior—concerning these issues could not be changed. Hence, even if it might appear at first sight that full-blooded Epicureanism would not lead to any practical changes even in those debates in bioethics where its answers to the thanatological questions it addresses could be deciders this does not show that in practice it would not have practical import after persons were persuaded of its truth.[41] Moreover, one would be remiss not to point out that even if full-blooded Epicureanism was not a decider in any bioethical debate, and even if its truth would not lead to any practical revisions in medical practice, it would still be valuable for both bioethicists and others to be aware of its truth. After all, would it not be better to be *outside* of Plato's cave, rather than imprisoned within it?[42]

A NOTE ON METHODOLOGY

Before moving to provide an outline of this volume a note on its methodology is in order. The arguments within this volume are, methodologically at least, firmly within the mainstream of contemporary analytic philosophy insofar as they are based on appeals to intuition. This might strike some as problematic, especially since the evidential role of intuition in contemporary philosophy has recently been subject to sustained criticism.[43] Yet the sting of this putative problem might be drawn by explaining the methodology and aim of this volume more clearly.[44] First, the subjects of philosophical analysis in this volume (e.g. "harm") are not understood as existing as Platonic forms (e.g., the Form of Harm), as natural kinds (e.g., harm "in the world" as it exists independently of minds), or as concepts in the Fregean sense, abstract entities that are somehow graspable by rational intuition (e.g., "harm" itself).[45] Instead, they are understood as what Goldman has termed "personal psychological concepts"—mental representations of categories, where "the concept is fixed by what's in its owner's head rather than what's in the heads of other members of the community".[46] This understanding of the nature of the subjects of philosophical analysis not only undercuts any objection to their evidentiary nature that might arise from their variability across persons, but since it is thoroughly naturalistic it fits well with the Epicurean thrust of this volume. But it might come at a price: After all, one might object, on this understanding of the target of philosophical analysis such analysis seems reduced merely to offering an analysis of the concept of X as this is held by the analyzer, and so will primarily be of interest only to the analyzer and to those who share her understanding of X (ie., as X1). This is a reasonable objection, but its force will be muted if it transpires that the understanding of X as X1 is widely shared. Not only would the audience for the analysis then be broad, but those persons who do not accept the understanding of X as X1 could also find it to be of interest. They could, for example, use it either to identify commonalities between this understanding of X and their own (i.e., as X2) to determine if there is be room to reconcile X1 and X2, or else (now that the ligaments of X1 are clearer) to show why X2 is preferable. (Perhaps it will require less bullet-biting than X1.)[47] When responding to this objection to the methodology of this volume in this way it must be admitted that the pro-hedonic intuitions that are expressed and defended in it are not as widely shared as others. Despite this, they certainly constitute a perennial and significant sub-set of intuitions concerning well-being, and so (for all of the reasons outlined above) this volume should be of interest both to those who accept them and those who do not.

OUTLINE OF THIS VOLUME

There is, then, plenty of reason from both a theoretical and a practical standpoint for someone interested in bioethics to be concerned with the arguments in this volume. This volume will begin by arguing that there is no reason to believe that posthumous harm is possible and then, more strongly, that there is reason to believe that posthumous harm is *not* possible. This—rather than the classic Epicurean question of whether death can be a harm to the person who dies—is the starting point for this volume for two reasons. First, the question of whether or not posthumous harm is possible is relevant to a wide variety of contemporary debates in bioethics, and so it makes sense for a volume that is examining theoretical issues concerning death to (in part) illuminate issues in bioethics to begin with this question. Second, approaching these two questions in this order is in line with (what was) orthodox methodology in philosophical thanatology. Following Joel Feinberg, it has often been assumed that the harm inflicted upon an agent by her own death would be a type of posthumous harm. It is widely assumed that a person's death would mark the first moment of her nonexistence, and hence any harm that it inflicted upon her would be occasioned at a time after she had ceased to exist. If this is so, then the answer to the question of whether a person could be harmed by her own death would be given by the answer to the question of whether posthumous harm is possible. Hence, it has made sense to address the question of whether posthumous harm is possible prior to addressing arguments that pertain directly to the question of whether an agent can be harmed by her own death. Although (as will be noted in Chapter 5) it should not simply be assumed that the questions of whether posthumous harm is possible and whether an agent could be harmed by her own death are linked in this way, that this has been the structure of the debate to date gives (some) reason to arrange this volume to reflect this.

Chapter 1 begins by arguing that the Feinberg-Pitcher account of how posthumous harm is possible—the account that is dominant in both discussions of the metaphysics of death and hence in the bioethical literature that draws on this—is mistaken. With this in hand Chapter 2 turns to argue that the major alternative accounts of how posthumous harm is possible (developed by Barbara Levenbook, Dorothy Grover, Daniel Sperling, and Paul Griseri) are also mistaken. Of course, this only shows that there is no reason to believe that posthumous harm is possible; it does not show that it is impossible. Going some way to establish this further claim is the goal of Chapter 3, in which two initial arguments for the view that posthumous harm is impossible will be discussed and found wanting. This Chapter will then begin to develop and defend a hedonistic account of well-being, on which it will be impossible for a person to be harmed by events that occur after her death.

That posthumous harm is impossible does not, however, show that persons will be unaffected by events that occur after their deaths. It is possible that a person could be wronged without thereby being harmed, and, since this is so, it is possible that one who thwarts a person's wishes after her death could thereby wrong her. And this is directly relevant to many debates within bioethics. One of the dominant arguments in the debate over the ethical status of presumed consent policies for organ procurement, for example, is concerned with whether or not a policy of presumed consent would lead to fewer instances of thwarting persons' autonomous wishes concerning the treatment of their postmortem bodies than its alternatives. This argument is couched not in terms of whether persons would be *harmed* by the thwarting of these wishes, but whether they would be *wronged* by this, insofar as such thwarting evinces a failure appropriately to respect their autonomy. To address this concern with the possibility of posthumous wrongs it will be argued in Chapter 4 that just as persons cannot be harmed by events that occur after their deaths, so too is it impossible to wrong the dead. Establishing that persons can neither be harmed nor wronged by events that occur after their deaths does not, however, establish that their deaths themselves cannot be harms to them. To establish this third aspect of full-blooded Epicureanism two versions of Epicurus' classic argument that death cannot be a harm to the person who dies will be developed and defended in Chapter 5; these will be buttressed in Chapter 6 by a defense of Lucretius' symmetry argument for this Epicurean position.

The view that death cannot be a harm to the person who dies has obvious implications for bioethics, most obviously for the debates over the rationality and morality of suicide and euthanasia. However tempting it might be directly to apply this Epicurean conclusion to these debates it must be acknowledged that its application to them poses problems for it. In particular, if death is really "nothing to us" as Epicurus claimed—that is, if we are neither harmed *nor benefitted* by death—then it appears that the claim that suicide could be prudentially rational for some persons would be difficult (if not impossible) to justify. Yet if the application of the Epicurean view concerning the putative harm of death might be more *difficult* to apply directly to the question of suicide than it at first appears, it seems that it is too *easy* to apply it to the debate concerning the morality of euthanasia. Thus, just as those who believe that the question of whether suicide can be prudentially rational in some circumstances might be inclined to reject the Epicurean view for its apparent implications that this is not the case, so too might one who believes that euthanasia poses difficult moral questions be inclined to reject the Epicurean position for its apparently simplistic approach to the issue. These issues will be addressed in Chapter 7. In addressing the Epicurean view in the light of these two bioethical debates this Chapter will provide a bridge between the theoretical part of this volume and the discussion of its practical applications for bioethics. With this bridge in place, rather than continuing to address the Epicurean view in the light of the concerns of bioethics, Chapters 8 and 9 will change tack, and will examine some important bioethical issues in the light of the Epicurean view. In Chapter 8 it will be argued that the dominant arguments within the debate over the moral status of policies of presumed consent—those that focus on whether such policies would result in "fewer mistakes" with respect to adhering to the wishes of persons concerning the treatment of their postmortem bodies than the alternatives—should be dismissed. Those "fewer mistakes" arguments that are based on a moral concern with avoiding the infliction of posthumous harm should be dismissed because such harm is chimerical, while those that are based on a concern with respecting the autonomy of the dead can be dismissed because they rest on misunderstandings of what is required by respect for autonomy. The conclusion of Chapter 8 is not, however, merely a negative one. Although the "fewer mistakes" arguments that have been marshaled concerning policies of presumed consent are orthogonal to the debate which they currently dominate, it will be argued that there is good reason to believe that such policies *could* be morally legitimate. Indeed, that there is reason to believe that their stronger cousins—policies of organ *taking* (or, as it is more frequently but inaccurately called, organ conscription)—*are* morally legitimate.[48] Having noted this, however, it will then be argued that the arguments for organ taking rest on two unjustified assumptions. With this in hand this Chapter will conclude with an argument that once these assumptions are acknowledged then, were a morally justifiable system of organ taking to be instituted, it would clear the ground for the development of markets in human organs. The application of the Epicurean view to contemporary bioethical issues will continue in Chapter 9, where it will be used to illuminate the debates over the ethics of assisted posthumous reproduction, the ethics of research on the dead, and the ethics of posthumous patient confidentiality. This volume will then conclude with both a summary of its key points and an outline of the ways in which full-blooded Epicureanism requires further elaboration and defense.

1   Posthumous Harm and Interestbased Accounts of Well-being

In 1428 the remains of John Wyclif, who died in 1384, were exhumed and burned by the Catholic Church to punish him for his criticisms of the doctrine of transubstantiation.[1] But the view that the dead can be harmed is not confined to the religious leaders of the fifteenth century.[2] It is still common for people to feel sorry for a decedent if his projects fail after his death or to believe that the waning of a person's reputation is bad for her.[3] In the medical realm, the belief that the dead can be harmed informs the debate over the ethics of using either a policy of presumed consent or a policy of conscription to procure human transplant organs from cadavers, the debate over the ethics of posthumous reproduction, debates that concern issues of posthumous medical confidentiality, and debates over the use of the dead in research. The account of how persons can be subject to such posthumous harm that has been most influential in both the metaphysical and bioethical discussions of this issue is that which has been developed by George Pitcher[4] and Joel Feinberg, and this has played a central role in each of the bioethical debates mentioned above.[5] The Feinberg-Pitcher view of how posthumous harm is possible has, for example, been both accepted by persons using it to ground objections to using a system of presumed consent to procure human transplant organs,[6] and criticized by persons who favor the posthumous taking of transplant organs.[7] It has also been used to support respecting the confidentiality of a person's medical records after her death[8], the claims of women who wish to retrieve semen from their dead partners so that they can posthumously father children,[9] in the context of discussing the management of postmortem pregnancy,[10] and to ground objections to using the dead as research subjects without their antemortem consent.[11]

Yet although the Feinberg-Pitcher account of how the dead can be harmed has had widespread influence both within bioethics and beyond it is mistaken. Before moving to argue for this conclusion, however, three points should be noted. First, even if the Feinberg-Pitcher account of posthumous harm is mistaken this does not entail that posthumous harm is impossible, for an alternative—and tenable—account of how such harm could occur could be developed.[12] (Such accounts will be criticized in the next two chapters.) However, the arguments that will be developed in this chapter against the Feinberg-Pitcher account of how posthumous harm is possible will go some way towards undercutting alternative accounts of posthumous harm, also. This is because they will in part show that the intuitions that give plausibility to the view that posthumous harm is possible can be accommodated without having to appeal to it. As such, the argument of this chapter differs considerably from others offered against the Feinberg-Pitcher account of posthumous harm, for it does not focus on showing that the Feinberg-Pitcher position has counterintuitive implications.[13] Rather, it will seek to show that since accepting the intuitively plausible claims that are widely taken (by both its proponents and critics alike) to support the Feinberg-Pitcher position do not commit one to doing so there is no reason to accept their view at all. Second, even if it is not possible to harm the dead this does not mean that one should no longer be concerned with the putative interests of the dead, for it is possible that one might wrong someone without harming her. Thus, if this is so, then those bioethical debates in which the concept of posthumous harm plays a role could still continue, albeit with a focus on whether certain acts or practices would *wrong* the dead, rather than *harm* them.[14] To address this it will be argued in Chapter 4 that just as the dead are immune from all harm, so too are they invulnerable to being wronged. Finally, as was noted in the Introduction, it is assumed in these arguments that agents cease to exist after the deaths of their physical bodies (or those parts of them that are relevant to the ascription of death) in any state in which they can have conscious experiences. Note, though, that if this view is false (if, for example, certain Christian beliefs concerning life after death are true), this does not in itself undermine the view that posthumous harm is impossible. This is because the Epicurean defender of the impossibility of posthumous harm could simply modify his argument to one that was concerned with the impossibility of harming persons after they case to exist—whenever that might be.[15]

THE INTUITIVE CASE FOR POSTHUMOUS HARM

Before outlining the Feinberg-Pitcher argument for the possibility of posthumous harm it is advisable first to outline why one might believe that the dead could be harmed. This is important, for this belief is faced with two immediate problems that, absent such a case, would undermine its plausibility from the outset.

The first of these problems ("the problem of the subject") derives from the Epicurean puzzle concerning the alleged harm of death.[16] According to Epicurus, a person cannot be harmed by his death. When a person is alive, he is not dead, and so his death has not harmed him. After he is dead, however, the person no longer exists, and so there is no subject for the alleged harm of death to befall.[17] This last Epicurean observation similarly applies to the view that a person can be harmed after his death. If a person is dead, he does not exist, and so no harm can befall him, for there is no subject for the harm to affect.

The second difficulty ("the problem of backwards causation") faced by the proponent of the view that a person can be harmed after his death is that to endorse the possibility of posthumous harm appears to commit one to endorsing the metaphysically dubious view that backwards causation is possible.[18] Both individually and together these two problems undermine the initial plausibility of the possibility of posthumous harm. There are, however, two sets of intuitions that can be marshaled to support the claim that the dead can be harmed. The first of these derives from a rejection of the hedonic view of well being. The second derives from the claim that the dead can be wronged.

The Anti-Hedonistic Intuition

The first aspect of the intuitive case for the possibility of posthumous harm is based on the intuition that a person can be harmed by an event in her lifetime that thwarts her interests, even if she never discovers that this thwarting has occurred, and even if her subjective experience of her life is unaffected by it. If it is plausible that the thwarting of a person's interests under such circumstances can harm her, then, by extension, the claim that persons can be harmed by events after their deaths that thwart their interests is similarly plausible.[19]

A version of this first aspect of the intuitive case for the possibility of posthumous harm has been offered by both Feinberg and Derek Parfit.[20] Feinberg compares two cases to show that the dead can suffer harm. In the first, Case A, a woman devotes thirty years of her life "to the furtherance of certain ideals and ambitions in the form of one vast undertaking." Unfortunately, one month before this woman dies "the empire of her hopes" collapses and she is disgraced. However, the woman's friends conceal this from her and she dies contented.[21] In the second case, Case B, the facts are the same as in the first, but both the collapse of the woman's undertaking and her disgrace occur a year after her death. Feinberg writes "it would not be very controversial to say that the woman in Case A has suffered grievous harm to her interests although she never learned the bad news." He goes on to note "Those very same interests are harmed in Case B to exactly the same extent, and again the woman does not learn the bad news, in this case because she is dead." From this, Feinberg concludes that there is no relevant difference between Case A and Case B. Thus, if one holds that the woman in Case A has been harmed by the thwarting of her interests one must also hold that the woman in Case B has similarly been harmed, even though the harm that she suffers occurs after her death.[22] A similar example has been developed by Derek Parfit.

In Parfit's example a man's interests in the well- being of his offspring are thwarted as they suffer misfortune. One finds that his education "makes him unemployable, another has a mental breakdown, another becomes a petty thief." [23] However, the man is in exile, and does not come to learn of these events. Despite this, Parfit claims, we intuitively want to say that this man has been harmed by the misfortunes of his children even though he did not know that his interests in their well being had been thwarted, and even though this thwarting had no effect on his subjective experience. Thus, concludes Parfit, if we accept that this man is harmed even though the thwarting of his interests had no effect on him, then we must also accept that the similarly subjectively ineffective thwarting of the interests of the dead can harm them, too.

Wronging the Dead

The second aspect of the intuitive case for the possibility of posthumous harm draws on the common view that the dead can be wronged. To show that it is plausible to hold that the dead can be wronged Feinberg adds a further twist to his example of the woman who is harmed by the collapse of the "empire of her hopes". In the revised version of this example, Case C, the woman's projects fail and she is disgraced owing to the actions of a "group of malevolent conspirators, [who] having made solemn promises to the woman before her death, deliberately violate them after she has died." [24] These conspirators bring about the collapse of the woman's institution and her disgrace by spreading damaging lies about her, revealing secret plans, and betraying her trust. [25] Feinberg contends that, intuitively, the woman in Case C is not merely *harmed* by these conspirators, but they also *wrong* her. Since this is so, it seems that the dead can be wronged. Feinberg writes,

> When a promise is broken, someone is wronged, and who if not the promisee? When a confidence is revealed, someone is betrayed, and who, if not the person whose confidence it was? When a reputation is falsely blackened, someone is defamed, and who, if not the person lied about? [26]

From this, Feinberg argues that since it is intuitively plausible to hold that the dead can be wronged then the view that they can be harmed should similarly be intuitively plausible, "especially when the harm is an essential ingredient of the wrong." [27] Moreover, Feinberg argues, since the nonexistence of the dead is no bar to their being wronged the "problem of the subject" cannot be a genuine problem, for if it were it would preclude the attribution of this property to them. Thus, Feinberg concludes, just as one can hold that the dead can be wronged, so too can one hold that they can be harmed. [28]

THE FEINBERG-PITCHER ARGUMENT
FOR POSTHUMOUS HARM

With the intuitive case for the possibility of posthumous harm in place it is now time to turn to the arguments that Feinberg and Pitcher have developed to defend it. [29]

Pitcher begins his account of how the dead can be harmed by distinguishing between describing someone after his death as either an antemortem person or a postmortem person. To describe someone after his death as an antemortem person is to describe him "as he was at some stage of his life—i.e., as a living person." To describe someone after his death as a postmortem person is to describe him "as he is now, in death—mouldering, perhaps, in a grave."[30] Noting "no one would want to argue seriously that a post-mortem person can be harmed after his death," Pitcher argues that the dead can be harmed insofar as antemortem persons can be harmed after their deaths.[31] With this clarification in hand, Pitcher claims that an event or a state of affairs will harm someone "when it is contrary to one or more of his important desires or interests." Thus, since an antemortem person's "important desires or interests" might be thwarted after her death, an antemortem person might be harmed after her death. Since Pitcher is clear that the subject of the postmortem harm is the antemortem person whose interests are thwarted postmortem, he avoids the problem of the subject. He also seems to avoid the problem of backwards causation. Pitcher recognizes that it is natural to construe his view to be that a person dies unharmed, and is only harmed once the event or state of affairs that thwarts his important desires or interests takes place. However, he disavows this understanding of his position. Instead, for Pitcher, an ante-mortem person is harmed *during his lifetime* by the fact that the thwarting of his interest that occurs after his death was going to occur. Consider the claim that an event that occurs after a person's death makes it true that he was harmed by it while he was alive. According to Pitcher, this should be understood in the same way as the claim that an event that destroys the world during the presidency after Ronald Reagan's makes it true that Reagan's presidency was the penultimate one of the United States.[32] Claiming that Ronald Reagan was the penultimate president of the United States does not commit one to endorsing backwards causation. By the same token, Pitcher claims, holding that the thwarting of a person's interests after his death harms him as an antemortem person does not commit one to endorsing backward causation.

ASSESSING THE ARGUMENT FOR POSTHUMOUS HARM

It is clear why the view that posthumous harm is possible is so pervasive among philosophers, and hence so widespread within those debates in bioethics that concern the treatment of the dead. The thought experiments developed by Feinberg and Parfit that support its possibility are compelling, and the arguments that Pitcher has developed to circumvent both the problem of the subject and the problem of backwards causation are elegant and persuasive.

Yet despite their plausibility Pitcher's arguments fail to demonstrate that posthumous harm is possible, for his example of it being made true that Reagan was the penultimate president of the United States does not support his claim that "An antemortem person can be harmed by events that happen after his death."[33] The property of "being the penultimate president of the United States" is a *sequential* property. That is, it is a property that a person would possess if he or she were to be the United States president at a particular point in the sequence of United States presidents. Harm, however, is *not* a sequential property. Rather, a person is harmed by an event if that event results in his well being being lower than it was (or would have been) prior to the event (or than it would have been had the event not occurred).[34] Harm thus cannot be ascribed to someone solely on the basis of his being in a particular position in a certain sequence, as can the property of holding a particular position in the sequence of United States presidents. Since this is so, the fact that events after a person's death can result in *sequential* properties being ascribed to her as she was antemortem cannot be used to show that *non-sequential* properties, such as harm, can similarly be ascribed to her as she was antemortem on the basis of events after her death.[35]

However, even if Pitcher's analogy between ascribing the property of being the penultimate president of the United States to Reagan on the basis of events that occurred after his presidency and ascribing the property of harm to an antemortem person on the basis of events that occur after he is dead fails, this does not show that *no* analogy could be developed to show that the retroactive attribution of harm to a person is unproblematic. And, indeed, other analogies between the posthumous ascription of harm to a person and the retroactive ascription of other properties to agents have been developed to show that the proponents of the view that posthumous harm is possible are not committed to endorsing the possibility of backwards causation. Dorothy Grover, for example, has argued that the property of being a killer can be ascribed to someone on the basis of events that occur after they die. A person, Mary, shoots Joe who, rather than dying instantly, shoots back and kills Mary. Joe then dies after Mary. Joe's death thus makes it true that Mary was a killer, although this property could not be ascribed to her before her death.[36] Similarly, as both Feinberg and Pitcher recognize, a future event could make it true that a person's current interest was thwarted, or (as Solomon and Luper independently note) her current desire fulfilled.[37]

As these examples make clear it is not necessary to endorse the possibility of backwards causation to accept that present events can make it true that persons who existed in the past now possess properties that they did not possess until the present events occurred.[38] Yet, as the above objection to Pitcher's argument demonstrates, showing that certain properties can be retroactively ascribed in this way is not enough to show that attributing posthumous *harm* to persons need not commit one to endorsing backwards causation. One must *also* show that harm is the same type of property as those whose retroactive ascription to persons is metaphysically unproblematic. It was argued above that Pitcher failed to show that the properties of being the penultimate president of the United States and of being harmed were the same type of property and this point can be generalized to accommodate the above examples. In the above examples it is uncontroversial that later events justify the ascription of the properties in question to the relevant persons or interests. It is uncontroversial that if an event destroyed the world during the United States presidency that came after Reagan's, then Reagan would be penultimate president of the United States. It is uncontroversial that if Mary killed Joe, then Mary is a killer, and it is uncontroversial that if an event thwarts a person's interests, then that interest is thwarted. The ascription of these properties to their subjects is uncontroversial because it is clear that this does not require the possibility of backwards causation. However, it is *not* uncontroversial that an event that occurs after a person's death can harm her. And the ascription of harm to a person in this case is controversial partly because it is *not* clear that such an ascription of harm would not require the possibility of backwards causation. Thus, that the properties of being the penultimate president of the United States, being a killer, and being thwarted can all be ascribed on the basis of later events without endorsing backwards causation does *not* show that the proponents of the view that posthumous harm is possible are not committed to endorsing the possibility of backwards causation. This is because it is not clear that harm can be ascribed in the same way as these properties. Owing to this disanalogy, then, the above examples do not show that one can endorse the possibility of posthumous harm without endorsing backwards causation. Accordingly, neither Pitcher nor the proponents of the examples outlined above have provided rational support for the intuitive case developed by Feinberg and Parfit in favor of the possibility of posthumous harm.[39]

ACCOMMODATING ORPHANED INTUITIONS

Pitcher's (and other's) failure to support the possibility of posthumous harm orphans the intuitions that were generated by Feinberg's and Parfit's thought experiments, for his (and Feinberg's) account of how posthumous harm is possible can no longer accommodate them. Given the strength of these intuitions one might be tempted to try to develop an alternative account of how posthumous harm is possible.[40] This temptation, however, should be resisted. Instead, one should adopt that close cousin of Ockham's

Razor, the Principle of Philosophical Parsimony. According to this Principle, if one can account for one's intuitions without having to develop a sophisticated philosophical framework to do so, then one should accept the simpler account that is available to one. Thus, rather than succumbing to the temptation to develop an account of how posthumous harm is possible to replace Pitcher's account to accommodate the intuitions concerning Feinberg's and Parfit's examples that were orphaned by its rejection, one should instead first see if these intuitions could be accommodated without having to endorse the possibility of posthumous harm. Fortunately for the sake of philosophical parsimony, they can.

Accommodating Feinberg's and Parfit's Anti-Hedonistic Intuitions

Feinberg certainly seems right to claim that the woman in Case A is harmed because her interests are thwarted. However, as this example is constructed it is clear that the success of this woman's enterprise and her enjoyment of a good reputation are not the only interests that she has. She also has an interest in not being deceived, an interest in the effective exercise of her autonomy, and an interest in being respected by her friends as an autonomous person. All of these interests are thwarted after the collapse of "the empire of her hopes" when her friends deceive her into thinking that her enterprise is still successful and that she enjoys a good reputation. By controlling the information to which she has access, this woman's friends usurp her autonomy, acting so as to ensure that it is they, and not she, who control what type of actions she performs. (That is, they control whether she performs actions that she considers it appropriate to perform if her enterprise is flourishing and her reputation is intact, or whether she performs actions that she considers appropriate for a situation where her enterprise has collapsed and her reputation is in tatters.)[41] Through this usurpation this woman's friends prevent her from effectively exercising her autonomy to achieve her own ends, and in so doing they fail to respect her as an autonomous person.

Given this, Feinberg's claim that the woman in Case A is harmed because her interests are thwarted seems correct. He also seems correct to claim that the collapse of this woman's enterprise and her subsequent disgrace lead to this harm, for her friends would not have deceived her as they did had these events not occurred. However, accepting these two claims does *not* commit one also to accepting the claim, implicit in Feinberg's analysis of persons' intuitions concerning Case A, that the thwarting of this woman's interests harms her *even though this has no effect on her life*. Instead, given the above account of why the woman in Case A can be said to have been harmed, this apparent harm comes about because her interests in not being deceived, in exercising her autonomy, and in being respected by her friends as an autonomous person have all been thwarted.[42] That is, the life that this woman *actually* leads (i.e., when her interests in not being deceived, in exercising her autonomy, and being respected as an autonomous person are thwarted) could be held in some respects to be worse than the life that she *would have* led were (some of) her interests not to have been thwarted by her friends' deception.[43] This claim is not that the woman in Case A would have enjoyed a greater degree of well being had her friends not deceived her. Instead, it is simply the claim that the woman in Case A can be said to be subject to harm as a result of this deception, and that this explains the intuition that she was harmed after her enterprise collapsed and her reputation was destroyed, even though she did not know of these events and did not subjectively experience harm as a result.

The intuition that this woman has been harmed is thus based on the view that owing to her friends' deception her life is in some respects worse than it would otherwise have been. But since this is so, Case A does not support the view that a person can be harmed by events that occur after her death, as Feinberg believes. Unlike the life of the woman in Case A the lives of persons whose interests are thwarted postmortem will *not* be affected by such thwarting. It can be accepted that, like the woman in Case A, antemortem persons will not know whether their interests are thwarted postmortem, and their subjective experiences will not be affected by such thwarting. But *unlike* the woman in Case A their lives will not be affected by such thwarting and so there is no clear basis on which to attribute harm to them. The plight of the woman in Case A is accordingly very different from that of the woman in Case B, for the woman in Case B is invulnerable to the type of harm that befell the woman in Case A. Thus, contra Feinberg, if it is intuitively plausible to think that the woman in Case A was harmed this need not commit one to holding that the woman in Case B was harmed, too.[44]

The intuitions concerning Feinberg's Case A can thus be explained in a way that shows that they do not necessarily support his view that the dead can be harmed. The same cannot be said, however, for the intuitions concerning the similar case that Parfit developed in order to demonstrate the possibility of posthumous harm. The harm that persons intuitively ascribe to the father in Parfit's example cannot be accounted for in the way that the harm befalling the woman in Feinberg's Case A can be accounted for, since he is not subject to deception. As such, even if the intuitions that are pumped by Feinberg's example do not support the possibility of posthumous harm, those pumped by Parfit's example cannot be accounted for without accepting this possibility. But if this is so, then the Principle of Philosophical Parsimony fails to take effect and an alternative account of how posthumous harm is possible should be sought.

Yet although the harm which persons intuitively ascribe to the father in Parfit's example cannot be accounted for in the same way as that which is ascribed to the woman in Feinberg's Case A this example does not necessarily lend much intuitive support to the view that the dead can be harmed. It does not seem as clear that the man in Parfit's example is harmed by the thwarting of his parental interests as it seems clear that the woman in

Case A was harmed by the combination of her ill fortune and her friends' deceit.[45] In Case A the woman could be said to be harmed because certain aspects of her life were adversely affected by her ill fortune and subsequent deception. However, the life of the man in Parfit's example does not go worse than it would have done were his children not to suffer misfortune. As such, it is not clear that the thwarting of his interests harms him, and so it is not clear that this example supports the view that posthumous harm is possible.

Furthermore, there is reason to believe that the man in Parfit's example is *not* harmed by the misfortunes of his children. Consider, for example, a variant on this case wherein the man's son disgraces the family name. It is plausible to think that in reprimanding him his mother might express relief that her husband is in exile and will never come to learn of the disgrace, on the grounds that he is thus immune from the harm that this would otherwise have caused him.[46] Of course, one could respond to this objection to Parfit's example by claiming that by definition the thwarting of a person's interests harms him. But such a response would be unsatisfactory, for one would then have merely stipulated that the thwarting of the interests of the dead could harm them rather than demonstrated how this could be.

It seems, then, that persons who hold that the dead can be harmed on the basis of their intuitive responses to cases such as Feinberg's Case A and Parfit's exiled parent are faced with a dilemma. On the one hand, if the person in the example on which they are resting their intuitions seems, intuitively, to be harmed (as in Feinberg's Case A) then the intuition that this is so can be explained in a way that avoids the implication that the dead can be harmed. On the other hand, if the ascription of harm to the person in the proffered example clearly implies that the dead can be harmed (as in Parfit's example) then the intuition that harm should be ascribed will not be a strong one. In neither case, then, will such examples firmly support the view that the dead can be harmed.

Can the Dead be Wronged?

As shown above, one can undermine the intuitive support for the claim that the dead can be harmed that can be drawn from examples such as Feinberg's Case A and Parfit's exiled parent. Likewise, one can undermine the support that might be gleaned for this claim from the view that the dead can be wronged. Feinberg's claim is intuitively plausible: if a person is defamed or her confidences revealed then she is wronged. It thus seems equally plausible that if the dead can be wronged by having their characters besmirched or their confidences betrayed, then so too can they be harmed, "especially when the harm is an essential ingredient of the wrong."[47] Feinberg is right to note that if it is intuitively plausible that the dead can be wronged by being defamed or betrayed, and if it is true that "an essential ingredient of the wrong" is that the wronged person is thereby harmed, then the claim that the dead can be harmed gains considerable intuitive support. It is important to note, however, that Feinberg gives no argument in support of the claim that the dead can be wronged, but simply relies on the intuitive plausibility of the claim that they can. This is unfortunate, for, as will be argued in Chapter 4, there is no reason to believe that the dead can be wronged. However, it is possible to undercut the support that Feinberg provides for his view that the dead can be harmed from the intuitive plausibility of the claim that they can be wronged without having to show that the latter claim is mistaken. This can be done in two ways. First, it is possible for persons to be wronged without thereby being harmed. Thus, even if it is true that the dead can be wronged (and so the problem of the subject might not be a genuine problem) it does not follow that they can also be harmed. Second, although at first sight it is plausible to claim that the dead can be wronged the intuitions that support this claim (like those that support the claim that the dead can be harmed) can be accommodated without its endorsement.

It is clear that persons can be wronged without being harmed. If Hardcastle offers to drive Sebastian to his early morning lecture and fails to show up, Hardcastle wrongs Sebastian. However, if Hardcastle's neighbor Charles drives Sebastian in instead, and if Sebastian were not inconvenienced or upset by this state of affairs, Hardcastle did not harm Sebastian through wronging him.[48] Since this is so, it is possible to agree with Feinberg that the dead can be wronged, and yet to deny that this shows that they can be harmed. Of course, one might reply that harm is an *essential* ingredient of the type of wrongs that the dead might be subject to. Yet not only does Feinberg fail to provide a reason to believe this, there is good reason to suppose that harm is *not* an essential ingredient of any wrongs to which the dead might be subject. Consider again Parfit's example of the exiled father. Imagine that instead of suffering misfortune, this man is betrayed by his son in some way, although, again, owing to his exile, he does not come to know this and it has no effect on his subjective experiences. Although it is tempting to say that this man's son *wronged* him it is not so clear (as can be seen from the above discussion of this example) that he also *harmed* him. Even if one accepts that the dead can be wronged, then, this does not provide as much intuitive support as Feinberg believes it does for the view that they can also be harmed.

What, then, of the claim that the dead can be wronged? Just as the intuitions that surrounded Feinberg's Case A can be accommodated without committing one to the view that the dead can be harmed, so too can the intuitions that surround the cases that Feinberg discusses in the context of wronging the dead be accommodated without accepting that the dead can be wronged. The intuitions that concern the wrongness of defamation, for example, can readily be accounted for without claiming that the person defamed has been either wronged or harmed. To defame someone is to deceive others about aspects of the defamed person's life or character. As such, a defamer could harm (and wrong) persons other than the defamee if such persons act on the false information that he provides them with. To the extent that such persons acted on the defamatory information that he provided them with as he wished them to act it would be he, and not they, who would be directing their actions. To the degree that this is so, then, the defamer would usurp these persons' autonomy.[49] Such usurpation of autonomy both wrongs its victims, and might also harm them, insofar as it undermines their ability to satisfy their desires as they would otherwise have been able to, including their desires to act autonomously. Similarly, if defaming a person leads to his being avoided by persons with whom he wishes to have contact the defamation would have harmed him, and through this wronged him. Thus, one could morally condemn defamation *either* on the grounds that it wrongs the persons who are manipulated by those who perpetrate it, *or* on the grounds that such manipulation results in wrong being done to the defamee (where this is an inclusive "or"). Since this is so, one can hold that the defamation of a dead person is a wrong without committing oneself to the claim that such defamation wrongs *him*.

Yet even in cases where the intuition that a person has wronged the dead cannot be explained in terms of the wronging of the living, the claim that a person has wronged the dead can be understood as a claim about wrongdoing that *refers* to the dead, where such reference does not imply that the dead person so referred to has been wronged.[50] In such cases a claim about wronging the dead should be understood in a similar manner to how claims about wrongful attempts are understood. For example, when Brenda attempts to steal from Tony by putting her hand in his pocket, Brenda engages in wrongdoing even if Tony's pocket is empty and she cannot steal from him.

Since Brenda could not have stolen from Tony she did not wrong him. Rather, she merely engaged in wrongdoing whose full description (e.g., "trying to steal from Tony") would include a reference to Tony. Similarly, saying "Bill betrayed Ben, who died last year" could be understood not as a claim that Bill *wronged* Ben, but simply as the elliptical claim that Bill performed wrongdoing whose full description would include reference to Ben. ("Wrongdoing" is used here rather than "wrong acts" so as not to beg the question against certain consequentialist accounts of wrong acts. An act consequentialist could accept that Brenda engages in wrongdoing without accepting that she does a wrong act. This is because "wrongdoing" could be used here to indicate that the act in question is evidence that Brenda had a bad character, even though her failure to steal from Tony resulted in her failure to commit a bad act.) Thus, to accept that the dead can be involved in the full description of a wrong act (e.g., a defamation or a betrayal) need not commit one to the view that they can be wronged. Unless additional reasons are provided in support of the claim that the dead can be wronged, then, there is no reason to believe that they can be. As such, then, the view that posthumous harm is possible cannot be supported by arguing that since the dead can be wronged, there is no bar to them being harmed.

PORTMORE, POSTHUMOUS HARM, AND
THE DESIRE THEORY OF WELFARE

The above arguments have shown that the Feinberg-Pitcher account of how posthumous harm is possible is still faced with the problem of backwards causation. They have also shown that the intuitions (concerning both harms and wrongs) that led to its development can be accommodated without positing the possibility of posthumous harm, thus obviating the need for it. In addition to these objections that are aimed specifically at the Feinberg-Pitcher account of how posthumous harm is possible Douglas Portmore has developed a series of arguments that show that no account of how posthumous harm is possible that is (like the Feinberg-Pitcher account), based on the desire theory of welfare is tenable.[51]

Portmore notes that the desire theory of welfare—the view that a person's welfare depends upon the degree to which her desires are thwarted or fulfilled—is a contentious one.[52] Rather than arguing that accounts of how posthumous harm is possible that are based upon this theory of welfare should be rejected as this theory is itself mistaken Portmore argues for the weaker conclusion that even persons who are sympathetic to the desire theory of welfare should be skeptical of the accounts of how posthumous harm is possible that are based on it.[53] There are, according to Portmore, two reasons why even a proponent of a desire theory of welfare should be skeptical of the possibility of posthumous harm.

First, desire theorists of welfare must accept that it "is only the non-fulfillment of certain desires, those that pertain to one's own life, that negatively affect one's welfare".[54] The desire theory of welfare must be restricted to being concerned with the non-fulfillment of such pertinent desires because the objects of many persons' desires are so unrelated to them that their fulfillment or non-fulfillment cannot plausibly be considered relevant to their welfare. This, notes Portmore, has been shown by Parfit's famous example in which he meets a stranger who has a fatal disease who arouses his sympathy, leading him to want the stranger to be cured. Unknown to Parfit, the stranger is later cured. As Parfit observes, "On the Unrestricted Desire . . . Theory, this event is good for me, and makes my life go better. This is not plausible. We should reject this theory."[55] Which of a person's desires, then, will be the pertinent ones? Portmore believes that the "most detailed and plausible version of the restricted desire theory offered to date" is that which has been developed by Mark Overvold.[56] On this version of the desire theory of welfare a person's welfare is solely a function of her desires that have as their objects those states of affairs where her existing at time t is a necessary condition for their being fulfilled at t.[57] This version of the desire theory of welfare does not fall foul of Parfit's objection, for it is not a necessary condition for the fulfillment of his desire that the stranger be cured that he exist at the time at which this occurs, and so this desire is not a pertinent desire for the theory. Yet, as Portmore notes, this will provide only cold comfort for those who wish to base an account of posthumous harm on a desire theory of welfare. This is because although Overvold's version of this theory avoids Parfit's objection it does so at the cost of rendering posthumous harm impossible, "for any state of affairs that obtains subsequent to a person's death cannot be one in which the person is an essential constituent".[58] Of course, this does not in itself show that it is impossible for a proponent of a desire theory of welfare to endorse the possibility for posthumous harm. Brad Hooker, for example, has revised Overvold's version of the desire theory of welfare so that "the relevant desires are the ones in whose propositional content the agent is an essential constituent in the sense that the state of affairs *is desired under a description that makes essential reference to the agent*" to provide a version of this view that can allow for the possibility of posthumous harm.[59] On this revised version of Overvold's account of welfare a person could be harmed after her death, because, for example, her desire that *her* projects be successful after her death is now one that is pertinent to her welfare. Yet Hooker's revision of Overvold's account will not do. This is because, as Portmore argues, it will count as pertinent desires whose fulfillment or thwarting are clearly irrelevant to one's welfare, such as the desire that Parfit might have that his grandchildren will live in the same neighborhood as the stranger's so that they might play together.[60] Given the failure of Hooker's version of the desire theory of welfare it is, concludes Portmore, not yet clear whether a suitably restricted version of the desire theory of welfare could allow for the possibility of posthumous harm.

This first problem for accounts of how posthumous harm is possible that are based on the desire theory of welfare is not, of course, a conclusive one, for it leaves open the possibility that a suitably restricted version of this theory could still recognize that such harm is possible. The second problem that Portmore identifies for accounts of how posthumous harm is possible that are based upon this theory of welfare is more problematic for them: that only a person's desires whose fulfillment do not depend on any future states of affairs (i.e., her *future-independent* desires) are those whose fulfillment or thwarting are pertinent to her welfare.[61] Thus, since the possibility of posthumous harm only arises with the thwarting of a person's future-*dependent* desires, this latter restriction of her pertinent desires will eliminate the possibility that an adherent of the desire theory of welfare could accept the possibility of posthumous harm.

Portmore's argument for the claim that only a person's future-independent desires could be pertinent to her welfare is based on showing that no plausible account of what it is for a person to be in a harmed condition can be given by any desire theorist of welfare who accepts that a person's future-dependent desires could be pertinent ones. (A harmed condition is "a state that it is self-interestedly bad to be in".)[62] Portmore begins his argument by considering what he terms *"the Sophisticated View"* of what it is for a person to be in a harmed condition. Here, "S is in a harmed condition if and only if all the following apply: (1) S desires that P, (2) P is false, and (3) S will never voluntarily abandon her desire that P," where S is held to have voluntarily abandoned her desire that P iff she has abandoned it as a result of a process that she would not oppose.[63] Although this View of what it is for a person to be in a harmed condition allows for the possibility of posthumous harm Portmore notes that it has a counterintuitive implication: that in a situation in which one's desires have been shifting back and forth between having A and ~A as their object "whether one is in a harmed condition now depends on whether one's desires are going to shift n or n-1 times before one dies . . . ".[64] To avoid this implication the desire theorist who wishes to retain the possibility that a person's set of pertinent desires could include future-dependent desires could modify this View so that S is in a harmed condition when her desire that P has been involuntarily removed only if in the nearest possible world she never voluntarily abandons her desire. Thus, if one's desires oscillate between A and ~A one will not be in a harmed condition as a result of the occurrence of either A or ~A because in the nearest possible world where one's token death did not occur one would have voluntarily abandoned whichever desire transpired to be unfulfilled.

But, Portmore notes, this attempt to rescue this View has difficulties of its own. To show this he offers two examples, based on a situation outlined by Parfit where as a young man he had wanted to become a poet, but changed his mind and became a philosopher instead. In the first example Parfit's desire to be a poet was involuntarily removed by an evil doctor before he had a chance to change his mind. Given that he would, in the nearest possible world, have changed his mind anyway, Parfit was not in a harmed condition when he desired to be a poet when this was not to be. However, in the second example in the nearest possible world to that where his desire to be a poet was involuntarily removed by an evil doctor this desire would have been involuntarily removed by an alternative evil doctor. In this case, the revised View entails that Parfit was in a harmed condition as a young man. But this, notes Portmore, is counterintuitive, for the fact that the removal of Parfit's desire was overdetermined in the second case should be irrelevant to assessing whether he is in a harmed condition. All that should matter is that he would have abandoned his desire to be a poet voluntarily had he been left alone. As such, Portmore argues, the desire theorist should revise her View so that "S's desiring that P where P is false constitutes a harmed condition only if, in the nearest possible world where this desire is never involuntarily removed, S never voluntarily abandons her desire".[65] But, holds Portmore, since the extinguishing of a person's desires by her death counts as an involuntary removal of them, to answer whether

S is in a harmed state or not we would have to ascertain whether she would never have voluntarily abandoned her desire that P in a situation in which she never died.[66] Since the answer to this question will typically be that S *would* have voluntarily abandoned her desire that P, the adoption of this version of this View will have the result that many of a person's future-dependent desires are not pertinent to assessing her level of welfare.[67] As such, concludes Portmore, desire theorists should hold that a person's future-dependent desires are simply irrelevant to her welfare. Instead, they should endorse *"the Future-Independent View*: S is in a harmed condition if and only if all the following apply: (1) S desires that P, (2) P is false, and (3) S's desire that P is a future-independent desire, where a desire that P, held at a particular time t, is *future independent* if and only if, for any possible worlds w1 and w2, if w1 and w2 are qualitatively identical both at t and at every time prior to t, then P has the same truth-value at w1 and w2."[68]And, since this is so, the desire theorist of welfare should reject the view that posthumous harm is possible, for events that occur after an antemortem person's death can never thwart her future-independent desires.

CONCLUSION

From the above discussion it is clear that neither Feinberg nor Pitcher have given us any reason to believe that the dead can be harmed. The arguments that they developed to support this view have failed, and the intuitions that led them to argue for the possibility of posthumous harm can be accommodated without accepting that such harm is possible. Furthermore, and more generally, from Portmore's arguments it is clear that the desire theory of welfare cannot accommodate the view that posthumous harm is possible. Yet although the arguments developed in this paper show that the influential Feinberg-Pitcher account of posthumous harm is mistaken they do not show that one should endorse the further claim that such harm is impossible. Rather, they only show that, to adopt the words of cautious Scottish courts, the claim that the dead can be harmed is "not proven". Such caution is well-advised here, for alternative accounts of how posthumous harm is possible have been developed to replace that of Feinberg and Pitcher. These arguments will be addressed in the next Chapter.

2   Further Criticisms of the Possibility of Posthumous Harm

It was argued in the previous chapter that the Feinberg-Pitcher account of how posthumous harm is possible is mistaken. However, it was also noted there that showing this is not to show that there is no reason to believe in the possibility of such harm, for it might be the case that an alternative account of the possibility of posthumous harm could be developed in its stead. In this chapter, then, it will be argued that just as the Feinberg-Pitcher account of how posthumous harm is possible fails, so too do other accounts that have been developed to defend its conclusion. To show this is not, however, to support the conclusion that posthumous harm is impossible, but only the weaker conclusion that there is, as yet, no reason to accept its possibility. To support the stronger conclusion that posthumous harm is *not* possible it will be argued in the next chapter that for a person to be harmed her experiences must be adversely affected in some way, and since a persons' experiences cannot be affected by events that occur after her death she is immune from being harmed by them. Before moving to this further argument, however, it would be wise to continue to clear away the underbrush of arguments that purport to establish the possibility of such harm. To this end the main alternatives to the Feinberg-Pitcher account of how posthumous harm is possible—those developed by Levenbook, Grover, Sperling, and Griseri—will be outlined and criticized.[1] And, as was noted earlier, showing that there is no reason to accept the possibility of posthumous harm will have important implications for those many debates in bioethics in which it is invoked, ranging from those concerned with posthumous organ procurement to those concerned with the management of postmortem pregnancy.

LEVENBOOK'S ACCOUNT OF HARM AS LOSS

Levenbook's Argument

Believing the Feinberg-Pitcher account of the possibility of posthumous harm to be unsatisfactory Barbara Baum Levenbook developed an alternative account that is based upon understanding harm in terms of loss.[2] Levenbook begins her account of harm as loss by suggesting that murder is harmful to the person murdered "because it is an irreversible loss to the person who was murdered of a function or functions necessary for his worthwhile existence".[3] With this in hand, Levenbook claims that to be harmed a person "must lose something or be deprived of something," and that "The loss or deprivation must be bad for him".[4] Murder, then, is a harm to its victim because it causes him the irreversible loss of experiencing, where such experiencing would have been "minimally worthwhile".[5] Levenbook notes that losses are events, and thus must occur at particular times. Since a person who is murdered will continue to experience things up to the moment of his death the loss of his experiencing, Levenbook argues, will "be going on at the moment of his death and thus at the first moment that he no longer exists".[6] As such, then, Levenbook holds that "(1) that one can lose something at the moment that he ceases to exist and (2) that some event going on at that moment can be bad for him".[7]

With this account of harm as loss in place Levenbook extends its base assumptions (1) and (2), to read: "(1') that one can lose something after he ceases to exist and (2') that some event occurring entirely when one does not exist can be bad for him".[8] Levenbook argues that since (1) must be accepted to account for the harm of murder there is no justification for not extending it to (1'). Levenbook holds that the extension of (1) to (1') and (2) to (2') cannot be rejected on the basis that a person who is dead does not exist, and so cannot lose anything, for the same could be said about a person at the moment of death—and yet there it seems that there is a loser to suffer loss. She also holds that one cannot block the extension of (1) to (1') on the grounds that "the moment of death is a time that a person loses something when he has had it up until that moment and because he has had it until then and has it no longer" (i.e., [1] could be acceptable) whereas after this "no one can have anything" (i.e., [1'] is not acceptable).[9] This attempt to block the extension of (1) to (1'), Levenbook argues, should be rejected because it is not true that no one can have anything after the moment of death, and so no one can lose anything after that point, for, she holds, it is possible for Einstein to lose or retain his scientific reputation after his death.

What, then, of (2')—the assumption that an event that occurs at a time when a person ceases to exist can be bad for him? Levenbook defends this assumption by appealing to an argument developed by Harry S. Silverstein, which purports to show that this assumption (when understood as being an assumption about states of affairs rather than as being about events) can only be rejected at the cost of rejecting the plausible assumption that to continue to live is good for some persons.[10] Silverstein argues that if to continue to live is a precondition for someone to enjoy the goods of life, then to claim that to continue to live is good for him is not a comparative claim. But it *would* be a *false* claim, for if to continue to live is simply a precondition for a person to enjoy goods it cannot itself be a good. As such, Silverstein concludes, to claim that to continue to live is good for a person it must be understood as a comparative claim: that to continue to live is better for the person concerned than it would be for him to die. But this comparison, notes Silverstein, must be based on the presupposition that a person's death must have value for him, be this positive, negative, or neutral. Since it is thus possible for a person's death to have a *negative* value for him, then it must be possible for a state of affairs that obtains when a person does not exist to be bad for him. To illustrate this point Levenbook offers an example in which "two events occur shortly before Jones's death: the publishing by Smith of his memoirs of Jones, and the releasing of police tapes of Smith and Jones. After his death, the former causes Jones to have a reputation for selflessness and honesty, and sometime later the latter destroys this reputation".[11] Levenbook argues that if one holds that events that occur after a person ceases to exist cannot be bad for him, then one must hold the "untenable" position "that the event that consists of going from a state of affairs that is good for . . . [Jones] . . . to a state of affairs that is bad for him . . . " is not bad for Jones. As such, then, she concludes, (2') must be accepted. Thus, it is possible for a person to suffer posthumous harm, since a person can lose something after he ceases to exist, and such a loss can be bad for him.

Criticisms of Levenbook's Argument

Levenbook accepts that she has not "proved the possibility of posthumous harm beyond a reasonable doubt," for she recognizes that "There are, undoubtedly, real difficulties of a metaphysical and metaethical nature in the thesis that someone can be harmed after he no longer exists".[12] Unfortunately, despite this becoming modesty Levenbook does not recognize just how weak her case for the possibility of posthumous harm is. Levenbook's case rests on assumptions (1') and (2'), which rest in turn on her assumptions (1) and (2). Levenbook's assumption (1) has been trenchantly criticized by Joan Callahan. Callahan charges that Levenbook's discussion of a person losing things (such as, at the moment of death, his mental functions), and hence her discussion of the alleged harm of murder, is misleading. Callahan notes that "To say 'A lost his mental functions at the moment of death' is simply a (bad) way of saying 'The mental functioning of A ceased at his death'".[13] As such, then, if A's death is defined as "the moment at which A ceases to exist" then A's death would be "the termination of A and all his capacities, including his capacities to gain or lose".[14] Moreover, charges Callahan, Levenbook cannot gain support for her claim that a person can lose things after he ceases to exist by claiming that it is possible for Einstein to lose his reputation as a scientific genius after his death. This is because, notes Callahan, to talk of Einstein's scientific reputation is just to talk of what persons who *currently exist* believe about Einstein. It is not to talk of something that

Einstein has. As such, then, to say that Einstein has not lost his reputation as a scientific genius is not to say that this reputation is something that *Einstein* could lose after his death; it is just to say that there are beliefs *about* Einstein that persons who currently exist could come to lose.[15]

Callahan, then, has shown that Levenbook has failed to establish that assumption (1) should be accepted. She has thus also shown that Levenbook has also failed to establish that (1') should be accepted—and since Levenbook's case for the possibility of posthumous harm rests on (1') being true Callahan has effectively undermined it. Yet to establish further that Levenbook's case for the possibility of posthumous harm is untenable, it should be noted that her assumption (2') should be rejected, also. In defending this assumption Levenbook appealed to an argument offered by Silverstein, which was based on the view that the claim that to continue to live would be good for a person was a comparative claim. If it were not, Silverstein argued, then the claim that to continue to live would be good for a person would be false, for if to continue to live is simply a precondition for a person to enjoy goods it cannot itself be a good—and to hold that to continue to live is not itself a good for a person is counterintuitive. Despite its plausibility, however, Silverstein's argument fails to show that the claim that it would be good for a person to continue to live is a comparative claim, for it *does* make sense to claim that continuing to live is not a good for a person, even if the life of the person in question is going well. In making this claim one is not claiming that the continued enjoyment of the goods of life is not good for a person. Rather, one is simply noting, as Silverstein does, that insofar as to continue to live is merely a precondition for a person's enjoyment of these goods it is not *itself* a good for a person. And once one recognizes the relationship that holds between the goodness in itself (or lack thereof) of one thing that is a precondition for the existence of something else that is good, this claim ceases to be counterintuitive. Thus, since to claim that to continue to live is good for a person is a false non-comparative claim, rather than a true comparative claim, there is no need to presuppose that a person's death will have any value for him. As such, then, there is no reason to believe that it must be possible for a state of affairs that obtains when a person does not exist to be bad for him. To turn to Levenbook's example, then, it *is* tenable to deny that it could be bad for Jones that his reputation was ruined by the releasing of the police tapes of him and Smith. Levenbook's assumption (2') can thus also be rejected.

GROVER'S QUALITY OF LIFE ARGUMENTS

Grover's Argument

Like Levenbook, Dorothy Grover also finds the Feinberg-Pitcher account of the possibility of posthumous harm unacceptable, although she rejects it because she finds Feinberg's account of what it is to harm someone unsatisfactory. According to Feinberg, a person can suffer from posthumous harm if her interests are thwarted, where these interests are based on a person's wants, desires, and goals.[16] Grover objects to this account of harm on the grounds that persons can be harmed "when society 'encourages' in them certain kinds of attitudes, for example, low self-esteem," or when they "have not had access to the encouragement, education, cultural activities, etc, which provide the circumstances in which we have the opportunity—should we wish—to acquire or choose between many of our more 'sophisticated' desires," even if "such opportunities could have been made available".[17] Yet, continues Grover, although persons do seem to be able to be harmed in these ways, they are not harmed because they have desires or interests that were thwarted by their social situation—indeed, the very basis of the harm that they are subject to is that they were *unable* to develop certain desires or interests.[18] To rectify what she sees as the deficiencies of Feinberg's account Grover develops an account of harm on which a person could be harmed either if the present quality of his life is impaired, or if the possibility that he is in a position to choose (or refrain from choosing) a good quality life is undermined. On this view, "A is harmed by an event or circumstance X, when the occurrence of X has the effect of A having a significantly lower quality of life than A might reasonably (given the resources of his society and A's resources) otherwise have had—where a life of good quality is one where the person has knowledge that she or he is active with things that are interesting and worthwhile".[19] For Grover, the quality of a person's life will depend, in part, on the degree of knowledge that she has within it, the degree of autonomy that she possesses, the level of interest and value that can appropriately be ascribed to her activities, which she should find to be interesting and worthwhile.[20]

With this account of harm in hand Grover outlines how a person might suffer posthumous harm. Grover claims that "posthumous events can . . . undermine the quality of a person's life by undermining the quality of the decisions made," noting further that "When our reasonable expectations are undermined by others, we make decisions in less than ideal circumstances".[21] To illustrate this, Grover offers the case of Basil, whose death is imminent and who has the option of either forgoing the final revisions to his book manuscript to negotiate with a publisher himself, or else finish his revisions and trust to a friend's promise to get the book published posthumously. Had he chosen the first option the book would have been published. Basil, however, chooses the second option, his friend breaks his promise to him, and the book is not published. Here, Grover concludes that "Basil did not have the knowledge necessary for a good decision; as a result he did not accomplish what he would have otherwise accomplished. So Basil is harmed posthumously".[22] To support her conclusion that posthumous events can have effects on the quality of antemortem persons' lives Grover notes that "not all components of the so-called posthumous events occur posthumously"; promises that are broken posthumously, for example, are made to persons while they are still alive.[23]

Unfortunately, it is not entirely clear how Grover's account of how posthumous harm is possible is supposed to be understood. From her discussion of what it is for an event or circumstance to harm someone, her account of what it is for a life to be of good quality, and her example of the (allegedly) posthumously-harmed Basil two possibilities suggest themselves. It could be the case that Grover holds that a person is harmed by an event that occurs after his death if that event lowers the quality of his life by making at least one of his activities less worthwhile than it would have otherwise been, by thwarting his accomplishing something that he would have otherwise achieved. This understanding of Grover's account of posthumous harm (which can be dubbed the "Accomplishment View") gains additional support from her final example, which she uses to distinguish her account of posthumous harm from Feinberg's. This is of Sam, a medical scientist who believes that a drug that he has isolated can cure lung cancer. After Sam dies other scientists discover another cure for lung cancer and ignore Sam's results. Still later, it is discovered that Sam's work is pertinent to developing a vaccine for AIDS, and his contribution to this is publicized.[24] Grover claims that whereas on Feinberg's theory of posthumous harm Sam is harmed because his interests (i.e., in discovering the cure for lung cancer) are thwarted, on her view the initial harm that he suffered as a result of the thwarting of his interests in partly ameliorated because "the value of one's actions can be enhanced by completely unanticipated achievements".[25] Alternatively, it could be the case that Grover believes that a person could be harmed not by a posthumous event preventing his actions from having value by preventing him from accomplishing something, but by the degrees of knowledge and autonomy that he possessed during his lifetime being diminished by the actions of others that occur after his death. (This can be dubbed the "Knowledge and Autonomy View".)[26]

Criticisms of Grover's Argument

While both of these different ways of understanding Grover's view of how posthumous harm is possible can glean textual support from her work neither is convincing. Consider first the Accomplishment View: that a person could be harmed by events that occur after his death that prevent his actions from having the value that they might have had. Since Grover wishes to distinguish her view from Feinberg's the value that a person's actions might have had will not be limited on her account to the value that they might have generated for him as a result of fulfilling his interests. Instead, the value of a person's actions should be understood as being derived from the value that they transpire to have for others, independently of the interests of the person whose quality of life is in question. At first sight, this is plausible; even if Sam were to have absolutely no interest in discovering a vaccine for AIDS his work would still have value if it led to this. However, that a person's actions can have value for others in a way that is not only unanticipated by the person concerned but also has no connection with his own interests does not support Grover's claim that were an event to preclude a person's actions having value in this way then it would harm him by adversely affecting the quality of his life. It is implausible to hold that a person's quality of life could be adversely affected in a way that could ground the claim that he was harmed by it by an event that precluded his actions from having value in a way that had no connection with his interests. Consider, for example, the case of the Scottish poet William McGonagall. Although he took himself to be a serious poet, McGonagall's poetry was so bad that its value lay in the fact that it was hugely (although unintentionally) comic.[27] McGonagall's writing, then, had (and still has!) value. But it was not the value that he wanted it to have—indeed, the value that it possesses is a value that he utterly repudiated. Now, imagine that for some reason McGonagall kept his poetry secret throughout his life, intending that it be published after his death so that the people he knew would feel sorry for not having realized that they had a literary genius in their midst. Unfortunately, in this example, after his death his manuscripts were lost, and so his poetry was never made public. Given the comedic value of his work, had McGonagall's manuscripts been published his act of writing them would have had great value to others. In precluding this, then, their loss precluded his writing acts from having this value. As such, on Grover's account of how posthumous harm is possible, the quality of McGonagall's life was adversely affected by the posthumous loss of his manuscripts, and so this harmed him. But this is mistaken. Indeed, given how seriously McGonagall took himself and his poetry it seems that persons who believe that posthumous harms and benefits are possible should instead conclude that McGonagall was *benefited*, not harmed, by the loss of his manuscripts, for this protected him from becoming a laughingstock.[28]

To be plausible, then, Grover's Accomplishment View must tie the value of the person's acts that are in question to the interests of the person whose acts they were. If this is not done, then she will be committed to the implausible conclusion that a person could be posthumously *harmed* by an event that occurs after her death that precludes her acts from having value to others in a way that *undermines* the fulfillment of her actual interests. But, if the Accomplishment View is revised so that it ties the value of a person's actions to their role in leading to the fulfillment of her interests it will simply become an interest-based account that is very similar to the Feinberg-Pitcher account. And, as such, it would then be vulnerable to the objections that were leveled against the Feinberg-Pitcher account of posthumous harm in the previous chapter.[29]

Given the failure of the Accomplishment View of how posthumous harm is possible what of the Knowledge and Autonomy View: that a person could be harmed by the degrees of knowledge and autonomy that he possessed during his lifetime being diminished by the actions of another that occur after his death? In discussing the example of Basil, whose friend's breaking of a promise to him prevented him from succeeding in getting his book published, Grover writes that

> A reason posthumous events can have such an effect [i.e., can harm] is that not all components of the so-called posthumous events occur posthumously. Promises can be broken posthumously, only if promises were made when the parties concerned were alive. Similarly, posthumous betrayal and slander can occur only if assumptions of trust are the norm among the living. When trust is the norm, posthumous breaking of a promise, betrayal, or posthumous slander can play havoc with the cognitive status of the deceased person's beliefs, and with the decisions and activities of the deceased.[30]

Recalling that Grover had earlier written that the quality of a person's life will depend, in part, upon the level of autonomy that he enjoys, it appears that, for Grover, the quality of a person's life could be adversely affected by his having a lower level of autonomy within it than he could have enjoyed. For Grover, it also appears that a person's autonomy can be adversely affected by a betrayal of trust, for such a betrayal "can play havoc" with the beliefs, and hence the decisions and activities, of the person betrayed. If this is Grover's view, then her claims concerning autonomy are certainly correct. If one person betrays the trust of another by, for example, making a promise to her that he does not intend to keep, he will be exerting control over the information that she bases her decisions on. To the extent that such control over the information that the betrayee bases her decisions on results in the betrayer's exerting control over the type of actions she performs, it will be he, and not she, who is directing them. The betrayee, then, will thus suffer from a diminution in her self-direction, her autonomy, with respect to her actions that are in question.[31] Turning back to the example of Basil, if his friend promised him that he would see that his book was published and yet never intended to ensure that this occurred then Basil's autonomy with respect to his consequent actions would be impaired. In making a promise to him that he had no intention of keeping Basil's friend acted so as to control the information on which Basil based his decisions, and so acted to bring it about that Basil would work on his book rather than negotiate with a publisher himself. It was thus Basil's friend, rather than Basil, who ultimately decided what type of actions Basil would perform, and so Basil suffered from a diminution in the degree to which he directed himself to perform them; he suffered from a diminution in his autonomy with respect to them.[32]

Yet although Grover is correct to note that subjecting a person to betrayal *can* compromise the degree to which she is autonomous with respect to her actions through playing havoc with her cognitive states this does not support her claim that posthumous betrayals *necessarily* adversely affect the autonomy of the antemortem persons who are their objects. To see this, note that the betrayal of a person's trust will adversely affect her autonomy with respect to her consequent actions if it is her betrayer, and not her, who ultimately decides which actions she should perform, and who leads her to perform them through manipulating the information upon which she makes her decisions. (Here, by withholding the information that he intends to betray her to another in the future—an intention that itself constitutes a betrayal of her trust). As such, then, a person's autonomy could be compromised through her being subject to betrayal if the (unrecognized) betrayal of her trust occurs *prior to* her performance of the actions in question. It will only be then that her actions can be said to be subject to the control of her betrayer.[33] Were a person's betrayer to intend to keep (for example) the promise that he made to her, then, during the time that this was so, he would not be acting to motivate her to perform the actions that he desired her to perform. He would not be usurping control over information that was relative to her decision, and so it would thus not be he, but she, who was controlling which actions she performed. Moreover, even once he did break his promise to her, she would not suffer from compromised autonomy with respect to her actions if she knew of this, for then it would still be she, and not he, who would be directing the acts that she performed.[34] Thus, although her exercise of her autonomy in these latter situations would likely to have diminished instrumental value for her, she would not suffer from any compromise in her autonomy *per se* with respect to her actions.[35]

With this in hand, then, it is clear that Basil's friend's posthumous breaking of his promise to see that Basil's book was published did not adversely affect Basil's autonomy with respect to his actions in the way that Grover believes. If Basil's friend never intended to keep this promise Basil's autonomy with respect to his actions was not compromised by his friend's failure to get his book published after he died (i.e., the posthumous event), but by his friend's deception of him while he was alive. As such, then, if one understands the compromising of Basil's autonomy to be a harm to him this would not be a *posthumous* harm. If, however, Basil's friend did intend to keep his promise while Basil was alive but broke it after his death (by, for example, being bribed to do so by one of Basil's academic rivals), then he did not deceive Basil during his life, and so he did not act to ensure that it was he, and not Basil, who ultimately decided what type of actions Basil would perform. As such, then, Basil's autonomy with respect to his actions was undiminished by this later betrayal—and, again, no posthumous harm was incurred.

Grover's Knowledge and Autonomy View of how posthumous harm is possible thus fails, for it is based on a misunderstanding of how being betrayed adversely affects a person's autonomy. One might, however, try to salvage this approach to offering an account of how posthumous harm is possible by arguing that insofar as a posthumous event such as a betrayal could adversely affect the *instrumental* value of a person's autonomy this could affect the quality of her life, and, as such, harm her. Yet although this approach might at first seem plausible, it too should be rejected. When an event adversely affects the instrumental value of a person's autonomy it does so by making it less likely that the desires or interests that the exercise of her autonomy was intended to satisfy or fulfill will be satisfied or fulfilled. Thus, to claim that a person could be harmed by an event after her death insofar as this would adversely affect the instrumental value of her autonomy is simply to claim that an event that occurs after a person's death could harm her by making it more likely that her desires or interests would be thwarted. This final autonomy-based attempt to offer an account of how posthumous harm is possible, then, is simply the Feinberg-Pitcher account of posthumous harm in disguise. And, as was argued in the previous chapter, this account of how posthumous harm is possible is mistaken.

SPERLING'S HUMAN SUBJECT ACCOUNT

Sperling's Argument

Since neither Levenbook's nor Grover's accounts of how posthumous harm is possible should be accepted, what of that developed by Daniel Sperling? Sperling begins his account by distinguishing between material and non-material ways in which people can exist. They can, he claims, exist materially as physical beings that are aggregates of cells, "and/or" they can exist in "a non-material way as a 'man', a 'person', a human being', etc."[36] Sperling holds that "some of the ways in which one exists—like human being or person—are fictions", such that "their creation is an imaginative construction or a pretence that does not represent actuality, but has been invented in order to symbolize some kind of moral or legal status their owner is endowed with."[37] With this claim in hand Sperling holds that one form of fictional existence that could be applied to men or women is that of the "Human Subject", where this is "the subject *holding* all human interests belonging to the person whose interests they are."[38] This subject, claims Sperling, is persistent over time, where this is understood as "there is no point in time where its existence ceases," it is "in time", and it is non-material.[39] Since, Sperling claims, some of a person's interests "apply" to periods of time before and after her actual life the existence of the Human Subject ranges over a period of time that extends both before and after the life of the person whose interests they are. The Human Subject does not have interests, though, but only holds them for the person whose interests they actually are.

Sperling claims that the existence of non-material objects such as the Human Subject is enshrined in our language, for we often both refer to persons that are no longer living and predicate properties of them, such as in the phrase "Napoleon is now being eulogized". Similarly, claims Sperling, when we say things such as "we love Socrates" we presume that Socrates (in the form of the Human Subject) still exists to be loved.[40] As such, concludes Sperling, "for the purpose of our talking, thinking, and ascribing properties to the dead or the subject whose person is no longer 'alive' (including the property of holding certain interests), it is sufficient to argue for the existence of a non-material subject holding interests for that person".[41] With these claims in hand Sperling argues that posthumous harm is possible because when a person's interests are thwarted the subject harmed "is the Human Subject and not the *ante-mortem* person who no longer exists after death". In this way, then, Sperling believes that he avoids both the problem of the subject and the problem of backwards causation that beset the Feinberg-Pitcher account of how posthumous harm is possible.

Criticisms of Sperling's Argument

The first point to make about Sperling's argument for the possibility of posthumous harm is the simplest one: Why should we believe that Human Subjects exist? Sperling's response to this question is to point out that we often refer to persons who are no longer living and predicate properties of them, and that we often claim to have certain emotional attitudes towards them, also. These phenomena, claim Sperling, indicate that the existence of a Human Subject is not counterintuitive to us. But this is not so. Instead, all that the phenomena he lists show is that we refer to, predicate properties of, and even have (or believe that we have) emotional attitudes towards things that we believe do not exist.[42] Thus, rather than supporting Sperling's view, these phenomena undermine it. Furthermore, Sperling's direct arguments for the existence of a Human Subject are unpersuasive. Sperling holds that just as people can exist in non-material ways as imaginative constructs such as "human being" or "person" which have been invented "to symbolize some kind of moral or legal status their owner is endowed with," so too can the Human Subject similarly exist to hold the interests of persons after they die. But there are two problems with this account. First, human beings are not "imaginative constructs", but are simply (and materially) bipedal primates in the family *Hominidae*. Second, while Sperling is on firmer ground claiming that persons are imaginative constructs, this does not mean that the concept of "person" does not pick out some cluster of properties that objectively (i.e., non-imaginatively) exist, and which would do so even if the concept of "person" ceased to be used. In response to this Sperling could claim that the same is true of the Human Subject. Given that it is objectively true that a person P's interests were $I_1. \ldots I_n$, then insofar as the Human Subject serves as a placeholder for these interests after P died it would, like the concept of a person, be an imaginative construct that picked out a cluster of properties that objectively exist. There is, however, an important disanalogy between the concept of a person and the concept of the Human Subject. This is that while the concept of a person has been constructed to pick out those properties of human beings that are held to have moral or legal significance the concept of a Human Person has been constructed *only* to explain how posthumous harm is possible while avoiding the problem of the subject and the problem of backwards causation. As such, then, it is based on the *assumption* that such harm is possible—and so its positing cannot support an *argument* for this without being circular. Moreover, in holding that it is not the person whose interests are thwarted or fulfilled that is harmed but the Human Subject who is holding them for him is puzzling, for it is not clear how a non-material construct can itself be harmed or benefitted—and it is especially unclear how such a construct can be harmed by the thwarting of interests that it is merely holding for another entity.[43] Sperling's account of how posthumous harm is possible thus fails.

HARM AND IMPLICATION IN EVIL

The final account of how posthumous harm is possible that will be considered in this chapter is that which has been developed by Paul Griseri. Griseri begins by claiming that a person can be harmed by being implicated in evil, even if she herself did not perform the evil acts.[44] To exemplify this he offers the example of a great pacifist leader whose supporters attempt to revenge his murder by the members of a different racial group by killing persons from that racial group, "even though those killed as a supposed revenge had no part in the original assassination".[45] This leader, Griseri claims, has been harmed by the actions of his followers even though he himself had no part in them and they went directly against his teachings. Griseri does not offer any clear argument as to why he is justified in claiming that the pacifist leader in his example suffered from posthumous harm inflicted upon him by his vengeful followers. However, two strands of argument can be teased out of his remarks, one explicit and one implicit.

   Griseri claims explicitly that "a dead person is harmed morally when our understanding of their former conception of the world is impaired by events subsequent to their death".[46] To support this Griseri argues that the performance of certain actions will lead to persons viewing the acts in question as being possible objects of choice. For example, a person who responds to a murder by engaging in retaliatory revenge will in so doing contribute to "creating or confirming a certain habitual way of seeing the world".[47] Were persons not to engage in such retaliation, however, it might be the case that retaliatory revenge would not be considered to be an option, even if in practice it could be. The avenging of the pacifist leader through retaliatory action, then, would serve to create, or at least to reinforce, a view of the world in which such retaliation is a viable option. *Ex hypothesi*, the pacifist leader's view of the world was one in which such retaliatory revenge was not an option in the sense that it would not even have been considered and dismissed. For his followers to respond to his death in this way, then, would be for them to undermine the possibility that his conception of the world and the appropriate ways to respond to events within it would be that which is generally accepted, and to move towards replacing it with their own.

Yet although this might be an accurate account of what would follow from the vengeful actions of the pacifist leader's followers it is not clear how this would harm the dead pacifist leader, *unless* Griseri's view is that in acting in such a way that his conception of the world could be replaced by theirs his followers are (however unwittingly) acting so as to thwart his interests, and that this thwarting harms him. But, if this is so, then Griseri's account of how posthumous is possible will collapse into the Feinberg-Pitcher account with all of its attendant problems.

What, then, of the alternative account of how posthumous harm is possible that was implicit in Griseri's discussion? On this account a person can be harmed by being implicated in evil, even though he himself has performed no evil act, nor acted to encourage others to do so. The hallmark of such a harm is that the person so implicated in evil would be a fit subject of pity, as, for example, the players of a football team might be pitied for the violent actions of their supporters, "because they have been caught up in wrong through no fault of their own".[48] To be a fit subject for such pity, Griseri claims, a person must have some serious connection with the evil acts in question, such as, in the case of the pacifist leader, identifying with the persons who came to avenge him as his flock.[49] That is, he must possess what Larry May has characterized as *metaphysical guilt*, guilt that "arises out of each person's shared membership in groups that shape their identity, such that each member is implicated in the activities of any other member of the group".[50] Yet although this might be necessary for a person to be morally tainted by the actions of others, it is not sufficient. As Marina A. L. Oshana has argued, the attribution of moral taint to a person is made not only on the grounds of her membership within a group; she must also know that she is a member of the group in question, and have expressed solidarity with it in the past through taking vicarious shame or pride in the actions of its members.[51] Moreover, it seems that the attribution of moral taint is made with a purpose: to call for the person so tainted to respond to the wrongdoing of the other members of her group through attempting to atone for them. That is, insofar as a person is associated with a particular group and has acknowledged this association, the attribution of moral taint to him for the wrongdoing of its members is a call on him to acknowledge that what was done was wrong. In this way, then, attributing moral taint to persons functions to reinforce norms, and to motivate persons to repair the damage done when they are transgressed.

If Oshana's account of moral taint is an accurate one, there are (at least) three problems with Griseri's implicit argument for the possibility of posthumous harm. If moral taint is attributed to persons as a call for them to acknowledge and atone for the wrongdoing of other members of a group with which they identify, then it seems that—contra both Griseri and Gaita—such taint would not be attributed to persons for acts that others performed *after* their deaths. It would, for example, be odd to claim that Germans who died before the rise of Nazi Germany were tainted by the acts of the Nazis, although it would not be so odd to claim that the immediate generations of Germans that followed them were.[52] Even though persons might be tainted as a result of the actions of others, then, the transitivity of such taint is restricted to persons who are alive either during or after the performance of the acts in question. As such, its possibility does not support the possibility of posthumous harm as implication in evil. A similar point can be drawn from the observation that the attribution of moral taint to a person is made on the basis of her membership in a group. While such attributions might make sense for persons who are alive, they do not make sense for persons who are dead, since the dead do not exist.[53] As such, they cannot be members of groups in the way required to ground moral taint, and so cannot be subject to it. Finally, insofar as a person's moral taint would be constituted by the attitudes that both she and others take towards her, dead persons cannot suffer this stain. Clearly, a dead person cannot consider herself to be tainted. And, drawing from Callahan's criticisms of Levenbook, above, even if persons considered someone who was dead to be implicated in evil acts that were performed after his death, and hence tainted by them, claims about this taint would be claims about the beliefs that living persons had about him. They are thus not claims about what non-relational properties the person in question has.

CONCLUSION

It has been argued in this Chapter that the main alternatives to the Feinberg-Picther account of how posthumous harm is possible (those that have been developed by Levenbook, Grover, Sperling, and Griseri) are no more successful in showing the possibility of such harm than the account that they seek to replace. As was noted in the Introduction to this Chapter to reach this conclusion is not, though, to conclude that posthumous harm is impossible; it is only to conclude that, as yet, there is no reason to accept its possibility. To support the stronger conclusion that posthumous harm is *not* possible it will be argued in the next chapter that for a person to be harmed her experiences must be adversely affected in some way. If this hedonistic account of harm is correct, then it is clear that not only is there no reason to believe that posthumous harm is possible, but there is good reason to believe that it is not. Posthumous harm would thus be no less mythical than fairies or leprechauns.[54] And, as will be explored later in this volume, recognizing this will have serious implications for the many debates in bioethics in which the concept of posthumous harm plays an important role.

3 The Impossibility of Posthumous Harm

So far it has been argued (in Chapter 1) that the dominant account of how posthumous harm is possible, that developed independently by Pitcher and Feinberg, is mistaken. It has also been argued (in Chapter 2) that the primary alternatives to the Feinberg-Pitcher account of how posthumous harm is possible (those developed by Levenbook, Grover, Sperling, and Griseri) are also mistaken. However, while the arguments in those two chapters support the claim that there is no reason to believe that posthumous harm is possible, they do not (as was noted in both) support the stronger claim of the full-blooded Epicurean thanatology of this volume: that posthumous harm is *im*possible. To fill this lacuna it will be argued in this Chapter that we should adopt a hedonistic account of well-being, on which a person's well-being will depend solely on the pleasures or pains that she experiences.[1] Before moving towards this hedonistic account of well-being, however, two alternative arguments for the view that posthumous harm is impossible will be outlined, together with Steven Luper's objections to them. It will be argued that this exchange fails to move us in either direction with respect to the question of whether or not posthumous harm is impossible, for while Luper's responses to these arguments in favor of this view are flawed, so too are the arguments themselves. Thus, to show that posthumous harm is impossible this Chapter will move beyond these arguments to defend hedonism.

DEATH, GOODS, AND THE EXTINCTION OF DESIRES

Luper recognizes two arguments that could be offered in favor of the view that posthumous harm is impossible. The first is based upon the claim that "death precludes our having any subsequent goods, and later events cannot preclude our having goods that are already out of reach," for "We can attain or retain a good only while we exist . . . ".[2] Luper lends intuitive support to this argument by noting that "For example, it would be good for us if we were to become smarter or morally better. . . . but nothing that occurs after we die will have any impact on our intellectual or moral progress".[3] The second argument against the possibility of posthumous harm is based on the view that the permanent removal of a desire either thwarts it, or else "ensures that it cannot be harmfully thwarted".[4] Since all of a person's desires are removed by her death events that occur after her death cannot harm her, either because they cannot thwart her desires *simpliciter* because they have already been thwarted by her death, or because they cannot harmfully thwart them.[5]

If these two arguments are sound, then posthumous harm is impossible. Luper, however, argues that neither of these arguments should be accepted. Luper argues that the proponents of the first argument fail to distinguish between *personally defined* projects and *impersonally defined* projects. A personally defined project is a project "we define in terms of ourselves," such as the desire "to write a great novel, or to be the first to swim across Lake Michigan".[6] An impersonally defined project is a project that we wish to see come to fruition (such as the project "of curing lung cancer within ten years"), and it does not matter to the person who has it whether or not she is the person who brings it to fruition.[7] Luper holds that the success or failure of a person's personally defined projects will depend solely on events that occur during her life; whether she actually writes a great novel, for example, or is the first person to swim across Lake Michigan. As such, he accepts that nothing that could occur after a person dies could typically have any effect on the success or failure of her personally defined projects—and so with respect to these she is typically immune from posthumous harm. However, Luper argues, the success or failure of a person's impersonally defined projects could depend on events that occur after her death. For example, a person might cure lung cancer after the death of the person who had this as an impersonally defined project. As such, then, with respect to her impersonally defined projects a person could be subject to posthumous harm. Furthermore, holds Luper, even some of a person's personally defined projects could succeed or fail depending on the events that occur after her death. A person's desire that she have a good reputation after her death is a personally defined project whose success or failure depends upon events that occur after her death, as is her desire that her will be honored by her heirs, or that she write a novel that becomes famous after her death.[8] As such, then, he claims, "there are intuitively plausible examples of goods we can be robbed of by events that take place after we no longer exist, and hence plausible examples of posthumous harms".[9]

Against the second argument for the impossibility of posthumous harm Luper accepts that the removal of many desires does thwart them, for if an event permanently removes a desire that a person has to complete a project that only she can complete, her desire will be thwarted.[10] Insofar as a person's death thwarts such desires by removing them, then, it renders her immune to any posthumous harms concerning them for events subsequent to her death cannot thwart desires that have already been thwarted. Luper also accepts that there are two types of desires that cannot be harmfully thwarted once they have been removed. The first of these consists of desires that a person has voluntarily abandoned, such as her childhood desire to become a fireman.[11] The second consists of desires whose existence is conditional on their own persistence.[12] The satisfaction of these self-dependent desires at time t will only be good for the person whose desires they are, and their thwarting at time t will only be bad for him, if he continues to have them at t. Such desires will be ones whose satisfaction is good for the person satisfying them only insofar as he enjoys satisfying them. However, argues Luper, "not all desires are thwarted when removed, and not all desires are incapable of being harmfully thwarted after being removed," for "There are intuitively plausible examples of harm brought about by the thwarting of a desire we no longer have . . . ".[13] To support these claims Luper returns to the example of the impersonally defined project that a timely cure for cancer be found, holding that even if something acted against a person's will to remove her desire that cancer be cured subsequent events could still occur to satisfy that desire. As such, then, removing a person's desire need not thwart it. Moreover, since a person's impersonally defined projects could be thwarted by events that occur after her death such events could harmfully thwart her desires even after they have been removed (i.e., by death). Thus, concludes Luper, neither of the above two arguments for the impossibility of posthumous harm succeed.

RESPONDING TO LUPER

Luper's response to the first argument for the impossibility of posthumous harm is based upon the view that a person could be harmed either by the posthumous failure of some of her personally defined projects (i.e., those that could be affected by posthumous events) or by the posthumous failure of her impersonally defined projects; he supports this view by citing examples of events that are commonly held to inflict posthumous harm upon persons. Similarly, Luper's response to the second argument for the impossibility of posthumous harm is based on the view that certain events could harm a person after her death by harmfully thwarting her desires, even if she no longer has them. Luper's response to the first argument for the impossibility of posthumous harm thus amounts to little more than the claim that since certain events that occur after a person's death do, intuitively, harm her, posthumous harm is possible. But this does not so much establish the possibility of posthumous harm so much as it merely asserts this. In a related vein, although Luper is correct to argue that the elimination of a person's desire does not entail that that desire cannot be thwarted at a later date (and hence that the first aspect of the second argument for the impossibility of posthumous harm is mistaken), he does not argue for the further (and crucial) claim that such thwartings could harm the person whose desires were thwarted. Instead, as with his response to the first argument he addresses, he simply supports this view by asserting that certain such thwartings are intuitively harmful to the person concerned. In fairness to Luper, however, this strategy is not an unreasonable one given the content of the arguments that he is addressing. The first argument for the impossibility of posthumous harm that Luper outlines is based on the claim that "death precludes us from having *any* subsequent goods," from which it is concluded that posthumous harm is impossible.[14] As such, then, this argument amounts to little more than an assertion that posthumous harm is impossible, for this conclusion follows directly from the (unargued-for) first premise. Similarly, the second argument for the impossibility of posthumous harm that Luper outlines amounts to little more than the assertion that once a person is dead her desires cannot be harmfully thwarted, and so she is immune from posthumous harm.

Neither these two arguments in favor of the impossibility of posthumous harm, nor Luper's responses to them, then, are satisfactory. At this point in this volume (and in the debate in general), then, an impasse has been reached: there is no reason to believe that posthumous harm is possible, and yet there is no reason to believe that it is impossible, either. What is clear, though, is that the question of whether posthumous harm is possible turns on the question of whether it is possible for a person to be harmed without experiencing the harm in question. If it is, then posthumous harm is at least possible; if it is not, then it is not. The crucial question, then, is whether a person's well-being depends on her experiences only, or not. The responses to the Feinberg-Pitcher account of how posthumous harm is possible that were offered in Chapter 1 (e.g., that concerning the putative harms that the woman in Case A was subject to) were compatible with the view that a person's well-being is dependent upon something *other than* her experiences, and, as such, they left the door open for further arguments in favor of the possibility of posthumous harm to be developed. It is now time to close that door, and to show that not only is there no reason to believe that posthumous harm is possible—there is reason to believe that it is *not*.

TOWARDS HEDONISM

The title of this section is well-chosen, for what follows will not be fully-fledged defense of the view that a person's well-being depends solely upon her actual experiences. Rather, in this section it will be argued that a plausible account of hedonism can be developed that can accommodate all of the intuitions that are generated by the thought experiments that are usually invoked to show that a person's well-being depends on something other than her experiences. If this account of hedonism is correct, then it will automatically follow that posthumous harm is impossible, for the experiences that an antemortem person has cannot be affected by events that occur after his death.[15]

To begin, then, consider one of the most famous thought experiments that have been taken to show that a person's experiences are not the only factors that contribute to the degree of well-being that she enjoys: Nozick's experience machine.[16] The experience machine could "give you any experience you desired. Superduper neurosurgeons could stimulate your brain so that you would think and feel that you were writing a great novel, or making a friend, or reading an interesting book. All the time you would be floating in a tank, with electrodes attached to your brain".[17] As attractive as the experience machine might sound, it is generally agreed that people would prefer not to plug into it.[18] This reluctance is equally generally held to indicate that a person's well-being is not constituted solely by her experiences, but by something other than her experiences alone.[19] And, if it is true that a person's well-being is constituted by something other than her experiences alone then the possibility of persons being subject to posthumous harm is a live one. Although an event that occurs after her death could not affect her antemortem experiences it *could* affect whatever else contributes to her well-being (e.g., that her interests not be thwarted) on whatever non-hedonistic account of well-being is correct.

Although he is not concerned with defending the view that posthumous harm is impossible Joseph Mendola has argued against the anti-hedonistic conclusion that the example of the experience machine is supposed to support on the grounds that it would not be held that persons within a Berkeleyian universe would lack any degree of well-being. Since there is no real difference between Nozick's experience machine and a Berkeleyian universe, Mendola argues, it seems that the example of the experience machine does not support the non-hedonistic approach to well-being as clearly as it is often taken to.[20] Yet although this comparison of Mendola's could be used to help indirectly support the case for the impossibility of posthumous harm it must be admitted that there is a disanalogy between the experience of a person within the experience machine and the experience of a person in a Berkeleyian universe. Whereas the person within the Berkeleyian universe would interact with other (immaterial, but nonetheless real) persons, a person in the experience machine would not. Of course, Mendola could respond by noting that this would not matter, insofar as the experiences of a person in a Berkeleyian universe and a person in an experience machine could be identical; it is just that the latter would be unwittingly interacting with zombies (beings that appear identical to humans but which lack mental states), whereas the former would not. As such, for a person to claim that life in a Berkleyian universe would be preferable to life in an experience machine would be for her to claim that there is something valuable in and of itself about interacting with persons that have certain mental states, even if such states are in principle inaccessible to the interactee. And this, one might think, would be a very odd claim indeed. To make this apparently anti-hedonistic conclusion more plausible, however, consider the difference between a person's being with someone who truly loves her, and her being with a zombie whose behavior is identical; although there is no difference in behavior, it might seem reasonable for a person to prefer being loved and experiencing this, rather than merely experiencing being loved.

Yet while it might seem that this response to Mendola's comparison between the experience machine and a Berkelyian universe supports the non-hedonistic approach to analyzing personal well-being it does not. Although it is natural to think that a person's preference for being loved over merely experiencing being loved would be made on the basis of her concern for her own well-being this is not necessarily the case. Instead, a person could prefer that she be loved over merely experiencing being loved even if her experiences would be identical because she believes that being loved is intrinsically valuable, and so she values it independently of any effect that it could have on her experiences. And if a person intrinsically values a certain state of affairs she will value it for its own sake independently of any considerations of her own well-being. (A person might, for example, value the well-being of her children in this way.)[21] As such, then, that persons might prefer not to enter the experience machine does not in itself support the non-hedonic approach to analyzing well-being, for this approach is compatible with a hedonistic account of well-being that admits the possibility of things (e.g. knowledge of one's real situation) other than well-being being intrinsically valuable.[22] Furthermore, noting that persons might value states of affairs for their own sake independently of any consideration that these might have on their own well-being indicates a distinction that needs to be drawn to support the intuitive plausibility of hedonism (and hence the view that posthumous harm is impossible). This distinction is that between something being a harm *for* a person, and its being a harm *to* her.[23] Something is a harm *for* a person at *t* when it prevents the existence of a state of affairs that she holds (or held) at *t* to be valuable independently of considerations of her own well-being. Thus, something could be a harm *for* a person without thereby affecting her well-being. Something is a harm *to* a person, however, when it adversely affects her well-being. (The usual sense of harm is thus captured by claims about things that are harms *to* persons.) It is important to note here that to claim that something is a harm *for* a person is not necessarily to ascribe any properties to her. Rather, it is just to note that something has occurred that has prevented the occurrence of something that she holds, or would have held to be, valuable independently of considerations of her own well-being. As such, third-person claims that something is a harm for a person (e.g., "Poor Richard—he would have been devastated had he known *The Castle* pub would close . . . ") are to be understood as being similar to claims about the effect that it would have had upon her had it affected her experiences.

It might be objected that something that is a harm for a person must thereby be a harm to her.[24] The plausibility of this objection, however, stems from conflating first-person ascriptions of something being a harm for a person with third-person ascriptions of something being such a harm.

When a person correctly believes that an event that has occurred is a harm *for* her she will hold that it has prevented the existence of a state of affairs that she holds to be valuable independently of its effect of her own well-being. In believing correctly that this event is a harm for her, then, she is likely to suffer disappointment, sadness, or frustration. A person's belief that something is a harm for her is thus likely to be accompanied by its being a harm to her, insofar as this belief is likely adversely to affect her well-being. A third-person ascription of harm for a person, however, need not have this effect. For example, when in Evelyn Waugh's novel *Decline and Fall* Paul Pennyfeather's guardian chastised him for being sent down from Oxford University by telling him that he was glad that his (Paul's) father had not lived to witness his disgrace he is holding both that Paul's disgrace is a harm for his father (i.e., it was a state of affairs that Paul's father would have disvalued in itself), and that it is not a harm to his father (i.e., he is glad that his father was spared the adverse effect that this would have had on his well-being).

Distinguishing between something's being a harm for a person and a harm to her could support the claim that posthumous events could be harms for a person, but not harms to her.[25] To provide full support for this claim, however, an account of what it is for something to be a harm to a person must be provided. It is uncontroversial that a person will be harmed by an event if it causes him to have a bad experience.[26] Causing pain to a person, for example, is to harm him. It is also uncontroversial that an event could be a harm to a person if it causes him to have an experience that is worse than that which he would have had had it not occurred, even if the experience that he has is not itself a bad one. For example, if a person does not secure an unexpected promotion that he would have otherwise been granted as a result of a slander that he never finds out about, the slander would have harmed him, even if his life without the promotion is a perfectly good one. Given these examples it makes sense (independently of the aim of this volume), to develop an experientially-based approach to analyzing what it is for an event to be a harm to a person. At first blush, then, an event E causes harm to a person P iff it adversely affects the experiences that he has, whether by inflicting bad experiences upon him or by preventing him from having better experiences than those that he actually has subsequent to E's occurrence.

Three points should be noted concerning this (admittedly rough) account of what it is for an event to cause harm to a person. First, as the example of the person harmed by the slander that he never discovers shows, on this account of what it is for an event to cause harm to a person the person concerned need not know about the event in question. As such, then, this account is not committed to the claim that what a person does not know about cannot hurt him.[27] Second, since this account of what it is for an event to cause harm to a person focuses on the effects on the effect upon his experience, it is possible for a person to be harmed by an event that occurs when he does not exist. A person could, for example, be harmed by an event that occurred before he was born, if it caused his experiences once he was alive to be worse than they would have otherwise been.[28] Finally, this experiential account of what it is for an event to cause harm to a person leaves open what type of experiences count. As it stands it is, for example, compatible with certain types of "objective list" accounts of well-being, on which a person's well-being will depend upon him having certain experiences, whether or not he himself desires them.[29] It is also compatible with a more agent-centered objective approach to analyzing well-being, on which a person's well-being will depend upon his having certain experiences that are good for him, whether or not he recognizes this. And, of course, it is compatible with a range of subjective accounts of well-being, on which a person's well-being is dependent upon his having experiences that he takes to be good for him.[30]

With this rough account of what it is for an event to cause harm to a person in place, it is clear that it is subject to an immediate objection: that on this account even events that thwart a person's most important interests would not be harms to him until they affected his experiences. This point can be illustrated through the example of a woman, Brenda, whose beloved husband Tony was killed in an accident while exploring a jungle in a foreign country. On this account of what it is for an event to cause harm to a person Brenda is not harmed by Tony's death until it has an adverse effect on her experiences. (This need not be when she finds out about it; her social-climbing friends, for example, who only associated with her because of his social status might hear of his death before her and disinvite her from their parties.) But this is counterintuitive; surely Brenda is harmed *by Tony's death*, and not by the effects that Tony's death have on her experiences? The intuitive force of this example can, however, by quelled by drawing upon the above distinction between an event being a harm *for* a person, and its being a harm *to* her. Tony's death was certainly a harm *for* Brenda, in that it was something that she disvalues independently of its effects on her well-being. However, it is not a harm *to* her until it adversely affects her experiences. To lend support to this claim consider a situation in which Brenda dies of a disease before Tony's death has any effect on her experiences. It is not implausible to imagine one of Brenda's (genuine) friends, Beaver, being relieved that Tony's death never harmed Brenda on the grounds that she was, at least, spared being affected by it in her final days. As such, it is not as odd as it might at first appear to hold that while Tony's death was a harm for Brenda it was not a harm to her.

To be sure, this account of what it is for an event to be a harm to a person is only a very rough outline. To be complete an account of the ways in which an event's effects upon a person's experiences will cause harm to her must be supplied. Similarly, an account of the correct baseline from which it should be judged that a person's experiences are better or worse than they would have been absent an event that is held to have caused harm to her will have to be supplied, to complete the account of when an event causes harm to a person through causing her to have worse experiences than she would have done absent its occurrence.[31] Yet although this account of what it is for an event to cause harm to a person is admittedly in need of elaboration it is still intuitively plausible. Moreover, in distinguishing between something being a harm to a person and a harm for her, it is still possible to claim that certain events should be regretted on a person's behalf (e.g., the death of Tony could be regretted on Brenda's behalf by Tony's companions in the jungle) without claiming that they cause harm to her, and so the intuition that such thwarting of a person's interests is in some (admittedly vestigial) sense bad for her can be preserved. And if both this account of what it is for an event to be a harm to a person and this distinction between harm to and harm for are acceptable, then it is clear that it is impossible for a person ever to be harmed by an event that occurs after her death.[32]

OBJECTS AND CAUSES

In outlining the above hedonistic account of harm it was assumed that since an event or a state of affairs will only be harmful to a person if it adversely affects her experiences an event or a state of affairs will be a harmful one iff it *causes* harm.[33] That a hedonistic account of harm necessitates a causal account of harm in this way has, however, been challenged by Silverstein. Although Silverstein accepts that an event or a state of affairs x that is harmful to a person, A, is such in virtue of its making it the case that A has a negative experience, Silverstein holds that "The relevant connection between an A-relative evil, x, and A's negative experience—A's feelings of grief, for instance—is not that x does (or can) *cause* those feelings but that x is (or can be) the *object* of those feelings."[34] Silverstein distinguishes between x causing harm to A through being connected in a certain way to A's having negative feelings and x being the object of those feelings to make room for his account of how posthumous harm is possible that is based on the view that "for x to be an evil for A, x must make, or at least be capable of making, a relevant (i.e., a 'negative') difference to A's experience".[35] If Silverstein is right that one can both hold an account of harm on which an event or a state of affairs can only be harmful if it adversely effects the life of the person it harms, *and* hold that the event or state of affairs in question need not cause this harm to be harmful then the above argument against the possibility of posthumous harm moves too quickly, for it is based on the implicit denial that these two views are compatible with each other. To support the view that posthumous harm is impossible, then, one must show that there is no reason to accept Silverstein's view.

The first attempt to show that there is no reason to accept Silverstein's view that a person can only be harmed by an event or a state of affairs if it is *connected with his having a negative experience* is compatible with the view that the event or state of affairs in question is harmful even though it did not *cause* the experience has been developed by Rosenbaum. Rosenbaum focuses on Silverstein's claim that the "relevant connection" between an A-relative evil x is not that x *causes* negative feelings in A, but that it is the *object* of them.[36] Rosenbaum holds that the objects of a person's negative feelings need not exist, illustrating this with the fact that "Britons in the early 1940's feared an invasion . . . by the Nazis," although "that event never occurred".[37] Since this is so, he argues, Silverstein is mistaken to believe that the relevant connection between an A-relative evil x and A's negative experience is that x is the object of A's experience. As Rosenbaum argues, something can only harm a person if it exists—and the objects of a person's psychological attitudes do not necessarily meet this requirement.

Rosenbaum's objection to Silverstein is, however, mistaken. As Silverstein makes clear in responding to Rosenbaum his argument in favor of the possibility of posthumous harm rests on a *de re* conception of the objects of a person's psychological attitudes, whereas Rosenbaum assumes that it is based on a *de dicto* conception of them. As Silverstein notes, whereas on Rosenbaum's conception of "object" the claim "A Nazi invasion of Britain is the "object" of A's fear" is true provided that it is true that A fears a Nazi invasion of Britain, on his (Silverstein's) conception of "object" this claim will only be true provided that there *is* a Nazi invasion of Britain and A fears it. Thus, concludes Silverstein, unless Rosenbaum can show that his *de re* conception of object is in some way illegitimate, he has not provided a reason for anyone to reject his (Silverstein's) argument.

With this response to Rosenbaum in hand, Silverstein argues that the relevant connection between an A-relative evil, x, and A's negative experience is that x is the *object*, and not the *cause*, of A's experience. Silverstein begins by offering "Case 1", in which John learns of his wife's, Ann's, affair with his friend Phil from another friend of his, Jim. Once this occurs "John shifts immediately from being gloriously happy to being totally miserable".[38] Silverstein notes that both Ann's affair and Jim's informing John of it were "causal factors in the production of John's misery," although "only Ann's behavior . . . is the object of those feelings," and "surely the most plausible view is that only Ann's behavior is an evil for John".[39] Since this is so, concludes Silverstein, this Case supports his view that the relevant connection between the evil of Ann's affair for John is not that it *caused* his misery (for so did Jim's informing John of it), but that it was the *object* of his negative experiences concerning it. As Silverstein recognizes, however, Case 1 does not show that x's being a causal antecedent of A's negative feelings is not a *necessary* condition for it to be a harm to him, for at most it only shows that its being one of their causal antecedents is not a *sufficient* condition for it to be a harm to him.[40] To rectify this Silverstein develops "Case 2", in which Jim thinks that he has learned that Ann is having an affair with Phil through overhearing a conversation, but where the couple under discussion was actually Jan and Bill. Notwithstanding Jim's mistake, Ann and Phil are actually having an affair, and so when John "shifts immediately from being gloriously happy to being totally miserable" he does so as a result of learning the truth about his situation.[41] Case 2, argues Silverstein, shows that the relevant connection between an A-relative evil x and A's negative experiences is not that x must be a causal antecedent of them, for although Ann's affair was what harmed John it was not a causal antecedent of John's misery. Instead, concludes Silverstein, Case 2 shows that the relevant connection between an A-relative evil x and A's negative experiences is that x is the *de re* object of them.

Silverstein's argument from Case 2 rests on it being the case that the A-relative evil at issue is Ann's affair—and there's the rub. As was argued above, Tony's death was not a harm *to* Brenda until it adversely affected her experiences (although it was a harm *for* her independently of this). Without argument, then, there is no reason to accept Silverstein's crucial claim that Ann's affair is the A-relative evil at issue (i.e., the harm to John) in Cases 1 and 2. Instead, given the arguments above, it seems that the harm to John (i.e., what harmed John) was not Ann's affair, but Jim's informing him of it. Silverstein, though, does have an argument for what he takes to be "the most plausible view" of the situation, "that only Ann's behavior is an evil for John": "If we ask John himself 'Were you harmed by Ann [because of her affair], by Jim [because he told you what Ann was doing], or both?' the natural answer would be 'I was harmed by Ann, not by Jim; Jim simply informed me of the harm Ann was doing.'". Yet although Silverstein is right that this would be the most natural answer, this does not support his view as much as he thinks it does. The question posed to John ("Were you harmed by Ann . . . by Jim . . . or both?") is ambiguous. It could be understood to be a *metaphysical* question, aimed at establishing whose actions brought about the harm to John. Or it could be understood as an *ethical* question, aimed at establishing who is blameworthy for bringing about the harm to John. Clearly, answering "Ann" to this question will only support Silverstein's view if it is the answer to the metaphysical understanding of this question. But the most natural understanding of this question is the ethical one. (That is, asking John "Were you harmed by Ann . . . by Jim . . . or both?" is most naturally understood as asking him who was blameworthy for his harming.) That John would naturally answer "Ann" to this question, then, does not show (as Silverstein believes) that the A-relative evil in question is Ann's affair.

Thus far, then, there is no reason to believe that the relevant connection between an A-relative evil x and A's negative experiences is that x is the *de re* object (and not cause) of them. Moreover, there is (and in addition to the arguments offered above) reason to believe that this connection *is* a causal one. To see this, consider a modified version of Silverstein's Case 2—Case 2(a)—in which only Jan, and not Ann, is having an affair. In this case it is clear that Jim is not harmed by any affair of Ann's, even though it is the *de dicto* object of his negative psychological attitudes. Rather, he is harmed by

Jim's making him believe that Ann is having an affair. Although Case 2(a) does not fit with Silverstein's account of the relevant connection between an A-relative evil, x, and A's negative experiences, it is open to him to claim that where there is no *de re* object of A's negative experiences then they could have a *de dicto* object, with the relevant connection between the perceived evil x and A's negative experiences being a causal one. (That is, John's negative experiences in Case 2(a) were caused by his [false] perception that Ann was having an affair.) Yet although this is a coherent account of this connection it would be better to have a unified account of it that would apply whether the object of A's negative psychological attitudes was *de dicto* or *de re*. And such an account would be one in which this connection was a *causal* one. Thus, in Case 1 John's negative psychological attitudes were caused jointly by Ann's affair and by Jim's informing him of it, while in Case 2 they were caused by Jim alone—as they were in Case 2(a).[42] As such, then, the assumption that grounded the above hedonistic account of harm—that an event or a state of affairs will be a harmful one iff it *causes* harm—is (contra Silverstein) justified.

CONCLUSION

The arguments in this Chapter have moved the Epicurean project of this volume beyond the conclusions of the two Chapters that preceded it, having shown not only is there no reason to believe that posthumous harm is possible, but that there is reason to believe that it is impossible. It was argued in this Chapter there is reason to believe that hedonism is the correct account of well-being—and if this is so, then no events that occur after a person's death could be harms *to* her; that is, they could not be harms proper. This is not to deny that persons might have reason to feel regret on behalf of another if her projects fail after her death, or other events occur that she would have been upset by, for such occurrences could be harms *for* a person. However, since such occurrences would not be harms to her they would not be harms proper (they would instead be, as it were, only *expressively* considered to be harms) and so they would have no affect on her well-being. Despite this, it must be stressed that the arguments presented in this chapter do not conclusively prove the truth of hedonism—and they are not intended to. However, they do show that as a theory of well-being hedonism has been too-swiftly rejected within contemporary philosophy, and that a more robust defense than it is usually credited with can be supplied. And since part of this involves arguing that the correct connection between an A-relative evil x and A's negative experiences is that x is the cause of these experiences there is good reason to reject Silverstein's account of how posthumous harm is possible. As has already been noted in both this and the preceding pair of chapters that persons cannot be harmed by events that occur after their deaths has significant implications for many debates within contemporary bioethics—a point that will be explored further in Chapters 8 and 9. Before turning to such practical matters, however, two further theoretical questions must be addressed: the question of whether the dead can be wronged, and the question of whether a person can be harmed by her own death.

4   Can the Dead be Wronged?

In Alexander McCall Smith's novel *Friends, Lovers, Chocolate*, the following exchange takes place between Isabel Dalhousie, the editor of the (fictitious) *Review of Applied Ethics*, and Angus Spens, a journalist, after Spens had claimed that Lord Darnley, the husband of Mary Queen of Scots, had participated in the murder of Rizzio, her Italian secretary, out of jealousy:

> "Where exactly is your evidence, Angus" she challenged. "You can't go around defaming people like that. You do Darnley a great injustice."
>
> Angus laughed. "How can you speak like that? This all happened in—when was it?—fifteen sixty-something. Can you do an injustice to somebody who hasn't been with us for over four hundred years? Hardly."
>
> Again Isabel felt that she had to protest. As it happened, she was interested in the philosophical issue of whether you can harm the dead. There was more than one view on that. . . . But perhaps this was not the time.[1]

Isabel is certainly correct to note that there is more than one view as to whether the dead can be harmed—although, as has been argued in the first three chapters of this volume, only the view that they cannot should be accepted. However, she is mistaken to assimilate the question of whether the dead can be harmed to the question of whether they can be wronged, to have injustice done to them, for these are separate issues.[2] First, as was noted in Chapter 1, it could be possible to wrong someone without thereby harming her.[3] Second, a person can be harmed without being wronged; such would be the case of a person who has been justly punished.

Given the arguments in the preceding Chapters the conflation of the question of whether posthumous harms are possible with the question of whether it is possible to wrong the dead is one that those who believe that events can adversely affect persons after their deaths would do well to avoid. Since it could be possible for a person to be wronged without being harmed it is possible that events that occur after a person's death might *wrong* her, even if they cannot *harm* her.[4] Moreover, establishing that persons could be subject to posthumous wrongs is not only of theoretical interest. Just as the possibility of posthumous harm is important in addressing a wide variety of bioethical issues, so too is the possibility of posthumous wrong.[5] Indeed, insofar as the claim that certain actions (such as the posthumous removal of a person's organs for transplant against her wishes) could harm persons after their deaths could be used to ground the claim that such actions were wrong, to establish that persons could be subject to posthumous wrongs independently of their being subject to posthumous harm would provide a more direct moral argument against the acts in question.

Can, then, the dead be wronged? It will be argued in this Chapter that not only is there no reason to believe that they can be (as none of the arguments that have been marshaled in defense of the view that they can be are successful), there is reason to think that the dead cannot be wronged.[6] And, like the conclusion that the dead cannot be harmed, this will not only be of interest to persons with thantaological interests, but will also have important implications for many debates in contemporary bioethics.

DESERT AND INJUSTICE

Despite the widespread acceptance of the view that the dead can be wronged arguments in favor of this position are conspicuous by their virtual absence in the philosophical literature.[7] This absence might be explained by the apparently widespread view that it is simply uncontroversial that the dead can be wronged.[8] Feinberg, for example, appears to find this claim obvious, and indeed uses its alleged uncontroversial nature to support his argument that posthumous harm is possible.[9] This absence might also be explained by the equally widespread view that if the dead can be harmed they can also be wronged, and by the focus in the philosophical literature on establishing the first of these claims.[10] One argument that has been developed in support of the view that the dead can be wronged is the desert-based argument of Nelson P. Lande. In the context of arguing that the Bolshevik Oppositionists who were victimized by Stalin deserve to have their good names posthumously rehabilitated Lande argues that persons have a right to their good names, provided that these are deserved, and hence a right not to have an undeserved bad name. From this, Lande holds that if a person has lies told about him that compromise his good name, or truths about him that would enhance it are either severed from it or prevented from being attached to it, then he will have been treated unjustly. Thus, since the good names of persons who are now dead could be affected in these ways, the dead can be treated unjustly—and so the dead can be wronged.[11]

Lande's argument is as follows:

> (a) Suppose that someone possess a good name. (b) Suppose too that his good name is also, as it were, a *true* name, i.e., that he has actually

done what he is reputed to have done, and has not done anything that would seriously compromise his good name. (c) It would seem to follow, then, that he *deserves* his good name. (d) Hence he has a *right* to it, as well as a right not to have a bad name. (e) But whoever foists upon one (without his consent, of course) that which he has a right to not have foisted upon him, or takes from one, or prevents one from acquiring (again, without his consent) that to which he has a right, thereby treats him unjustly.[12]

Lande's argument here is invalid, as the move from premise (c) to premise (d) is unjustified: that a person *deserves* X does not entail that he therefore *has a right to* X. Lande, however, recognizes that this is a problem, noting that "To be sure, not all cases of one's deserving a given object are cases of his having a right to it. Cordelia may well *deserve* . . . a share of the kingdom, but only her sisters, notwithstanding that they are undeserving of it, have a *right* to it".[13] Having noted this, Lande defends his move from premise (c) to premise (d) by claiming that "Normally. . . . when one is thought to deserve a particular object . . . and when his acquiring that object would not violate anyone else's rights, then not only would it be quite natural to say that he is *entitled* to it, it would be equally natural to say that he has a *right* to it, such that interference therewith would constitute an act of injustice".[14] However, just as Lande's inference from (c) to (d) is mistaken, so too is his inference that if a person P deserves X and P's acquiring X would not violate anyone else's rights, then P is entitled to X such that he has a right to receive it. To see this, consider a situation in which a person dies intestate, leaving behind only his faithful and loving daughter and his goods in a kingdom in which there are no legal provisions for the automatic inheritance of goods by the surviving relatives of intestate persons. Although in this situation the daughter would still (*ex hypothesi*) deserve to inherit her father's goods, she is not thereby automatically entitled to them, for, even though her acquisition of them would not violate the rights of other persons, *without further argument* she does not have a moral right to receive them. Thus, although this orphaned daughter *might* be entitled to receive her father's estate given the provision of arguments in support of her claim to it (e.g., that there are good rule-consequentialist reasons for deserving children to inherit their parents' estates), this entitlement does not automatically follow from the fact that she deserves it and that her receiving it would violate no one else's rights.

To undermine further Lande's argument here it is useful to consider the examples that he offers to support it; that of a person deserving a gold medal for having placed first in a competition, and a person who deserves a night on the town for having worked hard all week.[15] Let us grant the plausible claims that in both cases the persons concerned deserve the goods that they seek to acquire, and it is also true that neither will violate another's rights by acquiring them. Moreover, it also seems true that in both cases the persons concerned are *entitled* (at least negatively, in the case of the night on the town) to the goods in question. But this entitlement does not follow from the two claims concerning these persons that Lande believes support it. Consider first the case of the person who is entitled to receive a gold medal for having placed first. This entitlement flows directly from his having placed first, and, thus according to the rules of the competition in which he was involved, being entitled to receive the gold medal. As such, then, this entitlement does *not* flow directly from the facts that he deserved the medal and that his acquisition of it would not violate another person's rights, for neither of these claims feature in the account of why he is entitled to the medal. (Indeed, it is possible to imagine cases in which the winner of a competition did not deserve to win, but was still entitled to the medal once he did. For example, a bad tennis player might win a match against a world-class opponent simply through luck, as a result of dust being accidentally blown into his opponent's eyes throughout the match.) That a person is entitled to a prize that he won in competition does not thereby show that he deserves it. Now consider the case of the hard working person who was, Lande claims, entitled to a night on the town. Unlike the winner of the gold medal this person was not involved in a game whose rules entitled him to a night on the town if he met certain criteria. However, Lande's claim that "it would be quite natural to say that he is *entitled* to it," and so "it would be equally natural to say that he has a *right* to it," seem plausible (at least if the right in question is understood as a negative right). This entitlement and the right that it entails can be explained, however, not by reference to the claim that the hard worker in question deserved a night on the town and that his having one did not violate anyone else's rights, but simply by noting that he is entitled to spend his money and his time as he wishes, provided that he does not violate anyone else's rights in so doing. As such, then, his entitlement is not to *receive* a night on the town, as the medal winner was entitled to receive the medal, but to be free from others interfering with his pursuit of one. Thus, although Lande is correct to note that it is natural to hold that both the medal winner and the hard worker are entitled to the gold medal and a night on the town, respectively, these entitlements are not grounded in their deserving these goods.

Yet although Lande fails to show that if a person P deserves to acquire a good X, and his acquiring it would not violate the rights of anyone else, P is entitled to X such that he has a right to it, and thus he fails to show that a dead person could be wronged by having his right to a good name posthumously violated, an alternative version of his argument could be developed to establish the same conclusion. To begin, note that the Lande's argument was supposed to establish the conclusion that a dead person could be wronged if his right to have his deserved good name rehabilitated by the agent whose duty it was to do so was not upheld. Thus, as with the medal winner and the hard worker, Lande's view is that the Bolshevik Oppositionists had the right to receive something, namely the rehabilitation of their good names, and were they not to do so they would have been wronged. Rather than focusing on trying to establish that the dead have the *positive* right to receive some thing X from the living on the grounds that they deserve to receive X, then, it seems that it would be easier to establish that they have the *negative* right not to be ill-treated by the living. This argument for the claim that the dead could be wronged could thus be based on the claim that it is wrong to treat a person in a way that he did not deserve to be treated. For example, in violating Hector's body even after Patroclus' funeral was completed Achilles treated him in a way that he did not deserve, given that Hector had not similarly overstepped the bounds of acceptable conduct.[16] As such, then, if a person's good name is undeservedly besmirched he will have been wronged by the person who so besmirched it—and this will be true whether he was alive at the time of this besmirching or not.

This argument for the claim that the dead can be wronged is simple, elegant, and (at first sight), persuasive.[17] However, it should be rejected. To claim that a person P did not deserve some Z being imposed or inflicted upon him is to claim that P did not deserve to have *some ill* Z imposed or inflicted upon him. To claim that P did not deserve to have Z imposed or inflicted upon him, then, is to claim that Z is an ill to P. For the claim that a *dead person* P did not deserve to have Z imposed or inflicted upon him after his death to be true, then, it must be the case that it can be shown that Z is an ill to P. What, then, could such an ill consist of, for a person who is dead? It is clear that Z cannot be an ill to P in virtue of being a harm to P, for it has been established in Chapters 1, 2 and 3 that the dead cannot be harmed. It also cannot be claimed that Z is an ill to P in virtue of being a wrong to P, for the question of whether the dead can be wronged is precisely what is at issue, and so to claim that this would be to beg the question. Perhaps, then, it could be claimed that Z is an ill to P in virtue of its being a harm *for* P, that is, Z is an ill to P in virtue of its adverse effects upon something that P held to be valuable independently of the effect of this on P's own well-being. But this will not do either, for, as was argued in the preceding Chapter, that something is an ill, or a harm, *for* someone does not show that it is therefore an ill or a harm *to* her—and it is the latter and not the former claim that is at issue here. Thus, unless there is a non-question-begging account of what it is for some Z to be an ill for P where P is dead and Z occurs after P's death, this alternative desert-based argument for the possibility that the dead could be wronged is at best incomplete, and at worst mistaken.

BLUSTEIN AND THE "DEAR DEPARTED"

Lande's arguments (and those can be developed in the spirit of them) are not, however, the only arguments available to those who wish to establish that the dead can be wronged. Some of the most persuasive and imaginative arguments for this view can be drawn from arguments that have been offered by Jeffrey Blustein in support of his view that we have a moral obligation to remember the "dear departed", "persons we have loved, cherished, and/or esteemed . . . who have now passed away."[18] Blustein offers three independent arguments to provide theoretical support for "the sense of a certain *demand* in connection with remembering the dear departed": The "rescue from insignificance view," the "enduring duties view," and the "reciprocity view".[19]

"According to the first argument," writes Blustein, "remembrance is a chief means by which we overcome the finality of death and through which we affirm that death has not obliterated the significance of the one who has died."[20] This significance, holds Blustein, would be both particular and general, for each person's life would be both significant to *them*, such that they took their lives seriously, as well as being significant as a *human* life. Drawing from James Hartley's view that "The rites of mourning respond to the *dignity of one's having existed*," Blustein notes that dignity calls on persons to respond to those who possess it with an attitude of respect.[21] Thus, argues Blustein, insofar as remembrance of a person is a response to her having existed, it will express respect for her. As such, then, holds Blustein, we should respond to the dignity of the dear departed through respectfully remembering them—a position that is but a short step from the claim that not to do so would be to wrong those whom we had failed to remember. If sound, this argument will clearly have direct implications for those bioethical debates concerning the treatment of the newly-dead in which appeals to dignity are common, such as, for example, those that concern the ethics of research on the dead.[22]

The second argument that Blustein considers to support the view that we have a duty to remember the dear departed is the Enduring Duties View. On this view, duties of remembrance are owed to persons as they were when they were alive, and so "their breach wrongs the person as he was when alive."[23] The view is based on the claim that the duties of "love and honor (among others)" that are owed to persons while they were alive persist as duties to remember them in ways that are expressive of those attitudes. Unlike the Rescue from Insignificance View, then, the Enduring Duties View grounds the obligation to remember the dear departed not on their dignity and value *qua* humans, but on the personal relationships that they had with others. More precisely, the Enduring Duties View draws on the following three claims:

> (1) We have special duties to persons with whom we have close personal relationships, including duties of love and honor; (2) death by itself does not cancel these duties; and (3) duties to remember in ways appropriate to the dear departed flow from or instantiate duties of love and honor, among others.[24]

Recognizing that (1) will be subject to the objection that since "ought implies can" we cannot have duties of love and honor for these attitudes are not subject to our volitional control Blustein argues that "although they may not be voluntary in any straightforward way" these attitudes are not beyond our control, for they are sensitive to reasons. In particular, Blustein continues, "persons who love and honor another are prone to attend to and be moved by certain reasons for action and to downplay, or exclude from consideration both other reasons that support the same action as well as at least some countervailing reasons".[25] From this, he contends that duties of love and honor can be explained in terms of the reasons that structure a person's consideration for the object of these attitudes, with one's having a duty of love or a duty of honor simply being that one recognizes and responds to the reasons that persons who love and honor recognize and respond to.[26] With this defense of (1) in place Blustein moves to defend (2), holding that with respect to duties of love and honor even if the bearer of the correlative rights has died the moral reasons for having these duties towards the now-dead persons as they were once alive are implied by the reasons that the rights in question were attributed to these persons when they were alive. Thus, since these reasons could survive, even though the bearer of the right that they supported did not, the duties that they support could survive, also. Finally, in elaboration of (3), Blustein holds that our remembrance of the dear departed "testifies to the depth and steadfastness of our emotional attachment to the person who has died".[27]

The duties of remembrance that the Rescue from Insignificance and the Enduring Duties views support are unconditional duties. By contrast, the duties supported by the third argument that Blustein outlines, the Reciprocity View, are conditional, for this view supports the position that we should accept the obligation to remember the dead *if* we are to impose the obligation to remember us on our successors. The Reciprocity View is based on the claim that persons have the posterity-directed desire to be remembered after they die. Blustein holds that the argument that supports the moral imperative to remember begins by establishing the conditions under which we are entitled to demand that our successors fulfill our desires to be remembered. Following Janna Thompson's discussion of "inherited obligations" Blustein invokes a general "reciprocity test", that "We can regard our posterity-directed desires as morally legitimate demands on future people . . . if and only if we would be prepared to accept similar obligations in respect to the desires, deeds, projects, or goals of our predecessors".[28] However, while passing this reciprocity condition is a necessary condition for persons to have inherited obligations, it is not a sufficient one, for it must also be established that our successors must accept this demand as binding—and this will be the case only if "they cannot reasonably reject the obligation we have imposed on them".[29] According to this view, then, the obligation that we have to remember the dead is based on the importance that we attach to our posterity-directed desire to be remembered, and on our preparedness to accept the obligation to remember the dead to ensure that we are entitled to impose the obligation to remember us upon our successors.

RESPONSES TO BLUSTEIN'S ARGUMENTS

Response to the Rescue from Insignificance Argument

Despite their persuasiveness, however, Blustein's arguments fail to establish that persons have an obligation to the dead to remember them—and hence they fail to establish that the dead can be wronged by persons who fail to do so. Consider first the Rescue from Insignificance Argument. This argument was based on the view that we owe to the dead the duty to remember them in order to express our respect for their dignity, either as particular humans whose lives mattered to them, or (inclusively) in virtue of their humanity. If we grant that we ascribe to persons the type of moral dignity that this argument is based on it certainly appears to establish that we have a duty to remember the dead. After all, if we love someone our love for them is not extinguished by their death; we still continue to love them as they were while alive, and to express this love we engage in certain "behaviors, actions, gestures, modes of address" after their deaths.[30] Thus, for example, if someone who professed love for another failed to perform acts of remembrance for her after she died we would question whether he genuinely loved her. To value something, then, is to commit oneself to perform acts that are expressive of this evaluation.[31] Hence, if we value other humans in the way that our ascription of moral dignity to them requires of us then we should remember them, for not to do so would be (like the professed lover who failed to commemorate his professed beloved) to fail to respond to their value that we have ascribed to them in the appropriate way.

Yet although this argument might establish that we have an obligation to remember the dead if we believe that they have dignity it does not establish that we have a duty *to the dead* to do so—and hence it does not establish that we would wrong them were we to fail to remember them. This argument does not show that we have a duty to remember the dead, but only that our remembrance of them is entailed by our ascribing a certain value to them while they were alive. Rather than establishing that we have a moral obligation to remember them, then, this argument only establishes that we should remember them given that we valued them in a certain way, where the "should" in question is a requirement of consistency, rather than of morality. Thus, while our failure to remember the dead would cast doubt upon our claim to value them in a certain way, it would not be a *moral* failure; it would not wrong the dead.

However, it might be that this response to Blustein's first argument for the claim that we can wrong the dead by failing to remember them moves too quickly. Blustein's argument is based on the claim that humans have a certain type of moral dignity in virtue of their humanity that we should (morally) recognize and respond to, and not merely on the claim that we (can) ascribe such dignity to them. As such, it is based on the claim that we have a moral duty to recognize and respond to the value of this dignity—and hence that we derivatively have a moral duty to remember them as an expression of this. There are two points to be made in reply to this. First, and most obviously, insofar as the Rescue from Insignificance View rests on the claim that humans are valuable in virtue of their moral dignity it rises or falls with the truth of this claim—and so absent an argument for it Blustein's argument for the view that we can wrong the dead by failing to remember them is importantly incomplete. Of course, noting this is by no means a serious criticism of Blustein's argument, both because it would be unfair to impose upon him the obligation exhaustively to defend all the philosophical assumptions that his views are based on, and because there is a voluminous literature that he can draw upon to support his point here.[32] It does, however, underscore the fact that he has not yet shown that the dead can be wronged.[33] Second, even if we accept that humans have the type of moral dignity that undergirds the Rescue from Insignificance View it is not clear that this dignity would support a moral duty to remember the dead in the way that Blustein believes. The Rescue from Insignificance View draws its intuitive plausibility from a comparison between the impersonal evaluation of humans as having dignity and the personal evaluation of particular loved humans, such that just as loving someone entails that one should remember them after their death, so too should respecting human dignity entail that one remember the dead. Yet while loving someone does entail that one should remember them after their death it is not so clear that respecting human dignity require that one remember the dead. Blustein holds that remembering someone after their death is a way of affirming that their death does not obliterate the significance of their life, where this significance can be understood personally or impersonally. Yet to hold that we should affirm that a person's death does not obliterate the significance of her life is ambiguous. It could mean that to affirm that we value humans as being significant (either in themselves as individuals, or *qua* bearers of dignity) we are conceptually required to remember them, for, like loving someone, responding to a person's individuality or dignity requires that we express her value through acts of remembrance. But, this requirement is not of morality, but of consistency. Alternatively, it could mean that to affirm that persons' lives are significant we are required to affirm that a person's death does not alter their moral status as they were when alive. On this latter understanding, someone's failure appropriately to respond to another human's dignity during her life (e.g., through murdering her) would still be a wrong after the latter's death, for this would not have altered the moral significance of her life. Noting that there are two ways of understanding what is required by an affirmation that a person's death does not obliterate the significance of her life does not in itself show that Blustein is mistaken to hold that we have an obligation to remember the dead. However, it does show that there is a second lacuna is his argument for this claim. Even if we accept that we have a moral duty to recognize and appropriately respond to the special moral significance of human life (i.e., if we can fill the first lacuna in the Rescue from Insignificance View) and so have an obligation to affirm that death does not obliterate this significance this does not commit us to accepting an obligation to remember the dead. We could discharge the obligation to affirm the continued significance of the dead merely by affirming that their deaths have not retroactively altered the moral significance that they had in life.[34]

Perhaps, though, the second of these replies to Blustein also moves too fast. This is because it is based on holding that a person's death does not obliterate the moral significance of her life *qua* human (that is, it is based on the impersonal moral significance of her life), whereas Blustein is primarily concerned with the claim that we have an obligation to ensure that a person's death does not obliterate the personal significance of her life; that her life mattered *to her*, and not just *sub specie aeternitatis*.[35] Yet although this is a legitimate criticism of the above reply it serves only to highlight a further difficulty with Blustein's argument. Blustein holds that we have an obligation to remember the dead to acknowledge that their lives had meaning *for them* on the grounds that "If it really matters that we exist and, therefore, that we existed, then it is imperative for the living to acknowledge this in some way . . . Otherwise we concede that death robs our lives of meaning after all".[36] The first point to note here is that our lives could have meaning to us whether or not we will actually be remembered by others.[37] Using Blustein's own criterion of whether we take ourselves seriously as the hallmark of whether our lives have meaning to us, it is clear that we can take ourselves seriously during our lives whether or not we will actually be remembered by others after our deaths, and so it is clear that death will not rob our lives of personal meaning even if we fail to be remembered. The second point to note here is that Blustein seems to be implying that if our lives are not acknowledged by our successors then they will lack (presumably impersonal) meaning. This renders the (presumably impersonal) meaning of our lives dependent upon their being acknowledged. But surely it is more plausible to hold that what is being acknowledged is that our lives *had* (impersonal) meaning—in which case the acknowledgment itself is irrelevant for their possession of this.

To sum up these responses to Blustein's Rescue from Insignificance argument for the view that we have an obligation to remember the dead (and hence could wrong them if we fail to do so): The initial criticism of this argument was to note that it does not show that we have a moral duty to remember the dead, but only that we are required by consistency to do so if we ascribe a certain value to them. Blustein could respond to this, however, by noting that we have a moral duty to respond to the value of human dignity, and hence we have a moral duty to remember the dead as an expression of this. But this possible response points to two lacunae in his view: (1) that he needs to provide an argument for the foundational claim that humans should be valued as having dignity in this way, and (2) that even if we accept that they should be, that we could appropriately respond to this value by affirming that their deaths have not retroactively altered the moral significance that they possessed while they were alive. Finally, Blustein could charge that this last point is mistaken, for its focus is on the impersonal significance of persons' lives, whereas he focuses on their personal significance to them. But, as argued above, for Blustein to focus on the personal significance that persons' lives have to them would be a mistake, for a person's life can have significance for her whether or not this is acknowledged by others through their remembrance of her—and so a focus on the personal significance of persons' lives cannot ground an obligation to remember the dead.

Response to the Enduring Duties Argument

Blustein's argument from Enduring Duties fares no better than his Rescue from Insignificance Argument in providing support for the view that we have obligations of remembrance to the dead. Blustein attempts to establish claim (1) of this argument (that "We have special duties to persons with whom we have close personal relationships, including duties of love and honor") by noting that "love and honor engage attitudes that are sensitive to reasons".[38] From this, Blustein claims that "Duties of love, duties of honor, and the like can be explained in terms of the reasons that structure a person's regard for the object of his love or honor," and that "In general, duties of love and honor exist because there are distinctive patterns of privileged and protected reasons that persons who love and honor recognize and respond to".[39] But this is mistaken: that persons who love and honor others recognize and respond to reasons that are not similarly salient to persons who lack these attitudes towards others does not show that those who love and honor have *duties* of love and honor. To claim this is mistakenly to collapse the recognition of a (*prima facie*) reason to X into a (*prima facie*) duty to X: that as an aficionado of Islay malt whisky I have a reason to drink Lagavulin does not mean that I thereby have a duty to do so.[40] Of course, that Blustein has provided us with no reason to believe that there are duties of love and duty does not mean that there are none, and so let us grant that there are for the sake of argument (while noting in passing that this lacuna in this argument means that it does not support the claim that we owe obligations to the dead). What, then, of claim (2) in this argument—that a person's death does not extinguish the duties of love and honor that are owed to her? Blustein supports this claim by holding that "although the bearer of the correlative right has died, moral reasons for having a duty toward the deceased are implied by the reasons for attributing the corresponding right to the persons when he was alive . . . [and] [t]hese reasons [can] survive . . . "[41] Two points can be made in response to this claim. First, as noted above, Blustein has not shown that there are any duties of love and honor, and so this discussion of their purported survival is unsupported. Second, even if we grant for the sake of argument that persons do owe duties of love and honor towards others, it is implausible to hold that these duties survive the deaths of the persons to whom they are owed—for how can one owe duties to something that does not exist?[42] We thus need further argument to establish that if there are duties of love and honor then they are the sort of duties that can survive a person's death.

Response to the Reciprocity Argument

Thus far, then, neither of the two arguments that Blustein offers for the unconditional imposition of the obligation to remember the dead (and hence for the view that the dead would be wronged were these obligations not to be met) are satisfactory. What, then, of the final argument that he gives for an obligation to remember the dead—the Reciprocity View? On this View we have a duty to remember the dead if we have a posterity-directed desire that our successors remember us if two conditions are met: (1) that we are willing to accept a similar duty with respect to remembering our predecessors who had the same posterity-orientated desire, and (2) that our successors could not "reasonably reject the obligation we have imposed on them".[43] The problem with the Reciprocity argument for the duty to remember our predecessors stems from the second of these claims. To hold that if our successors could not "reasonably reject" the obligation that we impose on them to remember us—and hence they have such an obligation provided we are willing to shoulder a similar one with respect to our predecessors—is not to argue that they *actually do* have such an obligation so much as it is simply to note the conditions that must be in place *were* they to have one. That is, were they actually to have this obligation then they could not reasonably reject it, but to hold that a person could not reasonably reject an obligation that is imposed upon them without explaining why this is so is not to establish that they have such an obligation so much as it is merely to claim that they do—and to do this is just to beg the question against those who deny that the obligation in question exists.[44]

RIGHTS AND INTERESTS

So far, then, the arguments in this Chapter have reached a similar conclusion to that reached in Chapter 2, after the discussion of Levenbook's, Grover's, Sperling's and Griseri's attempts to show how posthumous harm is possible was complete: that there is no reason to believe that the dead can be wronged. But this conclusion does not, of course, show that the dead *cannot* be wronged, for it is possible that an argument might yet be developed to establish that they could be. To preclude this possibility, then, an argument needs to be developed to establish that the dead *cannot* be wronged.

One argument for the conclusion that the dead cannot be wronged has been recognized by Lande, who then moves to criticize it:[45]

> (a) Only existents possess interests. (b) Only entities possessing interests possess rights. (c) Therefore only existents possess rights. (d) The dead no longer exist.[46] (e) Therefore the dead do not possess rights. [Therefore the dead cannot be wronged by the violation of their rights].[47]

Prior to criticizing this argument for the view that it is impossible to wrong the dead through violating their rights Lande follows Feinberg and Pitcher in distinguishing between antemortem and postmortem persons, noting that it is the antemortem person who would be the subject of a posthumous wrong. With this distinction in hand Lande notes that premise (e) of the above argument is equivocal, for it could be understood in any one of three ways:

> (e1): X's remains tomorrow will not possess any rights which will exist tomorrow, and which could be either honored or violated tomorrow; or

> (e2): the nonexistent x of tomorrow will not possess any rights which will exist tomorrow, and which could either be honored or violated tomorrow; or

> (e3): the existent x of yesterday did not possess any rights which existed yesterday, which will continue to exist tomorrow, and which could be either honored or violated tomorrow.[48]

Although both (e1) and (e2) are obviously true, Lande notes that (e3) is the only plausible version of premise (e). As such, he argues, this argument against the possibility of the dead being wronged through the violation of their rights should be rejected, for, he argues, (e3) is false. In support of this view Lande notes that "it would be quite natural to characterize . . . the improper execution of x's will as a violation of a right—presumably an existing right—of the once-living x's. . . . ," and that "it would be quite natural to characterize the mutilation of x's corpse as a violation of an existing right of the once-living x's . . . ".[49] Lande, however, does not only rely on intuitive support for his view that (e3) is false, and that the rights of persons can survive their deaths.[50] Lande holds that it is "certainly true" that some of a person's interests and desires will continue to exist, and so could be either thwarted or fulfilled, after her death, since "a desire, after all, is fulfilled once the state of affairs that had been the object of the desire materializes," and that for some desires (e.g., those desires directed at what Luper characterizes as impersonally defined projects),[51] "this can occur whether or not the subject is still alive".[52] From this, Lande concludes that "if the relationship between interests and desires . . . and rights . . . is sufficiently close, then it would be reasonable to infer that some rights, like some interests and some desires, can also exist posthumously".[53] Given premise (b) of the above argument against the possibility of wronging the dead through violating their rights it is not unreasonable for Lande to conclude that the relationship between interests and desires, and rights, is a close one. Moreover, Lande supports his claim that this close relationship exists by noting that both interests and desires, and rights, have objects, that rights can be respected or violated just as interests can be furthered or thwarted, and that such respecting or setting back, furthering or thwarting, can occur without the knowledge of the persons whose interests, desires, or rights are in question. Finally, he notes that "a right either actually is, or at the very least is based upon, an interest—albeit an interest of a particular sort, i.e., one which ought to be protected by a given authority".[54] From these considerations, Lande concludes that since some interests and desires can exist posthumously, and there is a close relationship between interests and desires and rights, then rights, like interests and desires, can also exist posthumously. Thus, (e3) is false and the above argument against the possibility of wronging the dead by violating their posthumous rights is mistaken.

Lande's response to the above argument against the possibility of wronging the dead by violating their posthumous rights is flawed. The mere fact that interests and desires, and rights, share *some* features does not mean that they share *all* of them. Simply outlining the features that they have in common does not itself establish that they have the features that are relevant to the above argument (i.e., posthumous existence) in common. Moreover, it is clear there are important differences between interests and desires, and rights. For example, whereas it is clear that a person's rights will (typically) impose duties upon others, her interests and desires in themselves will not. As such, then, Lande must provide an argument for his claim that, like a person's interests and desires, her rights also continue to exist after her death.[55]

Of course, in itself this does not show that Lande is mistaken to hold that (e3) is false. Despite what Lande appears to believe, his argument against this premise does not depend on it being true that a person's interests and desires, and rights, exist after her death. Instead, to be sound his argument against (e3) only needs it to be the case that a person's (putative) rights could be violated posthumously, just as her interests and desires could be thwarted posthumously.[56] Lande, however, has failed to establish even this. While it is uncontroversial that a person's interests and desires could be thwarted by events that occur after both she and they cease to exist (just as it is uncontroversial that events that occur after a person's death could make her a killer while she was still alive), it is *not* uncontroversial to hold that a person's rights could be violated after she ceases to exist. (Indeed, if this was uncontroversial there would be no argument over whether or not a person could be wronged after her death!) As such, then, for his argument against (e3) to be cogent Lande must provide further argument for his view that "the relationship between interests and desires ... and rights ... is sufficiently close" such that what can be said of the former can also be said of the latter—especially since, as was noted above, there are important differences between a person's interests and desires, and her rights.[57]

Lande, then, has failed to provide a reason as to why the above argument against the view that the dead can be wronged through violations of their (alleged) rights should be rejected. Without further argument to the contrary, then, it should stand. This argument, however, does not show that the dead cannot be wronged *simpliciter*; it only shows that they cannot be wronged *through the violation of their rights* as they have no rights to be violated. To expand the scope of this argument, then, and hence to complete this argument against the view that the dead can be wronged, it should be noted that, from the arguments in the previous Chapters, it is clear that the dead cannot be wronged through being the subjects of illegitimate harm, since they cannot be harmed. And as was argued in Chapter 2 (and as will be argued further in Chapter 8) they cannot be wronged by any inappropriate failure to respect their autonomy. Thus, just as the dead are immune from being harmed, so too are they immune from being wronged.[58]

CONCLUSION

All of the arguments that have been offered in the extant philosophical literature to establish that the commonly-held views that the dead can be both harmed and wronged are mistaken.[59] Recognizing this gives rise to two further questions. First, why, if they are mistaken, are these views so widespread? Second, if the dead can be neither harmed nor wronged, what reason do the living have for respecting their wishes?—a question which has clear implications for those debates within bioethics (such as those concerning the posthumous procurement of organs, research on the newly dead, and the moral authority of advance directives), where the wishes of persons who are now dead play a major role. Although answering the first question in full would take us too far afield (and, in any case, would be more speculative than definitive) it might be that there is an evolutionary explanation for why persons believe that the dead can be harmed or wronged.[60] It is possible that events that are taken to harm or wrong a person posthumously are believed to do so owing to their likely adverse effects on the genetic fitness of her offspring, and, through this, her own inclusive genetic fitness. If so, then it would not be surprising were natural selection to operate in favor of persons who possessed the adaptive adverse attitudes towards the perpetrators of such posthumous harms and wrongs. Persons' concerns about *both* the antemortem *and* the posthumous harms or wrongs that befall others could thus be seen as stemming from the worry "What if that happened to me, or my descendents?" If it is true that the widespread intuition that posthumous harm is possible can be explained sociobiologically, this would obviate the need to develop an account of posthumous harm that justifies it.[61]

Given this, then, it might appear that (absent religiously-motivated concerns) persons should not care about what happens to their bodies after their death, and so should not object to their (or others') organs being harvested for transplantation, their remains being used for research, or even to being used as gestational chambers in postmortem pregnancies. But such appearances are misleading. As was noted in the previous Chapter not only can events cause harm *to* a person, but they could be harms *for* her, if they prevent the occurrence of states of affairs that she holds to be valuable in themselves independently of how they might affect her well-being. A person who holds something to be valuable in itself in this way (such as, for example, the well-being of her children, or the continued success of her *alma mater*), would believe herself to have reason to take steps to ensure that that state of affairs transpires even after she is herself dead. Why, though, should other persons be concerned with honoring the wishes of the dead, if they can neither harm them nor wrong them by failing to do so? The answer, it seems, is that persons have a reason to honor the wishes of the dead to ensure the continuance of such honoring as a social practice, so that their wishes will in turn be honored.[62] Their justification for doing so need not (indeed, *should* not) be to ensure that they themselves will not suffer either wrong or harm if their own wishes were not honored. Rather, it would be to help ensure that other persons would (quasi-reciprocally) protect or promote the occurrence of states of affairs after their deaths that they hold to be valuable in themselves.[63] This justification for honoring the wishes that persons who are now dead had is not necessarily incompatible with the truth of pure hedonism. If pure hedonism was true and persons were mistaken to believe that there were good or bad value atoms apart from those of pleasure or pains these mistaken evaluative beliefs together with their beliefs about future states of affairs could lead them to experience pleasures or pains according to whether they believed that what they (mistakenly) held to be intrinsically valuable would be protected or promoted, or not. As such, then, even a pure hedonist would have a *prima facie* derivative reason to cultivate a social practice whereby persons' preferences for future states of affairs were honored.

This conclusion might initially come as something of a disappointment to one who was expecting a universally revisionary approach to those debates within bioethics in which notions of posthumous harms and wrongs play a role to follow from the revisionary approach to the metaphysics of these issues that is entailed by the full-blooded Epicureanism defended here. Yet this initial disappointment should dissipate once it is recognized that the fact that persons can be subject to neither posthumous harms nor posthumous wrongs *does* have revisionary implications within the debate over (for example) the procurement of cadaveric organs. This is because (as will be outlined in Chapter 8) it eliminates those arguments both for and against "presumed consent" policies of organ procurement that are based on attempts to minimize the number of mistaken removals and non-removals of persons' organs after they are dead in order to minimize the possibility that the persons whose bodies are subject to them will thus be harmed. Moreover (as will also be outlined in Chapter 8) the fact that persons can neither be harmed nor wronged after their deaths also seems to pave the way not only for a policy of presumed consent, but for the introduction of a policy of posthumous organ *taking*. And this is so *despite* the concern, noted above, that most people would have to preserve the current *status quo* pertaining to respecting the former wishes of persons who are now dead. Furthermore, as will be discussed in Chapter 9, that persons cannot be subject to posthumous harms will also have revisionary implications for the debates over posthumous reproduction (leading to those arguments which rest on its possibility to be immediately set aside). And, just as the fact that posthumous harms and wrongs are impossible will have revisionary implications for certain debates within bioethics, so too will the equally-revisionary claim that death is not a harm to the person who dies. It is to this further claim of full-blooded Epicureanism that this volume will now turn.

5   Why Death is Not a Harm to the One Who Dies

So far in this volume it has been argued that the dead can neither be harmed nor wronged. Given the truth of the first of these conclusions one might think that the truth of the final aspect of full-blooded Epicureanism (that death is not a harm to the one who dies) has also been established, for one might think that if posthumous harm is impossible then death cannot be a harm to the person who dies. That these first and last aspects of full-blooded Epicureanism go hand in glove is certainly Joel Feinberg's view, for he boldly states that "Either death and posthumous harms alike can be harms, or neither can be."[1] Yet it is possible both to deny that posthumous harm is possible and to hold that death can be a harm to the one who dies. Ben Bradley, for example, argues that while events that are alleged to bring about posthumous harm would do so retroactively, death "is bad at all those times at which things would have been going better for the victim had her death not occurred," where a person's death "is bad at a time to the extent that things would be going better for the victim at that time than they would have been had her death not occurred".[2] Thus, notes Bradley, since there is this directional difference between posthumous harms and the (alleged) harm of death it is possible to deny the possibility of the former and yet endorse the possibility of the latter.[3]

To establish the truth of full-blooded Epicureanism, then, additional arguments will be developed in this Chapter to show that death is not a harm to the person who dies. The starting point for these arguments will be that which was famously (or notoriously) developed by Epicurus. As was noted in the Introduction, however, the aim of this volume is not to offer an exact reconstruction of Epicurus' actual argument (or arguments), but, instead, to offer arguments that are Epicurean in spirit.[4] To this end two such arguments will be developed out of Epicurus' remarks concerning the harmlessness of death to the one who dies and defended against objections: The Hedonic Variant of the Epicurean argument for this view, and the Existence Variant.

THE EPICUREAN ARGUMENT

In his second *Kyriai Doxai* Epicurus presents a brief argument for the view that a person's death cannot be a harm to her: "Death is nothing to us, since a decomposed thing is insensate, and whatever is insensate is nothing to us".[5] This argument is developed more fully in his *Letter to Menoeceus*:

> Make yourself familiar with the belief that death is nothing to us, since everything good or bad lies in sensation, and death is to be deprived of sensation. Hence the right recognition that death is nothing to us makes the mortality of life enjoyable, not by adding infinite duration to it but by removing the desire for immortality. For there is nothing to be feared in living, for one who has truly comprehended that there is nothing to be feared in not living. So one who says he fears death, not because it will hurt when it is here, but because it hurts when it is coming, talks nonsense, since whatever does not hurt when it is present hurts for no reason when it is expected.
>
> So that most fearful of all bad things, death, is nothing to us, since when we are, death is not present, and when death is present, then we are not. So it is nothing to the living and nothing to the dead, since with regard to the former, death is not, and as to the latter, they themselves no longer are.[6]

This Epicurean argument can be understood in two ways; the Hedonic Variant and the Existence Variant.[7] The Hedonic Variant is based on the view that an event or a state of affairs can only harm a person if it has an adverse effect on his experiences. Thus, since a person who is dead cannot experience anything, death cannot be a harm to the person who dies.[8] More formally, the Hedonic Variant of this Epicurean argument is:

1. An event or a state of affairs is a harm to a person only if it adversely affects her experiences.[9]
2. Postmortem persons cannot experience anything.

Thus, given (1) and (2):

3. An event or a state of affairs can only harm an antemortem person by adversely affecting her experiences.

Thus, from (3):

4. A person can only be harmed by an event or a state of affairs that occurs prior to her death.
5. A person's death does not occur prior to her death.

Thus, from (4) and (5):

Therefore, a person's death is not a harm to her.[10]

In contrast to the Hedonic Variant of this Epicurean argument, the Existence Variant is based on the view that an event or a state of affairs can only harm a person when he exists. Thus, since a person who is dead does not exist, he cannot be harmed by the occurrence of any event or state of affairs—and so (given the assumption that a person's death marks the first moment of his non-existence) he cannot be harmed by his own death. More formally, the Existence Variant of this Epicurean argument is:

1. An event or a state of affairs can only harm a person when she exists.

Thus,

2. An event or a state of affairs that occurs when a person does not exist cannot harm her.
3. Persons are either antemortem persons (i.e., persons whose deaths have not yet occurred) or postmortem persons (i.e., persons whose deaths have occurred).
4. An antemortem person (i.e., a person whose death has not yet occurred) exists.
5. A postmortem person (i.e., a person whose death has occurred) does not exist.

Thus, from (1), (2), and (5):

6. Postmortem persons cannot be harmed by their own deaths.

And from (2), and (4):

7. Antemortem persons cannot be harmed by their own deaths.

Thus, from (3), (6), and (7):

Therefore, persons cannot be harmed by their own deaths.

Prior to elaborating upon and defending the Epicurean view that death cannot be a harm to the person who dies several clarifications need to be made about the arguments in both this chapter and the next. First, it should be reiterated that rather than providing an exegetical account of the arguments that Epicurus himself made in favor of the view that death cannot be a harm to the one who dies the aim of these chapters is to defend this conclusion. The arguments offered here are thus purely philosophical, rather than exegetical or historical.[11] Second, the conclusion that will be defended here is that death is not a harm to the one who dies. It is perfectly compatible with this view to hold that the process of dying might be harmful to the one who undergoes it; a lingering death from lung cancer, for example, will certainly be harmful to a person who suffers from it, in that it will adversely affect her experiences.[12] Third, it is also compatible with the view defended here to hold that a person's death can be a harm to others, through adversely affecting their experiences. Fourth, although the focus of the Epicurean view is the claim that persons cannot be harmed by their own deaths, the arguments developed in support of this claim also support the broader conclusions that no living being can be harmed by its own death.[13] Fifth, the Epicurean view that death is not a harm to the person who dies is based on the assumption that persons cannot experience anything after their deaths. If this assumption is mistaken—if, for example, persons will experience an eternity of either bliss or torment in an afterlife—the Epicurean arguments for this view will also be mistaken.

While both the Hedonic Variant and the Existence Variant of the Epicurean Argument will be developed in this Chapter, its focus will be on the former, and not the latter. This is because the second premise of the Existence Variant of this argument entails both

(2a)   An event or a state of affairs that occurs after a person ceases to exist cannot harm her.

and

(2b)   An event of a state of affairs that occurs prior to a person's existence cannot harm her.

(2a) commits its proponents to denying the possibility of posthumous harm. This is a controversial claim—although a correct one, as was argued in Chapters 1, 2 and 3. (2b), however, is mistaken, for it appears to commit its proponents to holding that an event that occurs prior to a person's birth cannot harm her, a claim that has been trenchantly criticized by Fred Feldman.[14] Distinguishing between events or states of affairs that are *intrinsically* bad for a person (given hedonism, his own pains) and those that are bad for him *overall* (those that would render him worse off "all things considered" were they to occur), Feldman argues that an event or a state of affairs could be harmful overall for a person even if he did not exist at the time of its occurrence.[15] To illustrate this, he offers an example in which his father lost his job before he (Feldman) was born. As a result of this, Feldman writes, "my parents had to move to another town, and that I was therefore raised in a bad neighborhood and had to attend worse schools. I would have been happier if he had not lost his job when he did".[16] As such, concludes Feldman, "the fact that my father lost his job was bad for me—even though I did not exist when it occurred".[17] One might respond to Feldman by distinguishing between the event of his father losing his job and the persisting effects of that event, and then claiming that only the latter, and not the former, harmed Feldman.[18] This response, however, would commit one to claiming that, for example, Claudius's pouring of poison into King Hamlet's ear did not harm the King, for only its effects did, or that a nuclear exchange that devastated a planet was harmless to persons born on that world who were conceived after its occurrence. (Indeed, it would commit one to the highly counterintuitive claim that high doses of radiation are harmless to humans, on the grounds that they are only harmed by its effects.) Given the implausibility of this response to Feldman, then, premise (2b) should be rejected— and hence premise (2) of the Existence Variant of this Epicurean argument (and thus this variant of the argument itself) should either be modified or rejected. Modifying this premise to avoid committing the proponents of the Existence Variant of this Epicurean argument to (2b) is, however, simple, for (2) only needs to be altered to admit the possibility that a person could be harmed by events that occur prior to her existence. As such, then, the modified version of this premise should read:

(2c) An event or a state of affairs must either be contemporaneous with, or occur prior to, the time at which a person exists for it to harm him.

This modification both avoids Feldman's objection to (2b), and, when combined with premises (3) through (7) of the above Existence Variant of the Epicurean argument leads to the conclusion that a person's own death cannot harm him. It does so, however, by implicitly relying on the view that an event or a state of affairs can only harm a person if it adversely affects her experiences—premise (1) of the Hedonic Variant of this Epicurean argument. As such, then, although the Existence Variant and the Hedonic Variant of this Epicurean argument are separate, the plausibility of the former is derived from that of the latter. Thus, since this is so, it is sensible to focus on the latter Variant since it is the more fundamental of the two.

HEDONISM REVISITED

It is analytic that a person's death does not occur before her death, and so premise (5) of the Hedonic Variant of the Epicurean argument is immune from criticism. Premise (4) follows directly from premise (3), which, in turn, follows from the conjunction of premises (1) and (2). Like premise (5), premise (2) is uncontroversial. To undermine this variant of the Epicurean argument, then, one must show that premise (1) is false. There are two ways in which one could attempt to do this. One could attempt to show that persons can be harmed by events or states of affairs that do not adversely affect their experiences. Alternatively, one could argue that this premise is ambiguous in a way that allows for the possibility that a person's death could harm her in that it deprives her of positive experiences that she would have otherwise had.

   This first attempt at undermining premise (1) was addressed in Chapter 3. There, it was noted that events or states of affairs that are paradigmatically harmful to persons (such as injury, insult, or illness) are ones which adversely affect their experiences. It was also noted there that accepting this account of harm does not commit one to endorsing the claim that what a person does not know about does not harm her, for it is possible that an event that a person is unaware of could adversely affect her experiences by causing them to be worse than they would have otherwise been. (A slander that is neither discovered nor suspected by its victim, for example, could cause her to fail to receive a promotion that she would have otherwise received.) With these points in hand it was argued that the anti-hedonistic intuitions that are generated by types of examples that are typically invoked to show that persons can be harmed by events or states of affairs that do not affect their experiences in any way either should be rejected, or could be accommodated within a hedonistic framework. To recapitulate, first, it is not as obvious as those who oppose hedonism believe that an event or state of affairs that has no effect at all on a person's experiences harms her, even if it thwarts her interests. It does not seem at all odd, for example, to hold that an author whose work and picture is mocked by a far-flung tribe is not harmed by this—indeed, it seems *more* odd to hold that such mocking *does* harm him. Second, even in cases where it is more intuitively plausible to hold that a person could be harmed by an event that does not affect his experiences in any way, the intuitions that these cases generate can be accommodated by distinguishing between an event or a state of affairs being a harm *to* a person, and its being a harm *for* a person, as discussed in Chapter 3. Recall that something is a harm *to* a person when it adversely affects his experiences. Such harms are harms *proper*; they are those harms that, when inflicted on a person, adversely affect his well-being. Something is a harm *for* a person when it thwarts his interests. A Londoner might, for example, hold it to be intrinsically valuable that London continues indefinitely to be a major population center. If this interest of his is thwarted by, for example, the city's abandonment as a result of global warming and civil war (as portrayed in Ronald Wright's novel *A Scientific Romance*), this would be a harm for him, in that it could be regretted on his behalf by a third party.[19] That this is so, however, has no effect at all on his well-being, for events or states of affairs that are harms for persons are not harms proper. (And so they are not relevant to the questions of whether posthumous harm is possible, or whether death is a harm to the person who dies). This distinction between something being a harm to a person and its being a harm for her enables one to accommodate the anti-hedonistic intuitions generated by Nozick's experience machine and Feinberg's Case A. This distinction enables one to accommodate the intuitions generated by the experience machine in that it enables one to accept that persons can hold certain states of affairs to be intrinsically valuable, even if they have no effect on their experiences, and thus that their thwarting could be a cause for regret on the behalf of the persons who value them. Similarly, it enables one to hold that the collapse of the "empire of her hopes" is cause for regret on behalf of the woman in Feinberg's Case A.

DEATH AND DEPRIVATION

Given the defense of this hedonistic account of harm that was offered in Chapter 3 (and briefly recapitulated here) it seems that not only is there no reason to reject premise (1) on the basis of its hedonistic underpinnings, but there is good reason to accept it owing to their plausibility. What, then, of the second way in which premise (1) of the Hedonic Variant of this Epicurean argument could be undermined: that it is ambiguous in a way that allows for the possibility that a person's death could harm her in that it deprives her of positive experiences that she would have otherwise had?[20] This objection is initially plausible. As noted in Chapter 3, the hedonistic account of harm that premise (1) is based upon leaves it open as to what could count as adversely affecting a person's experiences. It is, however, accepted on this view that a person's experiences could be adversely affected by events or states of affairs that she does not know about if they cause her experiences to be worse that they would have otherwise been.[21] As such, then, the account of harm that is the basis for premise (1) is compatible with the claim that an event could harm a person by depriving her of positive experiences that she would have had had it not occurred. Thus, on the face of it, it is compatible with the claim that a person's death could be a harm to her through depriving her of the goods of life that she would have otherwise experienced.[22] And, if so, then, the Hedonic Variant of this Epicurean argument is invalid.

To defend the Hedonic Variant of this Epicurean argument from this criticism it must thus be shown that premise (1) cannot be understood as being compatible with the claim that death could be a harm to the person who dies through adversely affecting her experiences by depriving her of those that she would have otherwise had. That is to say, it must be shown that what might be termed an *unrestricted* understanding of (1) (on which a person could be harmed by her own death, through adversely affecting her experiences by depriving her of the goods of life that she would otherwise have enjoyed) should not be accepted, but that a more *restricted* understanding of it (on which death cannot harm the person who dies in this way) should. To achieve this, the same strategy will be pursued here as was pursued earlier in this volume to show the falsity of the view that posthumous harm is possible. First, it will be argued that there is no reason to believe that death can be a harm to the person who dies through its depriving her of the goods of life, for none of the most prominent attempts to establish this claim succeed in doing so. With this in hand, it will then be argued that not only is there no reason to believe that a person's death can be a harm to her through depriving her of the goods of life that she would otherwise have enjoyed, there is good reason to believe that it cannot be a harm to her for this reason. As such, then, premise (1) of the Hedonic Variant should not be understood as allowing for the possibility that a person's death could adversely affect her experiences through depriving her of future good ones, and hence the criticism of this argument that is based on this understanding should be rejected.

Does a Person's Death Deprive Her of the Goods of Life?

The view that a person's death is a harm to her because it will preclude her from having future positive experiences is widespread.[23] Thomas Nagel, for example, holds that "If death can be an evil at all, it cannot be because of its positive features, but only because of what it deprives us of . . . ," going on to claim that "If we are to make sense of the view that to die is bad, it must be on the grounds that life is a good and death is the corresponding deprivation or loss, bad not because of any positive features but because of the desirability of what it removes".[24] To illustrate the way in which death could be bad for the person who dies by depriving him of goods that he would have otherwise enjoyed Nagel offers an example "of deprivation whose severity approaches that of death": that of an intelligent man who suffers "a brain injury that reduces him to the mental condition of a contented infant," whose remaining desires can be readily satisfied by a custodian "so that he is free from care".[25] Nagel holds that even though the man would not, once he has been reduced to the status of a contented infant, mind his condition, his reduction to this state would be widely considered to be a misfortune to him.[26] Moreover, argues Nagel, holding that this man's brain injury was a misfortune to him would be correct, for harm that has befallen him is a result of the difference between the experiences that he *could have had* had he not been so injured and those that he actually *will* have. Thus, claims Nagel, given that a person's death would, like this man's brain injury, deprive the person who dies of the positive experiences that she would have otherwise received, death is also a misfortune to the persons who have been so deprived.[27]

A similar deprivation-based argument for the view that death can be a harm to the person who dies has been developed by both Fred Feldman and, drawing on Feldman's work, Ben Bradley.[28] Feldman begins his argument by holding that events or states of affairs can be extrinsically harmful to a person (i.e., they are "connected with" later harms, even if they are not themselves harmful) even if they do not cause intrinsic harms (i.e., experiences that are painful in themselves) for her. To illustrate this, Feldman offers two examples. In the first, a young man is accepted by two colleges, A and B, and decides to attend A, where he spends four happy years. He does not study philosophy there because it is not offered. Had he gone to B, however, he would have studied philosophy, and would have enjoyed it immensely. In the second, a girl is born in Country A where she is not permitted to learn to read or write, but, instead, is taught how to do laundry and bring up children. She is reasonably satisfied with her restricted life, believing that she lives as a woman should live. However, this woman had a great talent for poetry. As such, claims Feldman, "it is a great pity that this woman had not been born in another country," for as a result of her being born in Country A "something very bad happened to her, even though she never suffered any pain as a result".[29] From these examples, Feldman develops a principle that is very similar to the unrestricted understanding of premise (1) outlined above:

> EI: Something is extrinsically bad for a person if and only if he or she would have been intrinsically better off if it had not taken place.[30]

With EI in hand Feldman argues that death can be an extrinsic harm to the person who dies. To illustrate this, Feldman offers the example of a boy who is undergoing minor surgery, but who dies while on the operating table. Although his death is painless, Feldman holds that we would still hold it to be a great misfortune to him—and that we would do so because his "life contains less intrinsic value for him, measured hedonistically, than it would have contained had he not died when he did".[31] Given this, claims Feldman, this boy's death was a harm to him. Drawing on Feldman's account of how an event can be extrinsically bad for someone Bradley argues that "the overall value of something for a person is the difference it makes to how things go for that person, taking into account both its intrinsic and instrumental value (and whatever other sorts of value it has)".[32] Bradley's account of the overall value that a state of affairs has for a person is thus to be understood in terms of counterfactual conditionals, interpreted using the concept of possible worlds.[33] On this view, "to say that if X were to have happened, Y would have happened, is to say that at the closet possible world in which X happens, Y happens," where the closeness relation is to be understood in terms of similarity, where that world which is more similar to the actual world is that which is closest.[34] From this, Bradley develops the **Difference-Making Principle**:

> **DMP.** The value of an event E, for a person S, at world w, relative to similarity relation R = the intrinsic value of w for S, minus the intrinsic value for S of the most R-similar world to w where E does not occur.[35]

Bradley holds that "DMP entails that, when death takes a good life from its victim, that person's death is bad".[36]

The final deprivation-based argument that will be considered here is that which has been developed by Bernard Williams. Williams claims that if it is "genuinely true of life that the satisfaction of desire, and possession of the *praemia vitae*, are good things" then "longer enjoyment of them is better than shorter, and more of them, other things being equal, is better than less of them".[37] To support this claim Williams notes that if a person desires something then she will prefer a state of affairs to exist in which she gets what she wants to one in which she does not. As such, a person will have reason to resist that which will preclude her from getting what she wants, and so, concludes Williams, "wanting something itself gives one a reason for avoiding death," and hence to regard it as an evil.[38]

Responses to these Deprivation-based Arguments for the Harm of Death

None of the above arguments in favor of the view that death can harm the person who dies through depriving her of the goods of life that she would have otherwise enjoyed are sound.

Let us begin with Nagel's argument. There are, as Glenn Braddock has noted, two possible responses that an Epicurean can give to his example of the man who has been reduced to the status of a contented infant, with which one an Epicurean offers being dependant upon which view of personal identity she adopts.[39] First, one could hold that given the dramatic psychological change that occurred owing to the brain injury in question there was, contra Nagel, no reduction of the intelligent man to the status of a contented infant, for he simply ceased to exist as an experiencing being at the time of the brain injury and was replaced by another being.[40] Alternatively, if one holds that the intelligent man does continue to exist, then one could hold that his brain injury is a harm to him in that it adversely affects his experiences, even though he himself in his reduced condition is unaware of this.[41] The second of these responses would undermine the force of Nagel's example as one that purports to show that a person's death can be bad for him through depriving him of the goods of life. If the intelligent man does not cease to exist as an experiencing being as a result of his brain injury, then his case is importantly disanalogous to that of a person who dies. As such, then, even though one might hold that his brain injury is a misfortune to him this cannot support the claim that death would therefore be a misfortune to the person who dies. The first of these responses, however, would not immediately undermine the force of Nagel's objection in the same way. This is because to complete this response to Nagel the defender of the Hedonic Variant of the above Epicurean argument would have to insist that insofar as the intelligent man has ceased to exist as an experiencing being he is effectively dead, and so (and contra Nagel's assumption) the brain injury did not harm him as death is not a harm to the one who dies. But this would be unsatisfactory, for merely to assert in this way that the intelligent man was not harmed by his brain injury is simply to beg the question against Nagel. Noting this, however, should provide only cold comfort to Nagel, for just as the Epicurean is reduced merely to asserting that the intelligent man was not harmed by his death, so too are they reduced merely to asserting that he was. As such, then, Nagel has offered no reason to believe that a person could be harmed by her own death.[42]

Similar responses can also be offered to Feldman's attempt to show that death can be a harm to the person who dies.[43] Just as Nagel's example of the man whose brain injury reduced him to the status of a contented infant could be undermined by the Epicurean simply by noting that it was disanalogous to a case in which a person dies, for as the man continued to exist as an experiencing subject after his injury, so too can Feldman's examples of the man who chooses College A over College B, and the woman who is born into Country A, be undermined in the same way. An Epicurean could hold that irrespective of whether one adopts the restricted or the unrestricted understanding of premise (1) one could accept that this man and this woman were harmed by attending College A, and being born into Country A, respectively. What is important in this debate, an Epicurean could hold, is to determine whether a person's death could be a harm to the person who dies through adversely affecting her experiences. Thus, to show that this is so one must show that an agent can be harmed by an event that deprives him of goods that he would otherwise enjoy by precluding him from experiencing *anything* after its occurrence. Since Feldman's two examples do not do this, they cannot be used to support the unrestricted understanding of premise (1) over its restricted counterpart.[44] And that they do support principle EI is irrelevant, for EI is compatible with both understandings of this premise.

At first sight, it might appear that Bradley's deprivation account of how death can be bad for the person who dies could be objected to along the lines of the first response to Nagel's deprivation-based account, above: that since the value of E for S at w relative to R at a time t would be contingent upon S's existence as an experiencing being at t, then since S ceases to exist as such at the moment of her death then her death could not be bad for her, even if she would have had a good life in the closest possible world where she did not die, for E could only have value for S if she exists as a being capable of experiencing value. And, since this is the case, then since DMP (wrongly) entails that a person's death is bad for her under such conditions it should be rejected. But this moves too fast as an objection to DMP. First, in holding that the value of E for S at w relative to R at a time t would be contingent upon S's existence as an experiencing being at t it is being assumed that the value of E for S at w relative to R must be indexed to a particular time, t. That is, it is being assumed that all harms are *temporal* harms; that E must be bad for S at a particular time. But it might be possible that there are timeless evils; it might be the case that there are some events that are genuinely bad for a person, but which are not bad for her at any particular time. And, if this is so, then a person's death need not be bad for her at any particular time—and so its badness need not coincide with the time of her existence as an experiencing being.

What, then, should we make of the assumption that all harm is temporal? To counter this Bradley has developed an example of "an apparently timeless evil" that focuses on the situation of Andy, a man who decides whether or not to get married by flipping a coin; if it lands heads, he'll get married, else not.[45] Just before he flips the coin he sustains a brain injury that results in his "living out the remaining twenty years of his life with no good or bad experiences," although he is still conscious.[46] Had Andy "flipped the coin and it came up heads, he would have experienced ten years of extreme happiness . . . followed by ten years of moderate unhappiness," (life L1), otherwise "he would have experienced ten years of moderate unhappiness. . . . followed by ten years of extreme happiness" (life L2).[47] In this example there is no determinate answer to the question of whether the coin would have come up heads or tails had Andy flipped it. As such, claims Bradley, "given these assumptions, there is no time such that we can say that Andy's injury is bad for him at that time".[48] Given the indeterminacy of whether Andy would have experienced L1 or L2 there is no *particular* time at which we could say whether the event of his brain injury was good or bad for him according to DMP, although it *was* an evil for him, for overall his life would have gone better had it not occurred. Hence, it seems that Andy's brain injury is a timeless evil for him. Thus, given that timeless evils apparently exist, a person's death could be timelessly bad for her. And, if this is so, then the first assumption that underlies the above response to DMP should be rejected, for it is not true that all harm must be temporal.[49]

Bradley recognizes that an Epicurean could respond by moderating her position to hold that although death could be a timeless evil even if this is the case it is still not as bad as other evils that "harm us in both timeless and timeful ways," a position that would still run counter to Aristotle's claim that death "is the most terrible of all things".[50] But since such moderate Epicureanism falls far short of the full-blooded Epicureanism that is developed and defended in this volume, it is fortunate that it need not be accepted to counter Bradley's example of Andy. As Bradley later acknowledges, the example of the unfortunate Andy does not show that there are atemporal harms, but only that in some cases it will not be possible to identify the particular *moments* at which an event harms a person.[51] It does not show that there is no time at which Andy's injury is bad for him, for it is clear that its badness for him is located during the remaining twenty years of his life. As William Grey nicely puts it, "To say that there is no precise or *locatable* time at which harms occur is not to say that there is no time at which they occur".[52]

What, then, of Williams's argument for the claim that death is a harm to the person who dies? Williams's argument could be construed, like those of Nagel and Feldman, as an argument in which having a life that contains the *praemia vitae* is better for a person that dying, and so insofar as a person's death would deprive her of the *praemia vitae* that she would have otherwise had it is a harm to her.[53] As such, it would be subject to the same criticisms. Given this, it is better to construe Williams's argument as being one focused on what it is rational for a person to avoid, rather than being an argument that is straightforwardly based upon the claim that death deprives a person of the goods of life. Thus, on this understanding of his argument Williams claims that death is an evil for the person who dies since it would be rational for her to try to avoid it. Williams claims that "from the perspective of the wanting agent it is rational to aim for states of affairs in which his want is satisfied, and hence to regard death as something to be avoided; that is, to regard it as an evil."[54] Although it is rational for most persons to try to avoid death, this does not in itself show that death is an evil. It is rational for a person to prefer X to Y if X has a positive value for her and Y has no value (either positive or negative) at all. As such, then, that a person would prefer to live rather than to die does not show that death is an evil for her, as Williams assumes; it merely shows that life is a good for her. Like Nagel and Feldman, then, Williams has failed to show that death is a harm to the person who dies.

THE EXISTENCE VARIANT AND PRESENTISM DEFENDED

Recall that premise (5) of the Existence Variant of the Epicurean argument that death is not a harm to the person who dies is "A postmortem person (i.e., a person whose death has occurred) does not exist." This premise, however, rests on the assumption that presentism is true—and this assumption needd to be defended. As such, a robust defense of this Variant of this argument requires that some recent objections to presentism that have been offered by Bradley in the context of defending his deprivation-based account of death's badness be outlined and rejected.[55]

Bradley notes that the ontological view that undergirds the Existence Variant of this Epicurean argument "might stem from a general principle about relations: in order for a relation to relate things, it must relate them at a time, and in order for a relation to relate things at a time, both *relata* must exist at that time."[56] Thus, the "badness-for" relation can only hold between a person and a state of affairs or an event at those times at which both the person and the state of affairs or event both exist. However, as Bradley observes, this principle is too strong, for there are many examples of relations that hold between things that exist and things that do not. For example, causal relationships often exist between events that do not temporally overlap, while the "is a great-great-grandson of relation often relates an existing person and a nonexistent person."[57] Bradley holds that counterexamples such as these to the general principle about relations outlined above pose problems for presentists, who (he assumes) share its underlying view that for a relation to relate things at a time both *relata* must exist at that time. Rather than endorsing presentism, then, Bradley holds that *eternalism* should be endorsed: the view that "past and future objects exist", even if they do not exist now.[58] In addition to this problem for presentists Bradley offers two more: that if presentism were true then we would not be able to refer to past objects, nor be able "to account for the literal truth of our history books".[59]

All three of these objections to presentism are misguided. First, it is not true that a presentist is committed to holding that the over-strong general principle that "in order for a relation to relate things, it must relate them at a time, and in order for a relation to relate things at a time, both *relata* must exist at that time". To hold that a presentist is committed to this claim is to hold that presentists have a general problem with the ascription of relational properties (such as "is a great-great-great grandfather of") to objects that do not exist. As such, then, to hold that presentist is committed to this general principle about relations is to hold that she is committed to the claim that "If, at t, x has the property P, then x exists at t."[60] But the presentist is not committed to this claim, for it is perfectly possible for a presentist to hold that Cambridge changes can be predicated of objects that no longer exist. Although such a predication might predicate of the object in question a phony *change*, it still ascribes to it a perfectly genuine *property*.[61] It is thus simply not true that a presentist could have trouble ascribing the sort of relational properties that Bradley outlines to objects that no longer exist.[62] Bradley's second objection to presentism is similarly misguided. Presentists do not necessarily see any bar to referring to past objects, such as Napoleon or Lucretius, for presentism is compatible with both the description theory and the causal theory of reference determination.[63] Rather, it is the *predication of properties* to such past entities that appears puzzling for them.[64] Finally, it is also not true that presentists necessary have difficulties with accounting "for the literal truth of our history books". If it is held that a proposition, if true, is true at all times, then if x is P at t it is eternally true that x is P at t, even at those times when x does not exist. But this is not necessarily a problem for presentists. Presentists can accept that "x is P at t" is true after the time at which x ceases to exist; they only have a problem with the claim that "x is P at t" when "t" is a time at which x no longer exists.[65] Hence, claims about Socrates that are indexed to times at which Socrates existed (i.e., the usual sorts of claims found in history books) are unproblematic for presentists.

CONCLUSION

The Hedonic Variant of the Epicurean argument that death is not a harm to the person who dies can be defended against the two most salient objections that have been leveled against it: that persons can be harmed by events or states of affairs that do not adversely affect their experiences, and that a person's death could harm her in that it deprives her of positive experiences that she would have otherwise had. Moreover, the Existence Variant of this argument can be defended against the claim that its premise (5) should be rejected, for the truth of presentism can be defended against recent objections that have been leveled against it in the context of discussing the Epicurean view that death is a harm to the person who dies.

That the deprivation-based argument is ineffective against this Epicurean view should come as no surprise to persons familiar with the Epicurean view of the good life. For Epicurus, the goal of life, its *telos*, was *ataraxia*, tranquility. This was understood as consisting of both the katastematic plea-sure of the absence of pain (both mental and physical), as well as the kinetic pleasure of the pursuit of this katastematic pleasure through the process of removing the lacks that would undermine it.[66] Given this understanding of the eudaimonic life, it is clear that, for an Epicurean, an event or a state of affairs can only be harmful to a person if it imposes mental or physical pain upon her. As such, then, an event that deprives a person of something that might typically be thought to be a good for her (such as a promotion at work) would not, for an Epicurean, be a harm to her, unless it also imposed upon her some mental or physical harm (e.g., through causing her to think of how her life might have gone, or by continuing her economic privation). For this reason alone, then, an Epicurean would not be persuaded by the deprivation-based argument against the view that death is not a harm to the person who dies.[67] Furthermore, since an Epicurean believes that the only goods in life are those afforded either by the static pleasure of *ataraxia* or the kinetic pleasure of the pursuit of this state, the only deprivations of goods that an Epicurean would consider to be worth the name would be those that deprived the persons subject to them of either mental or physical tranquility, or its pursuit. For an Epicurean, then, the only events or states of affairs that could deprive a person of the goods of life would be those which imposed upon him positive ills (i.e., those that cause him directly to suffer from a lack of mental or physical tranquility). But since the propo-nents of the deprivation thesis do not hold that death imposes ills of this sort upon persons, the Epicurean would, given his view of the eudaimonic life, have no reason to believe that a person's death deprived him of any-thing at all. Deprivation arguments for the claim that death can be a harm to the person who dies can thus gain no traction against an Epicurean who adheres to the Epicurean view of the good human life.

One need not, however, accept the Epicurean view of the eudaimonic life to be unmoved by the deprivation-based argument against the view that death is not a harm to the person who dies, for, as was argued above, this objection fails for reasons that are entirely unrelated to this aspect of Epicu-reanism. As such, then, one need not endorse an Epicurean view of pleasure to accept the Epicurean view of death—and hence one need not endorse this view of pleasure to acknowledge the relevance of this view for those bioethical debates in which the question of whether death is a harm to the person who dies will play a central role. Thus, having established in this Chapter that death is not a harm to the person who dies the ground is pre-pared both for considering this view in the light of two such debates (those concerned with the rationality of suicide and the morality of euthanasia), and also for considering these debates in the light if it. Prior to so doing, however, it would be wise to buttress this Epicurean conclusion, since, as was acknowledged in the Introduction, it is often regarded as being "very odd". To this end, then, the arguments that were offered in support of it by Lucretius will be considered in the next Chapter.[68]

6 Fearless Symmetry

It was argued in the previous Chapter that death is not a harm to the person who dies. This Epicurean conclusion has famously been reinforced by Lucretius, who argued that just as a person's pre-natal non-existence as an experiencing being was not a harm to her, so too will her postmortem non-existence also fail to be a harm to her.[1] Although this "Symmetry Argument" for the view that death is not a harm to the person who died has not attracted as much critical attention as the Epicurean argument that preceded it, it has still been widely rejected.[2] In this Chapter it will be argued that, like the Epicurean argument that preceded it, the Lucretian Symmetry Argument successfully establishes that death is not a harm to the person who dies. And, since this is so, there is good reason to accept the third claim of the full-blooded Epicureanism of this volume—and hence to apply it to those bioethical debates in which the view that death is not a harm to the person who dies would play a role.[3]

LUCRETIAN ARGUMENTS

In the third book of Lucretius' *De Rerum Natura* (*DRN*) there are two passages that independently provide the basis of the Symmetry Argument for the view that death is not a harm to the person who dies. The first is:

> And just as in time past we felt no distress—while from all quarters Carthaginians were coming to the conflict, when the whole world, shaken by the terrifying tumult of war, shivered and quaked under the lofty and breezy heaven, and was in doubt under which domination all men were destined to fall by land and sea; so, when we shall no longer be, when the parting shall have come about between body and spirit from which we are compacted into one whole, then sure enough nothing at all will be able to happen to us, who will then no longer be, or to make us feel, not if earth be commingled with sea and sea with sky.[4]

The second is:

Look also and see how the ages of everlasting time past before we were born have been to us nothing. This therefore is a mirror which nature holds up to us, showing the time to come after we at length shall die. Is there anything horrible in that?[5]

The first point to note about this Lucretian argument is that it is unclear, for it could take (at least) two possible forms, each of which supports a different conclusion.[6] On the first understanding of this argument—what might be termed the *ontological* version—it is construed as an argument that establishes the conclusion that death is not a harm to the person who dies, thus:

1. The time before a person is born is nothing to him; i.e., it was not a harm to him.

Thus, from (1):

2. If a person's birth occurs at t2 rather than t1, this later birth is not a harm to him.

3. The time after a person's death is for him relevantly similar to the time before he was born.

Thus, from (1) and (3):

4. The time after a person's death is nothing to him; i.e., it is not a harm to him.

Thus, from (2) and (4):

5. If a person's death occurs at t1 rather than t2, this earlier death is not a harm to him.

Thus:

Conclusion: Death is not a harm to the person who dies.

On the second understanding of this argument—what might be termed the *attitudinal* version of it—it is construed as an argument that establishes the conclusion that persons should not feel distress as the prospect of their postmortem non-existence as experiencing beings, thus:

1. When a person looks back to the period of time that existed prior to his birth, he feels no distress.[7]

Thus, from (1):

2. If a person's birth occurs at t2 rather than t1, this later birth does not cause him any distress.
3. The time after a person's death is for him relevantly similar to the time before he was born.

Thus, from (1) and (3):

4. When a person contemplates the time that will occur after his death, he should feel no distress.

Thus, from (2) and (4):

5. A person should not be distressed when he contemplates the possibility that his death could occur at t1 rather than t2.

Thus:

Conclusion: A person's contemplation of his own death should not cause him any distress.

Despite its Blakeian title this Chapter will focus on the first, ontological, version of this Lucretian argument. This is for two reasons. First, the focus of this volume is on establishing the tripartite claims of full-blooded Epicureanism, and then, with these claims in hand, demonstrating their implications for various issues in bioethics. As such, only the ontological version this Lucretian argument is directly relevant to the focus of this volume.[8] Second, if the ontological version of this Lucretian argument successfully establishes that death is not a harm to the person who dies then either (i) the conclusion of the attitudinal version of this argument should also follow, or (ii) the distress that a person might still feel on contemplating his own death is not amenable to banishment by rational argument.[9] The first of these possibilities, (i), will follow from the conclusion of the ontological version of this Lucretian argument if a person's contemplation of his own death is distressing to him because he believes that it will be a harm to him. Thus, insofar as the ontological version of this Lucretian argument shows that this will not be the case, a person who feels distress at the prospect of his own death for this reason should have his fear alleviated by it.[10] However, not all persons will feel distress at the prospect of their own deaths for this reason. A person might, for instance, feel distress on contemplating his own death for altruistic reasons, such as the effect that he envisions it will have upon those who care for him.[11] Alternatively, a person might feel distress on contemplating his own death because he believes that even if it is not a harm to him, his death is an intrinsic bad.[12] As noted by J.S. Mill, however, it is not clear that a person can show through argument that something is, or is not, intrinsically bad, and so it is not clear that a person who continues to feel distress at the prospect of his own death for this reason would be amenable to argument.[13]

CHALLENGES TO THE LUCRETIAN SYMMETRY ARGUMENT

Like the original Epicurean argument for the view that death is not a harm to the person who dies the ontological version of this Lucretian symmetry argument (henceforth, "the Lucretian argument") has not gone unchallenged. Nagel, for example, has contested it on the grounds that the symmetry that it rests upon is illusory:

> But we cannot say that the time prior to a man's birth is time in which he would have lived had he been born not then but earlier. For aside from the brief margin permitted by premature labor, he *could* not have been born earlier; anyone born substantially earlier than he was would have been someone else. Therefore the time prior to his birth is not time in which his subsequent birth prevents him from living. His birth, when it occurs, does not entail the loss to him of any life whatever.[14]

Nagel, then, claims that the symmetry between a person's pre-natal non-existence as an experiencing being and his (allegedly) similar postmortem non-existence as such a being that the Lucretian ontological argument trades on to establish that death is not a harm to the person who dies does not exist. While it is true that a person P could have died later, and thus the claim in premise (5) that a person could have died later than he did, is true, it is *not* true that P could have been born earlier, for the (approximate) time of a person's birth is essential to his identity—and so the claim in premise (2) should be rejected, for his birth could not have occurred at t1 rather than t2. Hence, since the Lucretian argument rests on the symmetry between premises (2) and (5), once this is shown to be illusory it should be rejected.

Another major objection that has been leveled against the Lucretian argument has been dubbed the "backfire problem" by Rosenbaum.[15] Rather than challenging the symmetry that the proponents of the Lucretian argument hold to exist between premises (1) and (4), and hence (2) and (5), the proponent of this problem urges that the correct response to it is not to hold that a person's pre-natal nonexistence as an experiencing being is nothing to him (and from this derive the Lucretian conclusion that a person's death is not a harm to him). Instead, the proponent of this objection urges, one should draw on the intuition that a person's earlier death at t1 *is* a harm to him, and conjoin this with the claim that the period of time *after* t1 is relevantly similar to the period of time *prior* to a person's birth to conclude that just as a person's earlier death harms her, so too does her later birth.[16] This is an approach that Feldman takes in responding to this Lucretian argument, when he writes that "there are . . . two ways in which we can rectify the apparently irrational emotional asymmetry . . . We can follow Lucretius and cease viewing early death as a bad thing . . . [Or] we can at least try to start viewing late birth as a bad thing. My suggestion is that

. . . the latter course would be preferable. . . . ".[17] Moreover, and quite apart from whether or not persons should follow Feldman's suggestion, it seems that if this Lucretian argument can be used to support two contradictory conclusions there is something amiss with it.[18]

Feldman has also developed a further objection against this Lucretian argument, holding that the possibility that a person could have been born earlier than she was is not symmetrical with the possibility that she could have died later than she did as the proponents of the Lucretian argument are committed to claiming. To show this, Feldman considers the example of Claudette, who was born in 1950 and died in 2000 as a result of an accident. Feldman holds that her premature death is extrinsically bad for Claudette, and that she would not be considered to be so misfortunate were she to die in 2035, having enjoyed an extra 35 years of (good) life. However, notes Feldman, it does not seem plausible to hold that Claudette suffered a misfortune as a result of not being born in 1915 given her death in 2000, even though this earlier birth would have also afforded her an additional 35 years of (good) life. With this example in hand Feldman holds that the Lucretian view that earlier birth is on a par with later death is mistaken, for it trades on the twin assumptions that if a person is said to die later her birth date is held constant, and so she gains more life, whereas if a person is said to be born earlier her death date is not held to be constant, but is intuitively adjusted so that her life span remains constant.[19] As such, then, concludes Feldman, there is an asymmetry between claims concerning a person's later birth and earlier death that justifies her regretting the latter but not the former. Thus, the Lucretian argument fails.

The final objection to this Lucretian argument can be drawn from Derek Parfit's *Reasons and Persons*. Parfit offers an example in which he is in hospital for "some kind of surgery" that is very painful, and which cannot be done without anesthetics. Since the operation is so painful, those who undergo it are caused to forget it by the administration of a drug that removes their memories of it. Parfit wakes up, and asks a nurse when his operation is to take place, and how long it will take. She informs him that she has information about him and another patient, but she cannot remember which is which. She can only tell him that he "may be the patient who had his operation yesterday. In that case . . . [his] . . . operation was the longest ever performed, lasting ten hours. [Or he] . . . may instead be the patient who is to have the short operation later today".[20] Parfit notes that it is clear that he would prefer to be the person whose operation is in the past, even though that operation is longer (and so more painful) than the one he would undergo were his operation to lie in the future. Parfit goes on to claim that this preference is "not irrational".[21] If Parfit is correct here then it seems that having a bias towards the future (that is, one prefers that one's pains to be in one's past and pleasures to be in one's future) can sometimes be rational. Given this asymmetry between one's past and future states, it seems that it could be rational to regard one's own death as a harm even if one does not regard one's later (i.e., later than it otherwise could have been) birth as a harm. In this further way, then, it seems that the Lucretian argument can be undermined.

RESPONSES TO NAGEL'S OBJECTION

Stoic Fate

Perhaps the most extensively discussed of these four objections to the Lucretian argument is Nagel's. Nagel's argument, however, is subject to an obvious criticism: that he simply assumes that whereas there is considerable leeway available concerning the timing of a person's death there is little leeway available with respect to the timing of her birth. And this assumption would not be accepted by everyone. Drawing on the Stoic conception of fate in the context of arguing that a person who weeps because he will not be alive in a thousand years' time is just as foolish as a person who weeps because he was not alive a thousand years ago, Seneca writes:

> You have been cast upon this point of time; if you would make it longer how much longer shall you make it? Why weep? Why pray? You are taking pains to no purpose. "Give over your thinking that your prayers can bend/Divine decrees from their predestined end". These decrees are unalterable and fixed; they are governed by a mighty and everlasting compulsion. Your goal will be the goal of all things.[22]

The view expressed here is that the duration of a person's life is fixed: neither the time of his birth nor the time of his death are alterable. For Seneca, then, Nagel is simply mistaken to believe that there is an asymmetry between the (relatively fixed) timing of a person's birth and the (open) timing of her death in that there is little leeway in the former, but considerable leeway in the latter, for *both* are fixed.[23]

Hetherington's Symmetry Arguments

One need not, however, accept the Stoic conception of fate to object to Nagel's anti-Lucretian argument on the grounds that the asymmetry that he posits does not hold.[24]

Stephen Hetherington, for example, has objected to Nagel's argument on the *anti*-Stoic grounds that he is mistaken to hold that "there is almost no correlative leeway in the precise time at which one's life begins".[25] Noting that Nagel focuses on birth as the start of life, Hetherington argues that the leeway that exists concerning one's "precise time of birth might not be so insignificant, relative to the length of the preceding pregnancy," for "an extra year of life at a life's end could stand to the preceding lifespan as much as being born a few days earlier would stand to the time between your being conceived and your otherwise being born".[26] For example, explains Hetherington, "to die at 81 rather than at 80 is to lengthen one's life by 1.25 percent; and to be born four days prematurely is to shorten one's mother's pregnancy by approximately 1.48 percent".[27] Moreover, argues Hetherington, Nagel cannot defend his position by changing the focus of his claim from birth to conception, for this argument could simply be adapted to respond to that modified position also. Thus, it is possible that an egg might be fertilized by the same time that actually fertilized it at a slightly earlier time, and "when considered in relation to the relevant range of times within which that particular egg and that particular sperm might have met and interacted . . . some such leeway in timing could be similar, in percentage terms, to the possible leeways described [in the original argument offered against Nagel's position]".[28]

Hetherington's defense of the Lucretian argument against Nagel is, however, flawed in two respects. Hetherington renders the percentage lengthening of a person's (P1) life when she dies later rather than sooner relative to the length of the life that she had lived prior to the start of the additional period of time that she was afforded by her later death. However, the relevant percentage that Hetherington offers with respect to the person (P2) who was born earlier rather than later does not identify the percentage by which P2's *life* was lengthened by her earlier birth, but the percentage by which P2's *mother's pregnancy with her* was shortened. This difference in the bases for the percentages that Hetherington offers concerning P1 and P2 is not surprising. While it is natural to assess the degree to which P1's life was lengthened in this way, this assessment is impossible in the case of P2, for she had no previous lifespan on which it could be grounded. This is a clear dissimilarity between P1 and P2. Thus, even though Hetherington shows that the percentage by which P1's life could be extended could be similar to the percentage by which P2's mother's pregnancy could be shortened these relative percentages are *not* symmetrical, for they are grounded on different bases of comparison. Hetherington is thus mistaken to claim that there is a percentage-based symmetry between a person's earlier birth and her later death that Nagel has overlooked.

It should also be noted that Hetherington's response to Nagel is based on the assumption that the appropriate way to compare periods of life that have failed to be actualized as a result of a person's later birth or earlier death is by comparing them in terms of percentages of preceding periods. But comparing these periods of time in such *relative* terms is not the only way in which these comparisons could be drawn, for they could also be drawn in *absolute* terms. That is to say, rather than noting that a person who died at 80 when he could have died at 81 failed to have his life lengthened by 1.25 percent as a result of his life's failing to actualize that extra year, one could instead simply note that he failed to have his life lengthened by a year. Similarly, rather than noting that a person who was born on time rather than four days prematurely thereby failed to cut short his mother's pregnancy by approximately 1.48 percent, one could instead simply note that he failed to have his life lengthened by four days. As such, then, *even if* the percentage-based comparisons that Hetherington draws were legitimate ones he would still need to provide an argument as to why the comparisons that he wishes to draw between a person's earlier birth and her later death should be made in relative, rather than absolute, terms. And there are two reasons why a successful version of such an argument will not be forthcoming. The first has been outlined above: that the relative percentages that will be offered with respect to the earlier birth of P2 and the later death of P2 cannot be appropriately symmetrical. The second is that the most natural way to understand both the Lucretian argument and the views of those who object to it is in *absolute*, and *not* relative, terms. In mentioning the Punic Wars between Rome and Carthage in the first passage quoted above (at *DRN* 3.832–42) Lucretius is making the point that a person does not lament her failure to have been born earlier; she does not lament the "loss" to her of the century and a half (or so) of life that one might believe she could have had had she been born earlier. As such, then, persons should not lament the occurrence of their deaths, even if they believe that such deaths would rob them of a similarly extended additional portion of life. The appeal of the Lucretian argument thus rests upon comparing in absolute terms the life that is allegedly "lost" as a result of a person's later birth, and that which is allegedly "lost" as a result of her earlier death. Moreover, those who believe that death is a harm to the person who dies are also likely to understand the periods of "lost" time in question in absolute, and not relative, terms. If one accepts this anti-Epicurean claim it will be intuitive to hold that a person's loss of a significantly greater period of life is more of a harm to her than the loss of a shorter period. As such, then, for such persons the loss of four days of possible life will not be equivalent to the loss of a year of possible life. The latter will be a much greater harm than the former, even if these periods of times are equivalent in the relative terms that Hetherington relies upon. Thus, even if Hetherington can provide an account of how to assess "gains" in life in relative terms that are appropriately symmetrical, without further argument as to why the "lost" periods of time that are occasioned by later birth and earlier death should be compared in such terms Nagel has no reason to accept his objection.

Earlier Birth and Personal Identity

If one does not accept the Stoic view of fate, then, given the failure of Hetherington's arguments, how else might one respond to Nagel's objection to the Lucretian argument? Like Hetherington, Rosenbaum has argued that Nagel is mistaken to hold that there is an asymmetry between a person's earlier birth and her later death. Rosenbaum takes issue with Nagel's claim that whereas a person could have died later than she did, she could not have been conceived earlier than she was (although Nagel recognizes that there is some small degree of leeway here—a concession that Hetherington tried to exploit).[29] Nagel's argument for this claim is:

> The direction of time is crucial is assigning possibilities to people or other individuals. Distinct possible lives of a single person can diverge from a common beginning, but they cannot converge to a common conclusion from diverse beginnings. (The latter would represent not a set of different possible lives of one individual but a set of distinct possible individuals whose lives have identical conclusions.) Given an identifiable individual, countless possibilities for his continued existence are imaginable, and we can clearly conceive of what it would be for him to go on existing indefinitely.[30]

It seems that Nagel is here relying on the Kripkean idea that a person's genetic origin is essential to her identity as a particular person.[31] As such, Rosenbaum reconstructs Nagel's argument thus:

> It is logically possible for a person's life to be conceived earlier only if it is logically possible for a person's life to converge to one specific ending from different (logically) possible temporal beginnings (in conception). Since the latter is not logically possible, then the former is not.[32]

Against this reconstruction of Nagel's argument Rosenbaum notes that it does not seem to be logically impossible that a person's life could begin at different points in time, even if the time of her demise is held constant. Moreover, argues Rosenbaum, even if one grants to Nagel the Kripkean view that a person's genetic origin is essential to her identity this does not show that it is *logically* impossible for a person to have been earlier—although he grants that it "could be physically impossible".[33]

Rosenbaum is correct here. But this does not show that Nagel's argument is mistaken, for he could retreat from the claim that it is logically impossible for a person to be born earlier (whereas it is logically possible for her to die later) to the claim that whereas it is physically impossible for a person to be born earlier, it is not physically impossible for her to die later. Making this (weaker) claim would both avoid Rosenbaum's objection, and preserve the asymmetry that Nagel believes holds between the time of a person's birth and the time of her death. Unfortunately for Nagel, however, it is not physically impossible for a person to be born earlier than she was. It is possible to conceive a child through in vitro fertilization (IVF) and freeze the resulting embryos for implantation at a later date. Persons who had their origins in such embryos could thus have been implanted earlier than they actually were, assuming that they were not immediately implanted. As such, then, even if the Kripkean point concerning genetic origin and personal identity is accepted, one need not endorse Nagel's claim that it is physically impossible for a person to have been born later than she was.

Kaufman's Defense of Nagel's Argument

This rejection of Nagel's argument rests on accepting the Kripkean claim that what matters with respect to the question of whether a person could have been born earlier than she was is that the person in question be identified solely by reference to her genetic origins. It is thus open for a defender of Nagel's argument to respond by arguing that "the features of person-hood" that are relevant to identifying persons in the context of addressing the question of whether they could have been born earlier "are not captured by genetic . . . considerations . . . " but involve something else.[34] This approach to defending Nagel is adopted by Frederick Kaufman. Kaufman notes both that the word "person" could be used to refer to a biological entity such as "a member of the species *Homo sapiens*," or "to an ongoing centre of self-awareness."[35] He notes that it is this latter psychological sense of "person" that "most concerns us when we deliberate about whether or not we could have lived at different times or different places; and the prospect of psychological extinction is surely what disturbs us when we think about death".[36] Kaufman then observes that on the Kripkean approach to genetic origin and personal identity (what Kaufman terms "metaphysical personal identity") a person's identity could remain constant even if she lived two completely different lives.[37] Thus, notes Kaufman, on this view a middle-class American could instead have been a rural Spaniard, had his parents emigrated to Spain prior to his birth. But that this is so, argues Kaufman, shows that the Kripkean approach to personal identity is not that which is relevant to the question of whether a person could have been born earlier than she was. Given the psychological person that he now is, argues Kaufman, the Kaufman who would have been raised in Spain had his (Kaufman's) parents moved there prior to his birth would be as alien to him as would an individual living 300 years in the future who happened to be genetically identical with the presently existing Kaufman. Thus, concludes Kaufman, "In some broad sense, my biography is necessary for me to be me".[38] With this conclusion in place Kaufman argues that Nagel is correct to hold that it would not be possible for a person to be born earlier than she was, for "a psychological continuum which, by hypothesis, starts earlier, would be a sufficiently different set of memories and experiences, and hence be a different psychological self".[39] As such, claims Kaufman, "imaginatively moving a person 'back' disrupts the psychological self with which we are concerned".[40] But, Kaufman argues, such disruption does not occur when a person's life is imaginatively projected beyond the actual date of his death. In so doing the psychological continuum that constitutes him as a person (on Kaufman's view) will not be disrupted. Instead, it will merely be added to. Given this, while it is possible for a person to have died later than he did, it is not possible for him to have been born earlier than he was. Nagel is thus correct to claim that a person while a person could have died later than he did he "*could* not have been born earlier," for "anyone born substantially earlier than he was would have been someone else".[41] Thus, concludes Kaufman, the symmetry upon which the Lucretian argument depends is illusory, and so it does not show that death is not a harm to the person who dies.[42]

Responses to Kaufman

Kaufman's argument, however, suffers from two serious flaws. First, he conflates the criterion of personal identity *over time* (psychological personal identity) with the criterion of personal identity *across different possible lives* (metaphysical personal identity).[43] This point can be made both by focusing on the transitivity of identity, and by focusing on what is involved in establishing psychological contiguity of the sort that Kaufman bases his argument upon. The first of these approaches has been adopted by McMahan, who notes that both the (actual) American Kaufman and the (possible) Spanish Kaufman would be (weakly) psychologically continuous with the same late-stage fetus. Both of them, then, would be identical to it. Given the transitivity of identity (on which if B is identical to A and C is identical to A, B is identical to C) the American Kaufman would be identical (in the relevant respects) to the Spanish Kaufman. Thus, it is simply not the case that a person's biography is necessary for her to be her, and so Kaufman has failed to show that a person could not have been born earlier than he was. The second approach to making this point against Kaufman has been adopted by Anthony Brueckner and John Martin Fischer. Brueckner and Fischer note that the type of psychological continuity that Kaufman is concerned with consists of psychological connections between temporally distinct different person-stages. The having of (real) memories is one example of such psychological connectedness; one person-stage is psychologically contiguous with an earlier one if the later person-stage possesses a memory of an experience that is contained in that which preceded it.[44] With this in hand they then develop an example concerning a life-long New Jersey resident, Mary. The "actual sequence of person-stages that constitute Mary's life history, starting with her birth at t1 and ending with her death at t2" is denoted by "M".[45] M contains no memories of any pre-t1 psychological states, and so if one tries to imagine Mary having been born ten years earlier in Majorca none of the psychological states that one will try to imagine Mary having had had she been born earlier in this way will be contained in M. From this, Kaufman would conclude that New Jersey Mary and Majorca Mary could not be the same person, and so New Jersey Mary could not have been born earlier than she was. But, as Brueckner and Fischer note, not only is this not surprising, it does not support Kaufman's claim that there is an asymmetry between the possibilities for earlier birth and later death.

To see this, note that when a person imagines Mary and her experiences in Majorca pre-t1 one is imagining a *possible* world, and not the *actual* world. This possible world contains many possible psychological states that never actually existed, none of which are psychologically contiguous with any actual psychological state, for no *merely possible* psychological state is causally related to any *actual* psychological state. As such, then, none of Mary's imagined pre-t1 psychological states are psychologically contiguous with any of her actual psychological states. However, note Brueckner and Fischer, the same point can be made with respect to the psychological states that one could imagine Mary having were she to die ten years later than she actually did. Such imagined, merely possible, psychological states would not be causally connected with any of Mary's actual psychological states, and so none of them are psychologically contiguous with them. As such, then, just as none of the possible pre-t1 psychological states that one could imagine Mary having are psychologically contiguous with any of the states in M, nor are any of the possible *post-t2* psychological states that one could imagine Mary having. Kaufman, then, has failed to show that there is any asymmetry between a person's earlier birth and her later death. And he has failed to do so because in offering examples in which worlds other than the actual world need to be imagined he is entering into a discussion of *metaphysical personal identity across worlds*, rather than focusing on discussing *psychological personal identity within a single world*. Thus, although on a psychological criterion of personal identity it is trivially true that Mary-in-the-actual-world could not have had any pre-t1 psychological states (or, indeed, any post-t2 psychological states) this does not show that *Mary* could not have had such states. As such, then, Kaufman has not shown that Mary could not have been born earlier.[46] Thus, contra Nagel, the Lucretian symmetry holds.

The second objection to Kaufman's argument has been pressed against it by John Martin Fischer and Daniel Speak. In distinguishing between a Krip-kean approach to person identity and the psychological approach that he prefers Kaufman distinguishes between persons understood as "metaphysical essences" (a "thin" conception of personhood), and persons understood psychologically (a "thick" conception of personhood).[47] Kaufman argues that persons are concerned about their deaths *qua* thick persons, not *qua* thin persons. If a person's metaphysical essence E were to have led a very different life than that which the (actually existing) thick person lived she would have no more concern about the death of E than she would "about the death of any other stranger".[48] Thus, argues Kaufman, since (from the argument that he developed earlier, outlined above) a thick person cannot have been born earlier than she actually was born there is an asymmetry between a person's possible later birth and her possible earlier death. Since persons in the relevant sense could not have been born earlier (although thin persons could have been) their later births do not deprive them of the goods of life that they might have otherwise possessed. However, since they could die later than they actually did, their deaths do deprive them of goods that they could have had. Thus, concludes Kaufman, Nagel is correct to hold that whereas earlier death is a harm to the person who dies, their later birth is not—and so Lucretius is wrong to consider these two possibilities to be symmetrical.

Fischer and Speak concede that "the actual time of one's birth cannot deprive the thick person of goods he or she would have had".[49] However, they question why this is the only relevant issue, contending that it is also relevant to the issue at hand that the thin person could have been born earlier, and hence could have been deprived of the goods of life that an earlier birth would have afforded her. To support this Fischer and Speak argue that an actual thick person could coherently form preferences about how she would have preferred her life to have gone. For example, on learning that she had been given up at birth by an Eskimo couple a middle-class child from Anchorage might regret that she had not been brought up in the Eskimo community, believing that her having been brought up as a middle-class American child thereby deprived her of significant goods.[50] Since this is so, argue Fischer and Speak, persons can form "judgments and preferences about which thick persons our . . . thin selves . . . are associated with," even if the lives of the thick persons in question have beginnings that are very different from those of their own (actual) thick selves.[51] Given that Kaufman has conceded that thin persons could have been born earlier than they were, then, and Fischer and Speak have shown that it could be judged that they could have been deprived of some of the goods of life by such earlier birth, it seems that a later birth, like an earlier death, could deprive a (thin) person of the goods of life. Thus, conclude Fischer and Speak, Kaufman has failed to support Nagel's view that there is an asymmetry between earlier birth and later death.

Although they do not appear to realize it, Fischer's and Speak's arguments against Kaufman have unfortunate implications for the Lucretian argument—although, since they are deprivationists these implications are likely to be ones that they are willing to accept. Before considering these implications, however, it should be noted that Kaufman has argued that Fischer and Speak are faced with a dilemma. For a person to be deprived of something it is necessary that she have (or could have) preferences concerning the good in question. A thin self, however, has no preferences—and so a thin self could never be deprived of anything. Conversely, that a person wishes that she have something is not sufficient for it to be the case that she has been deprived of it if she lacks it. Thus, that a thick self might wish that she had been raised as an Eskimo (for example) does not mean that she has been deprived of such an upbringing if she did not receive it. Kaufman reinforces this point by conjoining two further claims: (i) no actual thick self could have been a different thick self, and (ii) for a person to be deprived of something it must be possible that she could have possessed it. With these two claims in hand Kaufman concludes (from (i)) that since a non-Eskimo thick self could not have been an Eskimo thick self, then (from (ii)) no actual non-Eskimo thick self has been deprived by not being raised as an Eskimo.[52]

Kaufman is correct to note that a thin self has no preferences, and hence cannot be deprived of anything. Recognizing this, John Martin Fischer modifies his (and Speak's) earlier objection to Kaufman, holding that the subject of deprivation that he is concerned with "is not the thin self (*qua* thin self), but some more complex entity, such as the thin self conjoined with a capacity to step back from any particular thick self and evaluate such selves".[53] But this will not do, for if a thin self has no preferences—and *ex hypothesi* it has not—it will have no basis from which to evaluate any particular thick self. Given this, Fischer's second account of the type of self that is at issue is better: "a thin self, a particular thick self, and the associated capacity to step back and form preferences [concerning the thick self] . . . ".[54] Fischer's "potential subject of harm and deprivation" is thus a thick self with a capacity for self-referential evaluation.[55] How, then, can Fischer meet Kaufman's two challenges to the view that a thick self could be the subject of deprivation as a result of having a later birth? Given the arguments that he has already presented with Brueckner, Fischer can meet the second of Kaufman's challenges readily, for "it is coherently conceivable, and thus metaphysically possible, that one's thick self could have come into being considerably earlier than it actually did".[56] With (i) rebutted in this way, Kaufman's claim that no actually existing thick self could be the subject to deprivation imposed by a later birth is met. Given this, Kaufman's challenge to the claim that a thick self could be deprived in this way can also be met. Kaufman is correct to note that a (thick) person's having a preference for a good G is not in itself sufficient to establish the claim that she has been deprived of it if she lacks it. He is, for example, correct to note that although he strongly prefers to be rich, he has not been deprived of a fortune simply because he lacks one.[57] What, then, is needed in addition to a person's having an unsatisfied preference for G (or could have had a preference for G that was unsatisfied) for her to have been deprived of G? It is clear that to be deprived of a good G one would have received G had not some event intervened. From this, then, a person P will be deprived of a good G if (i) P prefers to possess G, or would have preferred to possess G, (ii) an event E precludes P from possessing G, and (iii) P would have possessed G had E not occurred. But this account of what it is for P to be deprived of G is too simple, for a person could be deprived of a good as a result of the conjunction of several events. Nestor, for example, could be deprived of a tasty treat by the actions of Hamish and Lillian if there are only two treats available and they take them before he is able to. Conditions (ii) and (iii), then, need to be modified to reflect this: (ii) events E1. . . . En preclude P from possessing G, and (iii) P would have possessed G had E1. . . . En not occurred. With this more robust account of deprivation in place (and putting the arguments in the preceding Chapter to one side for the sake of this debate between Fischer and Kaufman), Fischer could hold that a person could be deprived of the goods of life that he would have received had he been born earlier since all three of these conditions could be met. Thus, a person P who would have preferred that he be raised as an Eskimo and was precluded from this in virtue of his birth (i) prefers that he would have been raised as an Eskimo, (ii) was prevented from being so raised by his actual birth (E) (and had he been born into another non-Eskimo life had event E not occurred, then this event E1, E2 . . . or En would have prevented him from being so raised), and (iii) P would have been born as an Eskimo had event E (or E1, E2. . . . En) not occurred. Fischer, then, has shown that *if* a deprivation account of how death harms the person who dies is correct, a similar account of how a person's later birth could be a harm to her, too. And, since this is so, Kaufman is mistaken to accept Nagel's view that the Lucretian symmetry between the time before a person's birth and the time before her death does not hold.

RESPONSES TO THE OTHER CRITICISMS OF THIS LUCRETIAN ARGUMENT

The Backfire Problem

It was noted above that Fischer's and Speak's arguments against Kaufman have unfortunate implications for the Lucretian argument—and what these are should now be clear. In arguing that Kaufman's attempt to support Nagel's anti-Lucretian claim that there is an asymmetry between a person's later conception and earlier death is mistaken Fischer and Speak have argued that there is a symmetry between these two events, in that both could harm a person by depriving him of the goods of life.[58] Fischer's and Speak's responses to Kaufman's defense of Nagel's objection to the Lucretian argument, then, provide only cold comfort to its proponents, for they serve directly to support the third objection that they are faced with: the Backfire Problem.

As was briefly mentioned above, the Backfire Problem can be used to support two related objections to this Lucretian argument: (1) that it begs the question insofar as it rests on the assumption that a person's later conception is not a harm to him, and (2) that if this question is not begged then this argument can be used to support two contradictory conclusions—and hence something must be wrong with it. Both of these objections, however, can be met—and in so doing the status of the Lucretian argument within the canon of Epicurean arguments concerning whether death is a harm to the person who dies will be further illuminated.

The proponents of the first of these objections to the Lucretian argument are correct to note that it rests on the assumption that a person is not harmed by his being conceived later—and they are correct to note that if this assumption is rejected then this Lucretian argument will fail. To meet this objection, then, the proponent of this Lucretian argument must argue for the assumption that a person is not harmed by his non-existence as an experiencing being prior to the time of his conception. Given that the conclusion of this argument is the claim that death is not a harm to the person who dies, and its basis is the claim that the time prior to a person's conception mirrors the time after his death, the Lucretian could simply argue for this assumption by modifying the Hedonic Variant of the Epicurean argument for the view that death is not a harm to the person who dies. This modified version ("Version 2") of the Hedonic Variant of this Epicurean argument is:

1. An event or a state of affairs is a harm to a person only if it adversely affects her experiences.
2. Pre-natal persons cannot experience anything.

Thus, given (1) and (2):

3. An event or a state of affairs can only adversely affect an antemortem person's experiences.

Thus, from (3):

4. A person can only be harmed by an event or a state of affairs that occurs after her conception.[59]

Therefore, a person cannot be harmed at any time prior to her conception.[60]

With this Version 2 of the Hedonic Variant of the original Epicurean argument in place the proponent of this Lucretian argument is able to meet the first objection that was supported by the Backfire Problem.[61] She is also able to meet the second objection, for when the Lucretian argument is coupled with Version 2 of the Hedonic Variant of the Epicurean argument it will not support the conclusion that a person's later conception will be a harm to him, and so it will not support the symmetrical conclusion concerning his earlier death.[62]

Feldman's Objection

The proponent of this Lucretian argument can also offer ready responses to Feldman's objection. The first and most basic of these is to note that although Feldman developed the example of Claudette to respond to "Lucretius's challenge" he failed to distinguish between the ontological and the attitudinal versions of this Lucretian argument. Having noted this, it is clear that Feldman took himself to be addressing the attitudinal version of this Lucretian argument, for he was attempting to explain why "we *feel* that early death is a greater misfortune for the prematurely deceased than is 'late birth' for the late born".[63] As a sociological account of why persons feel do not feel any distress at the possibility that they had a late birth, whereas they might feel distress at the possibility that they could have an early death, Feldman's point might be sound. But since this is only an attempt to explain why persons might have the attitudes that they have concerning late birth and early death it has no bearing at all on the issue of whether persons are actually harmed by late births or earlier deaths—and so it has no bearing on the ontological version of this Lucretian argument.[64]

Parfit's Hospital Example

Parfit's claim that his hospital example shows that it is not irrational for persons to have a bias towards the future has been challenged by Kaufman. Kaufman argues that Parfit's hospital example does not support his conclusion that persons are biased towards the future on the grounds that although Parfit has shown that persons are indifferent towards some past pains and yet dread future ones such asymmetrical attitudes cannot be generalized. To show this, he notes that "we prefer some bad experiences in front of us, not behind us, such as the loss of our reputations or bereavement over the loss of a loved one. And we prefer some good experiences behind us . . . such as the joys of childhood . . . ".[65] Yet, while Kaufman is certainly correct that persons generally have the temporal biases that he notes, this does nothing to show that Parfit's claim concerning attitudinal asymmetry is mistaken. Persons would prefer to suffer both the loss of their reputations, and bereavement, in the future rather than in the past because this would (typically) mean that they would then get to enjoy the benefits of their good reputations and the company of the people that they care about in both the present and the future prior to the occurrences of these events. That a person would prefer to have such losses in her future thus does nothing to undercut Parfit's claim that persons have a bias towards the future, for it is compatible with it. Kaufman's noting that persons would prefer that the joys of childhood be in their pasts rather than their futures also fails to undermine Parfit's claim concerning person's bias towards the future, for, as Kaufman recognizes, experiencing such joys now "would entail the loss of our status as adults".[66] Experiencing such joys, then, would come with a cost. That persons prefer such joys to be in their past thus simply shows that they do not wish to incur the cost involved in having them in their future—presumably because they believe that they experiences in the future would be better overall were they not to do so. Again, then, that persons would prefer the joys of childhood to be in their pasts does not undercut Parfit's claim that persons have a bias towards the future, but is compatible with it.[67]

Yet although Kaufman's initial objections to Parfit's claim that persons are biased towards the future are unsuccessful he is correct to note that Parfit's focus is on person's *attitudes* towards the *pains that they have experienced* in the past and will experience in the future.[68] As such, then, Parfit's concerns are orthogonal to the defense of the ontological version of the Lucretian argument (although they might be relevant to defenses of the attitudinal version of it). They are, first, orthogonal to it because to address this version of the Lucretian argument one must focus not on the *attitudes* that persons take towards the two periods of time in question, but on the issue of whether a person's pre-natal and postmortem non-existences *are* (ontologically) nothing to him *qua* experiencing being. Secondly, they are orthogonal to it since Parfit is concerned to show that persons have asymmetrical attitudes towards past and future *pains*. However, such concerns are irrelevant to both versions of the Lucretian argument, for persons cannot by definition experience pains during those periods of time when they do not exist as experiencing beings (i.e., pre-natally and postmortem). Thus, like Feldman's sociological conclusions concerning why persons have the attitudes that they do concerning later birth and earlier death, any conclusions that could be drawn from Parfit's hospital example would be irrelevant to the ontological version of this Lucetian argument.[69]

CONCLUSION

The ontological version of this Lucretian argument, then, can be used successfully to bolster the Epicurean argument for the view that death is not a harm to the person who dies—although it cannot support this conclusion independently of its predecessor. However, it is important to recall that the claim that the time before a person P is born is nothing to him is to be understood in this Lucretian argument as the claim that P was not the subject of harm at that time (just as the claim that the time after P's death is nothing to him should be understood in this way too). This is important, because otherwise one mistakenly might infer from the fact that the proponents of this Lucretian argument are concerned to show that a person's earlier death is not a harm to him (just as his later birth was not) that they are committed to the claim that the time at which a person is born, or the time at which he dies, do not matter to him. But this latter claim does not follow from this Lucretian argument. This is fortunate, for the time at which a person is born can make a difference to the degree of well-being that she possesses during her life. For example, as Glannon has noted, "people born immediately after an influenza epidemic may be at significantly higher risk for developing schizophrenia as adults than babies born in years without high 'flu rates".[70] More prosaically, if a person's parents' careers only blossom into success after his education is complete his life might have gone better than it did, given that this blossoming would have resulted in his being brought up in a better neighborhood than he was actually brought up in, and receiving a better education. And, of course, given that the degree of well-being that a person enjoys will be partly dependent upon the environment in which he lives, it is plausible to hold that being born in certain times and places would be preferable to being born in others.[71]

With these remarks in place, it should also be noted that it is plausible to hold that the time at which a person dies could make a difference to her level of well-being—but this seems to be a path to problems for the Epicurean. Were the last six months of a person's life to be spent in extreme agony, for example, one might hold that from the point of view of someone concerned with her well-being she would be better off dying earlier (i.e., just before her agony starts) rather than later. And there's the rub, for although it seems plausible to hold that some people would be better off dead, the Epicurean is precluded from doing so by her commitment to the view that persons cannot be harmed *or benefited* by their own deaths. Thus, although the Epicurean could hold that a person could be benefited from a change in the time of her birth, she cannot hold that he could be benefited from a change in the time of his death. As such, then, it seems that an Epicurean is committed to denying that it is ever prudentially rational for a person to commit suicide or request euthanasia—even if he wishes to do so to avoid excruciating and unrelenting agony. Given that it seems to be true that (at least in some cases) it is prudentially rational for a person to commit suicide or to request euthanasia, a commitment to denying this should cause one to pause, and possibly reconsider the apparent plausibility of the Epicurean position. Given this pause, then, it is time to turn to consider the import that full-blooded Epicureanism has for the bioethical discussions of suicide and euthanasia.

7 Epicureanism, Suicide, and Euthanasia

It is common to hold that a person who is subject to a great deal of suffering that cannot be alleviated would be "better off dead".[1] So entrenched is this view that it is often held to justify both suicide and active voluntary euthanasia, with the devoutly-wished consummation of these acts being considered to be "a merciful release" that ends both "The heartache, and the thousand natural shocks/That flesh is heir to".[2] Indeed, even some Epicureans believed that suicide was rational in situations when one's suffering could not be overcome by, for example, the pleasures of recollecting past philosophical conversations that one has enjoyed.[3] But, as was noted at the end of the last Chapter, it is not clear that Epicureans can consistently hold that suicide is rational under those conditions. If death really is "nothing to us," then it seems that it cannot be an object of choice—and if death cannot be an object of choice, then it cannot be prudentially rational for a person to kill herself.[4] Given that the view that suicide can be prudentially rational under some conditions is so entrenched, the apparent inability of Epicureanism to accommodate this seems to point to a serious difficulty with the position. Thus, unless Epicureans can explain how suicide can be prudentially rational despite death's being nothing to us it seems that persons who believe that suicide can be rational have reason to reject the Epicurean position. But this is not the only difficulty that the Epicurean view encounters when applied to contemporary bioethical issues. Just as the view that suicide could be rational might lead persons to reject the Epicurean view on the grounds that it appears to have counterintuitive implications, so too might the view that the issue of active voluntary euthanasia raises difficult moral questions.[5] However, given the Epicurean view that death is not a harm to the person who dies one might think that euthanasia poses no difficult moral questions for Epicureanism. But this cavalier treatment of the morality of euthanasia is likely to strike many who are concerned with this issue as too glib. Thus, if this response to this issue really is a natural consequence of the Epicurean view, then, like those who believe that suicide can be rational, persons who believe that the issue of euthanasia poses difficult moral questions will have reason to reject it.

The issues of the rationality of suicide and the morality of euthanasia thus pose problems for Epicureanism that are mirror images of each other.

The Epicurean commitment to holding that death is nothing to us appears to make it *too difficult* for its adherents to account for the common view that it can be rational for a person to commit suicide. By contrast, this same Epicurean commitment seems to make it *too easy* for them to address the question of the moral status of euthanasia. As such, then, it seems that both persons who believe that it can be prudentially rational to commit suicide and persons who believe that the moral status of euthanasia is a genuine moral problem have reason to reject both standard Epicureanism as well as the full-blooded Epicureanism of this volume. The aim of this Chapter is thus to take arms against this sea of troubles on behalf of Epicureanism, to show both that it can accommodate the view that suicide could be rational, and also to show that it need not be as blasé about the moral status of euthanasia as it might at first appear.

MCMAHAN'S RECONCILIATION STRATEGY

Recognizing that the Epicurean view that death is not a harm to the person who dies seems to threaten the commonly-held views that killing is wrong, and "that suicide can be rational or irrational," Jeff McMahan has argued that these views could be compatible with the Epicurean view of death.[6] McMahan begins his argument for his *reconciliation strategy* by holding that if a person's life would be good then it would be good for that person for him to come into existence.[7] Since this is so, he continues, it would also be good for such a person to continue to exist, *provided* that his life is still worth living for him. With these two claims in place McMahan then notes that the latter claim is compatible with the Epicurean argument that death is not a harm to the person who dies. It is compatible with the Existence Variant of this argument for the beneficiary of the goods of life is an existing person, and it is compatible with its Hedonic Variant for the person in question is benefited by his continued existence owing to the experiences that he has. As such, then, continuing life could be good for a person, even if death would not be a harm to him.[8]

With this outline of the reconciliation strategy in place McMahan then criticizes it from the point of view of an Epicurean. McMahan holds that an Epicurean could argue that the claim that continuing to live is good is incompatible with the claim that death is not a harm to the person who dies (term this claim "PE", for "Perverse Epicureanism").[9] Such an Epicurean, McMahan claims, could do this through combining the conclusion that death is not a harm to the person who dies with the Comparative View.[10] The Comparative View

> is the view that any judgment about what is good or bad for a person must be implicitly comparative . . . The judgment that an act or event is *good* for someone implies that, if there is no relevant alternative that

would be equally good or better, then the relevant alternative or alternatives to that act must be *worse* for a person. Similarly, the claim that an act or event is *bad* for someone implies that, unless there is some relevant alternative that would be as bad or worse, then any relevant alternative must be *better* for that person.[11]

When the Epicurean conclusion that death is not bad for the person who dies is combined with the Comparative View the conclusion is that, *contra* the reconciliation strategy, a person's continuing to live cannot be good for him. Who, then, is correct—an Epicurean who endorses PE, or the proponent of the reconciliation strategy?

McMahan argues that it is the position of the (Perverse) Epicurean, and not that of the reconciliation strategist, that should be rejected. In support of this McMahan offers two independent arguments. First, noting that the Perverse Epicurean rejects the view that continuing to live is good on the grounds that she believes that this is incompatible with the view that death is not a harm to the person who dies, he argues that there is good reason to believe that this Epicurean's assessment of the value of life is mistaken. McMahan argues that the view that continuing to exist is a good for a person (provided that her life is going well) is supported by the common-sense position that it would be "wrong . . . to bring a person into existence if his life could be expected to be utterly miserable".[12] This position is rendered intuitive as a result of the plausibility of the joint claims that to cause such a person to exist would be bad for him, and that it is generally wrong to do what is bad for people. From this, McMahan argues, if it could be *bad* for a person to cause him to exist, then it must also be the case that it could be *good* for a person to cause him to exist. And if it could be good for a person to cause him to exist, then it could also be good for him to continue existing. McMahan acknowledges that this is a weak case to level against the (Perverse) Epicureans, and that more could be said in its defense. However, he claims, "even a weak case will do" for he buttresses this first argument with a second. McMahan observes that in typical cases the Comparative View seems to be true "as a matter of logic," for in typical cases the person for whom the goodness or badness of an act or event is in question will exist in both possible outcomes.[13] Despite this, claims McMahan, "in the two nonstandard pairs of alternatives (coming to exist or not coming to exist and continuing to exist or ceasing to exist) in which the person exists in only one of the alternatives, there is no reason to think that the Comparative View must be true. There is no reason to generalize from the standard to the nonstandard cases". As such, concludes McMahan, the Comparative View "should be rejected as a general necessary condition for something being good or bad for a person".[14] Thus, the Perverse Epicurean position (that a person's continuing to exist is not a good for her) that is based upon the conjunction of the conclusion of the Epicurean argument and the Comparative View should be rejected, and the reconciliation strategy accepted.

Yet although McMahan's reconciliation strategy successfully shows that an Epicurean (albeit not a *Perverse* Epicurean) can hold that a person's continuing to exist could be a good for her even if her death is not a bad for her this does not mean that he has thereby shown that Epicureanism is compatible with the commonsense beliefs "that killing is wrong, that suicide can be rational or irrational, and so on".[15] Presumably the reconciliation strategy could show that, for an Epicurean, killing would be wrong on the grounds that if a person's continued life is a good for her, then she has reason to continue living, and that it is *prima facie* wrong to preclude a person from performing an action that she has reason to do and that does not wrongfully harm others.[16] Similarly, the reconciliation strategy could presumably be used to determine when it would be prudentially *irrational* for a person to kill herself (e.g., when her life is worth continuing).[17] However, given the discussion above, since the reconciliation strategy still adheres to the Epicurean view that "death is nothing to us" it is not clear how it can reconcile this view with the commonsense view that sometimes suicide is *rational*, for it seems that *this* view is based on the claim that some persons would be better off dead. Thus, even if the reconciliation strategy should be accepted more needs to be said to show how the Epicurean view of death is compatible with the full range of common views concerning the rationality of suicide.

AN EPICUREAN APPROACH TO SUICIDE AND EUTHANASIA

Suicide

McMahan's reconciliation strategy thus cannot accommodate the view that it could be prudentially rational for a person to kill herself, for it adheres to the Epicurean view that death is "nothing to us," and hence neither a harm *nor a benefit*. And, as was noted above, this apparent inability of an Epicurean to accommodate the view that suicide could be prudentially *rational* appears to be a significant bar to accepting the Epicurean view of death. Hence, unless she can either explain how she can accommodate the common view that suicide could be rational for some persons under some circumstances, or else explain why such an account is not needed, things look bleak indeed for the Epicurean.

As the problem is stated, however, it seems that the Epicurean could readily provide various accounts of how it could be rational for a person to kill herself. It was noted in Chapter 5 that an Epicurean holds that death is not a harm or a benefit *to the person who dies*, but that it could be a harm or a benefit *to others*. As such, then, an Epicurean could hold that it would be rational for a person to kill herself if she believed that by doing so she would either benefit persons that she cared about, or harm persons that she disliked, where such benefiting or harming would be valuable for her independently of considerations of her own well-being. (Perhaps she would benefit her relatives by committing suicide if they would then receive her life insurance, or perhaps she simply wishes for them to cease seeing her suffering as it upsetting to them. Conversely, a person might commit suicide to deprive another of the pleasure of killing her, or else simply to make others regret how they treated her while she was alive.) Alternatively, the proponents of the Hedonic Variant of the Epicurean argument could hold that insofar as pain is intrinsically disvaluable a world in which there is less pain rather than more would be a better world, and hence one that persons have a reason to bring about. Thus, if a person experiences pain that cannot be overcome (either by medicine, or by her recall of past philosophical conversations that she has had) and this renders her life one of suffering, she has a reason to kill herself, for in so doing she would make the world better by reducing the amount of suffering within it. This Epicurean claim is not that a world which contained less suffering as a result of the suicide of a suffering person would be one that would be better in the sense of rendering a benefit *to* anyone's well-being (for the Epicurean is committed to claiming that the end of a person's suffering through death is not a benefit to her). Rather, it should be understood as the claim that such a world would be impersonally better than an alternative world (i.e., that in which the suicide did not occur) which contained more suffering.[18]

Yet although it might be rational for a person to kill herself either out of altruism or malice, or to secure a world in which there is (impersonally) less suffering rather than more, suicides motivated by such concerns are atypical. Thus, even though the Epicurean can explain why some suicides could be rational her explanations will leave untouched the typical case of suicide. Such a suicide will be one in which a person kills herself to end her own suffering for her own sake, not for the sake of others who might be distressed by it, or to bring about a world that she considers to be impersonally preferable to that in which she is suffering, and whose value to her is independent of any effects that its existence would have on her. But things might not be as bleak for the Epicurean as they seem. It is natural to understand the question of whether it is rational for a person to pursue a certain course of action in terms of the choices that she believes she has available to her, such that she has a reason to kill herself if she believes that to do so would be better (either for her, or in some other way) than the alternatives that she believes she has available to her. But a person might have reason to perform an action even if she is not assessing it comparatively in this way.[19] A person might, for instance, have a reason to choose one way of life over another that is also attractive to her even though the values that she could instantiate in each are incommensurable with each other. For example, a person might have a strong desire to join the Catholic priesthood, and a strong desire to get married and have a family. Since the values that he could pursue in each way of life are incommensurable with each other it would not be the case that if he chose the priesthood he would do so as he believed this to be a *better* way of life for him that having a family. Rather, it is the case that, given his value set, he believes that he has sufficient reason to enter the priesthood *independently* of any other alternative ways of living that he believes are available to him. That persons could have such *noncomparative* reasons for acting enables the Epicurean to explain how even typical cases of suicide could be rational. The fact that a person is suffering combined with her desire to end such suffering could give her a noncomparative reason to take action to end her suffering; a reason that exists independently of any alternatives that she might consider. As such, then, if the only way in which a person could end her suffering is to take a dose of drugs whose ingestion is incompatible with her continuing to live, then if her suffering is acute enough she will have a *prima facie* reason to take this dose.[20] Accordingly, an Epicurean could accept that it would, under some circumstances, be rational for a person to perform an action that she believes would bring about her death, *provided* that she does so because she believes that she has a noncomparative reason to end her life. That is, it would, for an Epicurean, be rational for a person to end her life *provided* that she does not think that she would be *better off dead*, but only that she *has a reason to end her life*.[21] An Epicurean could thus accept that even typical cases of suicide could be prudentially rational.[22] And that an Epicurean can come to this conclusion without having to endorse the common claim that the suicidal persons concerned would be better off dead is a strength, not a weakness, of her position—for given the Epicurean arguments advanced in Chapter 5 this common colloquialism fails to make sense.[23]

Euthanasia

As with the concern that an Epicurean would find it too difficult to accommodate the common view that suicide can be rational owing to her commitment to the view that death cannot be a benefit to the person who dies, the concern that an Epicurean would find it too easy to address the moral status of euthanasia can also be readily addressed—indeed, this concern can be addressed even *more* readily, since it is based on a misunderstanding. As was noted at the start of Chapter 4 it is possible for a person to be wronged without being harmed. As such, then, it is possible for a person to perform an action that is wrong but harmless. An action might, for example, be prohibited in a deontological system of ethics simply because it is wrong in itself even though it is acknowledged to be harmless (injunctions against homosexuality might be of this sort). Similarly, a rule utilitarian could hold that even though a particular act A is harmless, the type of act of which it is a token is generally harmful, and so A is a wrong act. Moreover, even an act utilitarian could hold that even though an act was harmless to the person acted upon, if its performance harmed others to a degree that outweighed the benefits that accrued from it, it would be a wrong act.[24] Thus, that an Epicurean would hold that euthanizing a person (whether actively or passively, voluntarily or involuntarily) would not be a harm *to the person euthanized*, then, does not in itself tell her anything about the morality of such an act. It is thus simply *not* true that determining the moral status of euthanasia would be too easy for an Epicurean, and her answer to this question too glib, for to address it properly she will have to engage with the same moral arguments as those who proffer this charge against her.

CONCLUSION

This Chapter addressed both the concern that the Epicurean view that death cannot be a benefit to the person who dies would make it *too difficult* for Epicureans to account for the common view that it could be rational for a person to kill herself, and the concern that the Epicurean view that death cannot be a harm to the person who dies would make it *too easy* for her to assess the morality of euthanasia. Both of these concerns have now been allayed. Given this, both persons who believe that suicide can sometimes be rational and those who believe that euthanasia is a thorny moral issue can accept the Epicurean view that death is not a harm to the person who dies. With these final objections to the Epicurean position advanced in this volume laid to rest, it is time now to turn to its implications for other contemporary bioethical issues, including (in the next Chapter) the ethics of using either policies of presumed consent or conscription to procure transplantable cadaveric organs, and (in Chapter 9) the ethics of assisted posthumous reproduction, the ethics of medical research on the dead, and the ethical issues associated with posthumous patient confidentiality.

8 Epicureanism and Organ Procurement

In the previous Chapter it was noted that one might believe that the Epicurean view that death is not a harm to the person who dies should be rejected on the grounds that this view would make it both too difficult for the Epicurean to acknowledge that suicide could in some circumstances be rational, and too easy for her to endorse the moral acceptability of euthanasia. There, the plausibility of this Epicurean view was assessed in the light of these two bioethical debates. In both this Chapter and the next, however, a different tack will be taken, with the arguments of various contemporary bioethical debates being assessed through the lens of full-blooded Epicureanism.

From the arguments in the last Chapter it is clear that even though the full-blooded Epicurean (as well as her more moderate counterpart) holds that death is nothing to us she is not thereby committed to rejecting the claim that persons whose lives are going well have reason to continue living. Instead, all but the Perverse Epicurean would agree with Lucretius that "For whoever is born must wish to remain in life, so long as soothing pleasure shall keep him there. . . . "[1] Given this, it is also clear that a full-blooded Epicurean should be concerned with those debates in contemporary bioethics that address the ethical restrictions that are imposed upon policy makers and healthcare professionals in their quest to improve and further human life. That is, an Epicurean should be concerned with both the prudential and ethical issues that surround the possibility of the development of life-extending technology, such as the question of whether immortality (or near immortality) is desirable, as well as the questions of distributive justice that its possibility would raise.[2] Similarly, she should also be concerned with debates that address policy measures that could currently be implemented in an attempt to extend human life, such as whether "libertarian paternalism" should be used to "nudge" persons towards making more healthy choices,[3] and which means of increasing the supply of human organs that are available for transplantation are morally legitimate.[4]

Yet while the full-blooded Epicurean should be interested in these bioethical issues her thanatology will not be directly relevant to all of them. (An Epicurean thanatologist, for example, would not have anything to say *qua* Epicurean thanatologist about the issues of distributive justice that would be raised by the discovery of an expensive but effective elixir of life.) It will, however, be both relevant and important to some of these issues, even if (as was acknowledged in the Introduction to this volume) its truth will not itself decide those debates that it is relevant to. One debate that the Epicurean view is directly relevant to is the question of whether it is morally legitimate to use policies of presumed consent—or even organs *takings*—to secure an additional supply of cadaveric organs for transplant.[5] And it is this issue that this Chapter will focus on.

EPICUREANISM AND POLICIES OF PRESUMED CONSENT

It is widely acknowledged that there is currently a significant shortfall in the number of human organs that become available for transplantation each year.[6] One proposed solution to alleviating this shortfall is to introduce a system of presumed consent, whereby a person is presumed to have consented to have her transplantable organs removed from her postmortem body unless she has explicitly indicated otherwise.[7] Such a system stands in contrast to the system of organ procurement ("presumed refusal") that is currently used in both the United States and the United Kingdom, whereby it is presumed that a person would refuse to have her transplantable organs removed from her postmortem unless she had explicitly indicated otherwise. Unlike the debates over the ethics of other proposed means of alleviating the organ shortage (such as introducing a market for human organs)[8] the debate over the ethics of introducing a policy of presumed consent has largely focused on a single issue, and one that clearly is of interest to a full-blooded Epicurean: Whether a policy of presumed consent or a policy of presumed refusal would lead to fulfilling the wishes of a greater number of persons with respect to the treatment of their bodies after they are dead.[9] Persons who favor introducing policies of presumed consent argue that they would be more likely to respect person's wishes than the practice of presumed refusal.[10] Conversely, persons who ethically oppose policies of presumed consent do so on the grounds that such policies would be worse with respect to the violation of person's wishes than the current practice. These persons argue either that such a policy would lead to the violation of the wishes of more people, or else that the wishes that it would violate would be especially important to the persons concerned.[11] Moreover, just as the lines of the debate over the ethical status of presumed consent policies are clear, so too are the reasons that are given by both sides as to why it is morally important to respect the wishes of persons concerning the treatment of their postmortem bodies. Such respect is required, the participants in this debate agree, either out of concern for persons' autonomy, or to ensure they are not harmed by the thwarting of their wishes concerning the treatment of their bodies.[12]

Given that (as was argued in Chapters 1, 2 and 3) not only is there no reason to believe that posthumous harm is possible, but there is good reason to believe that it is impossible, those "fewer mistakes" arguments that are based on the concern with avoiding harming persons by thwarting their wishes postmortem can be immediately dismissed. One might also be tempted similarly to dismiss immediately those "fewer mistakes" arguments that are based on the moral concern with personal autonomy on the grounds that (as was argued in Chapter 4) the dead cannot be wronged, and so even if it was possible to violate their autonomy postmortem to do so would not be a wrong to them. Thus, one might think, since the dead can neither be harmed nor wronged there can be no reason to be concerned about the postmortem thwarting of their wishes. However, while this argument is certainly a tempting one for a full-blooded Epicurean to make she should resist its appeal. The ethical concern with respecting the wishes of the dead is deeply entrenched within contemporary bioethical discussions, and especially within those pertaining to the ethics of posthumous organ procurement. It thus behooves the full-blooded Epicurean to explain fully why the "fewer mistakes" arguments that are based on the value of personal autonomy are irrelevant to the debate over the ethical status of policies of presumed consent. Moreover, given the revisionary nature of this claim, it is sensible for the full-blooded Epicurean to resist the temptation to rest his case in this area on the arguments against the "Knowledge and Autonomy" view of how posthumous harm is possible that were developed in Chapter 2, and, instead, directly to argue against the relevance of the "fewer mistakes" arguments to the debate over the ethics of posthumous organ procurement. With these introductory remarks in hand it should be noted that the argument that will be offered in this Chapter against the "fewer mistakes" argument will be based on the view that the moral concern with personal autonomy can be fully satisfied through ensuring that certain procedures are followed to allow persons to express their wishes concerning the disposal of their bodies. Given that following such procedures will satisfy the moral concern for personal autonomy, the number of mistakes that are made in either removing or not removing persons' transplantable organs from their postmortem bodies is irrelevant to the question of whether one has exhibited the appropriate concern for this moral value.

Yet this Epicurean argument against the relevance of the "fewer mistakes" arguments to debates over the ethical legitimacy of policies of presumed consent can be taken further than this. The proponents of the "fewer mistakes" arguments assume that it is ethically incumbent upon persons to respect the views of others concerning the treatment of their bodies after their deaths. But (and *especially* for a full-blooded Epicurean) it is not clear that this is so. Indeed, there are good arguments to be made that given the significant costs to others (i.e., those who need the organs to survive) of respecting such wishes there is no ethical duty to be concerned with persons' consent (or otherwise) to the harvesting of their organs at all, but that, instead, *all* useable organs should be considered available for transplant regardless of the desires of those persons in whose living bodies they were contained. Rather than being concerned with policies of presumed consent, then, perhaps a full-blooded Epicurean should be more interested in moving to implement policies of organ *taking*.[13] This abandonment of the ethical concern with securing persons' consent to the postmortem use of their organs is greeted with horror by many, especially classical liberals who regard it as being tantamount to organ theft.[14] And the ethical qualms of such persons might not be unwarranted for (as will be argued in this Chapter) the standard arguments concerning organ takings rest on two assumptions that (absent further argument) are currently unjustified. However, even if it transpires that the ethical qualms of the classical liberal opponents to organ takings are *not* warranted, they might not be as dismayed by the practical implications of such a policy as they are by its theoretical justification. As will be argued at the close of this Chapter, given the falsity of the assumptions that underlie current arguments for organ taking it is likely that in practice such a policy would naturally lead to the development of markets in human organs—a consummation devoutly to be wished by the classical liberal opponents of organ taking.

The strategy of this Chapter is as follows. First, the "fewer mistakes" arguments that are the focus of the debate over the moral permissibility of policies of presumed consent will be outlined. Second, it will be argued that the autonomy-based "fewer mistakes" arguments that have been developed to show that policies of presumed consent are ethically acceptable are mistaken. Indeed, it will be shown here that these arguments are actually irrelevant to the debate concerning the ethical acceptability of policies of presumed consent. With this in hand the main arguments in favor of organ taking will be outlined, and the assumptions that they are based on exposed and criticized. Finally, it will be argued that given the rejection of these assumptions if a policy of organ taking conscription were to be implemented, it would naturally lead to the development of markets in transplantable human organs.

PRESUMED CONSENT AND THE "FEWER MISTAKES" ARGUMENTS

Under a system of presumed consent it is presumed that persons would prefer to donate their organs for transplantation after their deaths. If persons do not wish to donate, they would have the opportunity in such a system to register their objection to having some or all of their organs removed, and their objection would be respected. (Systems of presumed consent are thus often referred to "opt out" systems, as persons "opt out" of having their organs removed.) Thus, under such a system of organ procurement if a person died without registering her objection to the removal of her organs postmortem it would be presumed that she had consented to have them removed were they suitable for transplantation. The presumed consent approach to organ procurement is in contrast to the current system of organ donation in place in the United Kingdom and the United States. Currently, both of these countries have systems of "presumed refusal" (often termed "opt in" systems), in which a person's organs will not be removed from her postmortem body unless she has explicitly consented to this being done.

The debate over the moral status of policies of presumed consent focuses on "whether or not a policy of presumed consent would do a better job than the current system at respecting people's wishes about what should happen to their bodies after death."[15] The proponents of presumed consent argue that acting on the presumption that persons would wish to have their organs removed for transplantation after their deaths would be more likely to respect persons' actual wishes than the presumption that undergirds the current system (i.e., that persons do not wish to have their organs removed postmortem for transplantation). C. Cohen, for example, notes that about 70% of Americans would be willing to have their organs removed postmortem for transplantation if they were suitable for this.[16] However, he observes, under the current system of presumed refusal the wishes of only a small percentage of these people would be acted upon. This is because very few people adequately indicate that they wish to donate their organs postmortem, and so their antemortem wish to do so is not considered.[17] Under a policy of presumed consent, though, persons' wishes would be respected at least 70% of the time.[18] As such, concludes Cohen, a policy of presumed consent is more likely than the current system of presumed refusal to respect persons' wishes.

In contrast to Cohen, R. M. Veatch and J.B. Pitt have argued that presumed consent is ethically unacceptable since it is likely to violate persons' antemortem wishes concerning the postmortem disposal of their bodies.[19] Drawing on the same data as Cohen, Veatch and Pitt note that 30% of Americans wish not to donate their organs postmortem. Some percentage of this group of persons would, observe Veatch and Pitt, fail to register their objection to having their organs removed after their deaths. Under a policy of presumed consent the organs of these people would, if they were suitable for transplantation, be removed from their bodies after their deaths. These persons' desires concerning what happens to their postmortem bodies would thus be thwarted. Moreover, argue Veatch and Pitt, under the current system of presumed refusal it is very unlikely that a person's organs would be removed postmortem if they had not explicitly consented to this. As such, they conclude, adopting a system of presumed consent rather than retaining the current system of presumed refusal is more likely to thwart the wishes of those who do not want their organs removed after their deaths.

Both sides of the debate over the moral status of policies of presumed consent thus focus on establishing one claim: That the method of organ retrieval that they morally favor would lead to the fewest number of mistakes in the postmortem retrieval of organs. That is, persons on both sides of the debate argue that their preferred method of organ retrieval would violate a fewer number of person's wishes concerning whether their organs can be transplanted postmortem than would the alternative method. (Such "fewer mistakes" arguments can be called the *quantitative* "fewer mistakes" arguments.) If this were the end point of the debate then it would seem that the proponents of presumed consent policies would be in a stronger position than their opponents.[20] As Michael Gill has noted, "not only . . . [do] . . . a majority of Americans prefer to donate their organs, but . . . it is plausible to believe that a person who does not want to donate is more likely to opt out under a system of presumed consent than a person who does want to donate is to opt in under the current system."[21] A person who does not want to have her organs removed for transplantation after her death is likely to oppose their removal for moral, prudential, or religious reasons that are very important to her. She is thus very likely to register her refusal to have her organs removed after her death. For example, a person who believes that she cannot be resurrected unless her body is intact is unlikely to delay registering her objection to the removal of her organs. By contrast, Gill argues, a person who wishes to donate her organs would be less motivated to register her desire for this, for the effects of her failing to do so would be unlikely to be as significant for her.[22] Given these motivational differences between persons who wish not to have their organs transplanted postmortem, and those who do, then, it is likely that fewer mistakes will be made in following the antemortem wishes of decedents were a policy of presumed consent to be adopted.

This quantitative "fewer mistakes" argument in favor of a policy of presumed consent rests, however, on an implicit premise that the opponents of this policy do not accept: That "mistaken removals and mistaken non-removals [of organs] are morally equivalent . . . ," and so all that matters is the number of each.[23] Some who oppose presumed consent polices claim that this premise is false, holding that rather than being on a par, mistaken removals are morally worse than mistaken non-removals. Those who oppose policies of presumed consent on these grounds charge that even though a policy of presumed consent might lead to fewer mistakes, the gravity of the mistakes that it would lead to (i.e., mistaken removals) would be such that the incidence of even just a few such mistakes would be morally worse than the occurrence of a greater number of lesser mistakes (i.e., mistaken non-removals). This *qualitative* version of the "fewer mistakes" argument, then, rests on the claim that the *type* of desires that are thwarted by mistaken removals of organs are qualitatively different from those that are thwarted by mistaken non-removals.[24]

AUTONOMY-BASED "FEWER MISTAKES" ARGUMENTS

Gill's Arguments

Both those who use "fewer mistakes" arguments to support the adoption of presumed consent policies and those who draw on such arguments to oppose them agree that we should endeavor to treat persons' postmortem bodies as they would wish us to treat them. The most common reason offered for this concern is that such treatment is required by respect for the autonomy of the persons whose bodies they were.[25] (As will be noted below, this claim does not commit one to holding the bizarre view that one should respect the autonomy of the dead. Rather, it should be understood such that respecting the autonomy of persons *while they are alive* commits one to taking their expressed autonomously-formed desires concerning the treatment of their postmortem bodies into account when deciding how to treat them.) An autonomy-based version of the "fewer mistakes" argument of this sort has been developed by Michael B. Gill to support the adoption of presumed consent policies. Gill begins his argument by taking issue with the autonomy-based qualitative "fewer mistakes" argument that is marshaled to oppose the implementation of presumed consent policies. Gill illustrates the core idea of this qualitative argument by comparing "our different attitudes toward punishing the innocent and not punishing the guilty." Gill notes that we do not believe "that all legal mistakes are morally equivalent," for although "Mistaken convictions and mistaken acquittals are both bad. . . . mistaken convictions are worse. It's worse to punish an innocent person than not to punish a guilty one."[26] Similarly, observes Gill, those who oppose policies of presumed consent on the basis of qualitative "fewer mistakes" arguments believe that the mistaken removal of a person's organs is much worse, morally, than the mistaken non-removal of a person's organs.[27] These opponents of policies of presumed consent, Gill claims, believe that mistaken removals of organs are morally worse than mistaken non-removals of organs because the former "violate the right of bodily control" while the latter do not.[28] As Gill puts it, those who oppose policies of presumed consent on these grounds

> . . . seem to believe that when we remove organs from the body of someone who did not want them removed, we invade her body against her wishes, which constitutes a blatant violation of her autonomy. Mistaken non-removals, in contrast, merely fail to help bring about a state of affairs the individual desired. And while it is unfortunate if we fail to help a person achieve one of her goals, this failure pales in comparison to the violation of a person's right to decide whether an invasive procedure is performed on her body.[29]

Against this autonomy-based qualitative "fewer mistakes" argument Gill argues that the mistaken removal of a person's organs is morally equivalent to their mistaken non-removal. Gill begins his argument for this claim by distinguishing

> . . . between two models of respect for autonomy . . . The first is what we can call the non-interference model of autonomy: it tells us that it is wrong to interfere with a person's body unless the person has given us explicit permission to do so. The second is what we can call the respect-for-wishes model of autonomy: it tells us that we ought to treat a person's body in the way that he wishes it to be treated.[30]

With these two models of respect for autonomy in place, Gill argues that the respect-for-wishes model should direct our treatment of persons' postmortem bodies. Gill argues that it would not be reasonable to use the non-interference model of respect for autonomy to govern our treatment of persons' postmortem bodies because this model implies that we should do nothing to them if the persons whose bodies they were left no specific instructions concerning their treatment. But such complete non-interference is impractical. We would not, for example, simply leave such persons' bodies where they fell. Given this, infers Gill, we should use the respect-for-wishes model of respect for autonomy to govern our treatment of persons' postmortem bodies. And on this model, Gill holds, "each type of mistake is on a moral par, for each type of mistake involves treating a person's body in a way that the person did not want."[31] Thus, concludes Gill,

> If . . . our goal is to respect the autonomy of brain-dead individuals, we have no choice but to operate under the respect-for-wishes model of autonomy. And according to the respect-for-wishes model, we ought to implement the organ procurement policy that results in the fewest mistakes. If, therefore, presumed consent will result in fewer mistakes than the current system, presumed consent will be more respectful of autonomy than the current system.[32]

Why Gill's Argument against the Qualitative "Fewer Mistakes" Argument Fails

Gill attempts to establish three related conclusions with his arguments: That the autonomy-based qualitative "fewer mistakes" argument should be rejected, that the autonomy-based quantitative "fewer mistakes" argument should be accepted—and that this latter conclusion supports adopting a policy of presumed consent. However, Gill's arguments fail to establish any of these conclusions.

There are two mistakes in Gill's argument that the qualitative "fewer mistakes" argument should be rejected. The first concerns his view that the "non-interference" model of respect for autonomy should be rejected and the "respect-for-wishes" model of respect for autonomy should be accepted. Gill is correct to note that if the non-interference model of respect for autonomy should be accepted and the respect-for-wishes model rejected then the autonomy-based qualitative "fewer mistakes" argument should be accepted over his own autonomy-based quantitative "fewer mistakes" argument. This is because if respect for autonomy requires only that a person's body is not interfered with rather than requiring that "we ought to treat a person's body in the way that he wishes it to be treated," then the mistaken removal of a person's organs (an interference with her body) would be worse from the point of view of one who was concerned with respecting autonomy than would their mistaken non-removal (which would merely be a failure to treat her body as she wished). However, in framing the argument this way Gill treats these models of respect for autonomy as though they are competitors. But they are not. The non-interference model of respect for autonomy is plausible as a model of respect for autonomy *only if* it is assumed that a person would not wish others to interfere with her body. The non-interference model of respect for autonomy is therefore simply a variant of the respect-for-wishes model of respect for autonomy in which the plausible assumption that persons do not want their bodies interfered with has been made explicit. At first sight, this first mistake in Gill's argument against the qualitative "fewer mistakes" argument does not undermine it, but, rather, seems to lend support to it. (Although, as will be argued below, this appearance is misleading.) Gill intends his argument to establish that the respect-for-wishes model of respect for autonomy and not the non-interference model of respect for autonomy should be used to guide decisions concerning which organ procurement policies should be implemented. Thus, insofar as the non-interference model of respect for autonomy is simply a variant of the respect-for-wishes model of respect for autonomy Gill's conclusion here can be accepted.

However, although Gill is right that the respect-for-wishes model of respect for autonomy should be accepted as that which should be drawn upon when considering which organ procurement policies to adopt (assuming that one believes that respect for autonomy is important) this does not support his rejection of the qualitative version of the "fewer mistakes" argument. Although all parties to the debate over the ethical status of policies of presumed consent should accept that the respect-for-wishes model of autonomy is the appropriate one to use in deciding how to treat persons' postmortem bodies this does not show, as Gill claims, that "each type of mistake [concerning organ retrieval] is on a moral par, for each type of mistake involves treating a person's body in a way the person did not want."[33] Gill fails to recognize that the respect-for-wishes model of respect for autonomy is perfectly compatible with the central claim made by the proponents of the qualitative "fewer mistakes" argument. That is, it is perfectly compatible with the claim that respecting certain wishes (e.g., the wish not to have one's organs removed) is more important than respecting others (e.g., the wish for one's organs to be transplanted into another after one's death). That both mistaken removals and mistaken non-removals of organs involve treating a person's body as she did not want it to be treated thus does *not* show that such mistakes are therefore on a moral par, as Gill asserts.

Gill's mistaken distinction between the two models of respect for autonomy that he outlined is thus not as innocuous as it might have first appeared. This distinction appears to have led Gill into believing that the qualitative "fewer mistakes" argument had to be coupled with the non-interference model, and the quantitative "fewer mistakes" argument had to be coupled with the respect-for-wishes model. If this presumption about Gill's thinking is correct, then this distinction appears to have led him to believe that all he had to do to show that the latter argument should be accepted and the former rejected was to show that the non-interference model of respect for autonomy would be an inappropriate one to use to direct the treatment of persons' postmortem bodies. Gill's initial distinction between the two models of respect for autonomy and their coupling with the two different approaches to the "fewer mistakes" argument, then, served to gloss over the fact that accepting the respect-for-wishes model of autonomy is perfectly compatible with accepting the qualitative version of the autonomy-based "fewer mistakes" argument. And since this is so, Gill's argument that established that the respect-for-wishes argument should be accepted failed also to show that his quantitative version of autonomy-based "fewer mistakes" argument should be accepted in place of its qualitative rival.

Objections to Gill's Quantitative Autonomy-based "Fewer Mistakes" Argument

Having shown that Gill's argument against the autonomy-based qualitative "fewer mistakes" argument fails, his autonomy-based quantitative "fewer mistakes" argument in favor of a policy of presumed consent will now be considered.[34] This argument is based on the claim that to respect the autonomy of those persons whose cadaveric organs would be suitable for transplantation one should implement policies that respect their choices concerning the treatment of their postmortem bodies. For Gill, then, respect for autonomy requires that policies concerning the retrieval of transplantable organs from cadavers be implemented that leads to the fewer number of mistakes being made, where a mistake is made if a person's postmortem body is treated in a way that she would have not wished it to have been treated. At first sight, this argument seems reasonable. It *seems* clear that respect for the autonomy of deceased persons requires that we attempt to minimize the number of mistakes that might be made (e.g., the mistaken removal of a person's transplantable organs when she opposed this) concerning the treatment of their postmortem bodies. After all, if one did not attempt to minimize the number of such mistakes then it seems that one would be failing to take seriously persons' wishes concerning the treatment of their bodies after their deaths. And if one did this then it would appear that one was failing to respect their autonomy.

Despite first appearances, however, this argument of Gill's is mistaken. Its plausibility rests on the view that if one fails to take steps to ensure that persons' wishes concerning the treatment of their bodies are not likely to be thwarted after their deaths then one will have failed to respect their autonomy. This view requires that for one person to respect the autonomy of another she must act to ensure that his wishes are not likely to be thwarted. (This claim is not, as Gill makes clear, the stronger claim that to respect a person's autonomy one must treat her postmortem body in the way she wanted it to be treated.)[35] But this is an implausibly stringent account of what it is to respect a person's autonomy, and overlooks the fact that there are three different ways in which respect for autonomy could be instantiated: *Strong absolutism* (in which a person's consent for her involvement in a procedure is necessary for it to be morally permissible for her to be involved in it); *weak absolutism* (in which a person's involvement in a procedure is impermissible if she has refused to be involved in it), and *proceduralism* (in which even if a person objects to being involved in a procedure requiring her to be involved in it could be permissible if her interests have been given the appropriate moral consideration). Which of these ways of respecting autonomy would be the appropriate one to adopt depends upon the situation at hand. Assuming that the value of a person P's autonomy conflicts with the value of the well-being of other persons the decision concerning which of these would be the appropriate approach to take to instantiate respect for P's autonomy would turn on the answers to five questions: (i) the degree of harm or wrong that P would incur were his autonomous decision not to be adhered to; (ii) the degree to which such a failure to adhere to P's decision would advantage or disadvantage the other persons that it concerned; (iii) whether a failure to adhere to P's decision would serve to prevent harm to others, or to provide them with certain benefits; (iv) whether failing to adhere to P's decision would result in his being required actively to provide some good or service; (v) whether the goods that would be produced by the failure to adhere to P's decision could be produced in another way, and, if so, what the costs of doing so would be. Taking each of these in turn, the greater the degree of harm or wrong that P would incur were his decision not to be adhered to, the greater the justification for adopting an approach to respecting his autonomy that would lean more towards strong absolutism than towards proceduralism. Conversely, the greater the degree to which others would be disadvantaged by adhering to P's decision in comparison with the harm that would befall him the greater the justification for adopting a proceduralist approach to respecting his autonomy. Moreover, there would be more reason to lean towards a proceduralist approach to respecting P's autonomy if a failure to adhere to his decision would serve to prevent harm to others rather than to provide them with a benefit, and there would be more reason to lean towards a strong absolutist approach if a failure to adhere to P's decision would require him actively to provide some good or service. Finally, if the good or service that is at issue could be provided in some way other than that which would require failing to adhere to P's decision this should incline one towards strong absolutism with respect to respecting his autonomy, and this inclination should be greater the lower the costs of so doing are.

Naturally, this account of what could be required by respect for autonomy is merely a programmatic one—and a highly formal one at that—and the precise approach that one should take in any given situation would be a matter for debate. Yet, even though this is so, given the arguments of Chapters 1 to 4 it is clear that a proceduralist approach to respecting autonomy would be a justifiable one to adopt with respect the question of how one should respect persons' autonomous wishes concerning the treatment of their transplantable organs after their deaths. Clearly (given the arguments of those Chapters) the question of (posthumous) harm can be put to one side in addressing (i), as can the question of whether persons would be wronged by the removal of their organs postmortem were they to object to this. Second, one should also incline towards proceduralism here given that a failure to adhere to persons' decisions not to have their organs removed postmortem would greatly disadvantage the other persons concerned (i.e., the potential recipients of their organs). The answers to the third and fourth questions also support proceduralism in this case. A failure to adhere to persons' decisions concerning their postmortem bodies is likely to prevent harm to those persons who would otherwise suffer from not receiving his organs, while (in answer to the fourth question) a failure to adhere to their decisions not to have their organs removed would not result in their providing some good to others (for they would not exist at the time of removal).[36] Finally, although the organs could be procured for transplant into any particular person could be secured in more than one way (through donation, for example, or purchase, as well as through policies of presumed consent) given the limitations of altruistic donation and the current prohibition on a market in human organs it is unlikely that any significant increase in the number of organs procured will occur without a policy of either presumed consent or organ taking.[37]

As such, then, within the context of this debate over the morality of policies of presumed consent one need not take steps to minimize the likelihood that a person's wishes will be thwarted to respect her autonomy. Instead, one need only take those wishes that she is autonomous with respect to seriously, and give them due weight in one's considerations.[38] Since this is so, an organ procurement policy would fully respect the autonomy of those who were subject to it if it included procedures whereby they could express their autonomously-formed wishes concerning the treatment of their postmortem bodies, and if such wishes would be given due consideration. It is thus possible fully to satisfy the moral duty to respect autonomy by allowing persons to opt-in to a system of organ donation when a policy of presumed refusal is in place, or to opt-out of a system of organ donation when a system of presumed consent is in place. Since taking persons' wishes concerning the treatment of their postmortem bodies seriously in this way would suffice for their autonomy to be respected, the number of mistaken removals or mistaken non-removals of person's organs is of no interest to persons concerned with respect for autonomy. As such, the autonomy-based "fewer mistakes" arguments (both qualitative and quantitative) that focus on which policy of cadaveric organ procurement is required by respect for autonomy are irrelevant to the debate over the ethical status of policies of presumed consent.

The "Fewer Mistakes" Arguments and Violations of Autonomy

Yet even though the autonomy-based "fewer mistakes" arguments that focus on *respect* for autonomy are irrelevant to the debate over the ethical status of presumed consent policies one might still attempt to defend the moral relevance of other autonomy-based "fewer mistakes" arguments to this debate by distinguishing between a *failure to respect* a person's autonomy, and a *violation* of her autonomy.[39] One might argue that even if mistaken removals and mistaken non-removals of persons' transplantable organs would not themselves evince a failure to *respect* the autonomy of the persons whose bodies were thus mistreated, they would still *violate* it. With this claim in hand, one might argue that if one is concerned with the moral value of personal autonomy one should still be concerned with autonomy-based "fewer mistakes" arguments, for one should identify which system of cadaveric organ procurement would result in the least number of such autonomy violations.

This approach to defending the relevance of autonomy-based "fewer mistakes" arguments to the debate over the ethical status of presumed consent policies has a promising start. One might violate the autonomy of another without failing to respect it, and one might fail to respect a person's autonomy without thereby violating it. To illustrate the first possibility one might forcibly prevent another person from autonomously crossing a bridge that one believes to be dangerous to ensure that he was not crossing it in ignorance of his danger, and thus unwittingly putting his autonomy at risk. This would be a local violation of another's autonomy that was performed out of respect for his autonomy. To illustrate the second possibility, consider a person who is utterly indifferent to the autonomy of his colleagues, and, were he to gain some advantage from violating it, would not hesitate to do so. His circumstances, however, are such that he is never faced with the possibility of securing an advantage in this way. In being willing to violate his colleagues' autonomy, then, this person fails to respect it, even though he never actually violates it. With a failure to respect a person's autonomy being distinguished from a violation of a person's autonomy a defender of the autonomy-based "fewer mistakes" arguments now has to show that a mistaken removal or mistaken non-removal of a person's transplantable cadaveric organs would indeed violate her (antemortem) autonomy.

This task is complicated by the fact that although it is common to write that a person's autonomy has been "violated" it is not immediately clear what is meant by this. There are, for example (at least) three (non-exclusive) ways in which a person's autonomy could be violated. First, a person's autonomy could be violated if her mental capacity for autonomy was adversely affected. For example, one might violate the autonomy of another by inflicting brain damage upon her so that her ability to direct her own life in accordance with her desires and values is now impaired. Alternatively, one might violate the autonomy of another by preventing him from using his autonomy to pursue his goals, for example, by imprisoning him. Finally, one might violate the autonomy of another by usurping control over his actions, whether covertly or overtly. A person who deceives another would violate her autonomy in this third way.

Unfortunately for the defenders of the autonomy-based "fewer mistakes" arguments, once these ways in which a person's autonomy can be violated have been outlined it is apparent that neither the mistaken removal nor the mistaken non-removal of a person's cadaveric organs would violate her autonomy. It is clear that neither type of mistake would adversely affect the capacity for autonomy that she possessed prior to the mistreatment of her postmortem body. Similarly, neither type of mistake would adversely affect her ability to exercise her autonomy prior to her death. Finally, neither type of mistake would evince either an overt or a covert usurpation of control over such a person's actions. Given this, then, the number of mistaken removals and mistaken non-removals that are made would be irrelevant to the question of whether or not the autonomy of the persons whose postmortem bodies are in question would be violated. Thus, just as the autonomy-based "fewer mistakes" arguments that focus on respect for autonomy are irrelevant to the debate over the ethical status of presumed consent in which they are invoked, so too are the autonomy-based "fewer mistakes" arguments that focus on possible violations of autonomy.

Presumed Consent and Respect for Autonomy

Having argued that persons cannot suffer from violations of their autonomy after they are dead it is necessary to clarify the role that the moral concern for respecting autonomy plays in the debate over the moral permissibility (or otherwise) of using policies of presumed consent to procure transplant organs. Just as one cannot violate the autonomy of dead persons, neither can one fail to respect it. As was argued above, to respect a person's autonomy is to take her desires seriously, such that they are given due weight in one's deliberations. However, since the dead have no desires, one can only respect (and, thus, can only fail to respect) the autonomy of the living. Since this is so, one might conclude that neither a moral concern with respect for autonomy, nor a moral concern with avoiding violating autonomy, are relevant to the debate over the moral permissibility (or otherwise) of policies of presumed consent.

This conclusion is not at odds with the view argued for above—that the autonomy-based "fewer mistakes" arguments (both qualitative and quantitative) are irrelevant to the debate over the ethical status of policies of presumed consent. However, one should not infer from this that the moral concern with respecting autonomy is irrelevant to the issue of how the bodies of the dead should be treated. As noted above, one can only respect the autonomy of another if one gives those desires that she is autonomous with respect to due weight in one's deliberations.[40] Accordingly, if living persons make their (autonomously formed) desires known concerning the treatment of their postmortem bodies, then respect for their autonomy requires that one give these desires due weight when one is considering *while these persons are alive* how one will treat their bodies after their deaths. To respect a person's autonomy in this way requires that one perform certain actions while she is alive to ensure that her desires are appropriately considered. For example, if a policy of presumed consent is in place, then, to give due weight in the *current* deliberations concerning the *future* procurement of organs to the desires of persons who do not want their organs removed from their bodies after their deaths it should be ensured that these desires are recorded. (Alternatively, if a policy of presumed refusal is in place, it should be ensured that the desires of persons who wish to become organ donors upon their deaths are recorded.) To fail to do this would be to fail to respect the autonomy of persons who have expressed their desires concerning the postmortem treatment of their bodies with the intention that these desires be taken into account when decisions are being made about organ procurement. In addition to requiring that persons' desires be recorded, respect for their autonomy precludes recording their desires *without intending to give them due weight* when deliberating whether to remove their organs after their deaths. To see this, note that if Bill asks Ben to do something for him in the future, and Ben agrees to do so, Ben fails to respect Bill's autonomy if he gives his agreement with no intention of keeping it.[41] Respect for autonomy, then, requires that persons be afforded the opportunity to make their wishes known concerning the treatment of their postmortem bodies, *and that these wishes be recorded with the intent that they be followed.*[42] Thus, unless a reason to treat a person's postmortem body in a manner other than that which she desired arises, and this reason prevails once her relevant desires have been given their due weight, a person's wishes concerning the treatment of her corpse should be followed.[43] To do otherwise would indicate that the intent to give due weight to the wishes of the person in question was lacking. (Note that if the intent to respect a person's wishes was lacking while she was alive then it is *at that time* that her autonomy failed to be respected. It is *not* the case that her autonomy would fail to be respected when she was dead and her antemortem wishes were not taken into account, for, as noted above, it is impossible to fail to respect person's autonomy once they are dead.) Thus, even though one cannot fail to respect a person's autonomy once she is dead, this does not mean that a concern for respect for autonomy is irrelevant to the question of how the bodies of the dead should be treated.[44] And this is so even though, as was argued above, none of the autonomy-based "fewer mistakes" arguments are relevant to the debate over the ethical status of policies of presumed consent.

FROM PRESUMED CONSENT TO ORGAN TAKING

It was noted above that unless there is a reason to treat a postmortem person's body in a manner other than that which she desires and this reason prevails once her relevant desires have been given their due weight, a person's desires concerning the treatment of her corpse should be followed. The proponents of organ taking, however, argue that given the current shortage of organs available for transplantation there is often a prevailing reason to *fail* to treat a person's postmortem body in the way that she desires it to be treated if she desires it to be left intact: that the organs that are contained within it could be used to save the lives of others.

The Standard Pro-Taking Argument

From the above observation it is clear that the standard argument in favor of organ taking is a consequentialist one. It typically begins with the twin observations that there is a chronic shortage of organs available for transplantation, and that this shortage could be eliminated, or at least significantly alleviated, through taking transplantable organs from the recently deceased without concern for securing consent either from the antemortem person whose organs they were, or from her surviving relatives.[45] It then concludes with the claim that since we have a moral duty to minimize suffering, and since eliminating or reducing the shortage of transplant organs through posthumous organ taking would achieve this, we have a moral duty to initiate the taking of transplantatable organs from neomorts (the newly dead). The case that the coupling of these observations can be used to make for the implementation of a policy of State organ taking is often bolstered by those who favor this through comparing such taking with other State-mandated practices. Thus, for example, it is argued that if the State can legitimately conscript people into military service for the benefit of society as a whole, then it should also be legitimate for it to take persons' organs after they are dead to provide a social benefit (i.e., a bank of transplantable organs to be distributed among those citizens who need them). Indeed, proponents of organ taking often argue that since it is held to be legitimate for the State to conscript people into the military, and since this harms them by coercing them into engaging in an occupation that they did not wish to engage in absent such coercion (and also subjecting them to the risk of even more serious harm), it is even *more* legitimate for the State to take organs from the recently deceased, since such taking is harmless to those subjected to it.[46] Similarly, proponents of organ taking often argue that since it is held to be legitimate for the State to require mandatory autopsies in certain circumstances for the benefit of the public (e.g., in cases where foul play is suspected, or a death might have been caused by certain types of communicable disease), then it should also be legitimate for it similarly to work for the public benefit by taking organs from neomorts. (It is important to note that these pro-takings arguments assume the legitimacy of these State actions. Given the considerable philosophical plausibility of anarchism, however, it is not at all clear that this assumption in warranted.) With these arguments in favor of organ taking in place its proponents then move to counter the two obvious objections that this policy faces: (1) That it would evince a failure to respect the autonomy of those persons who had explicitly stated that they did not want their organs to be removed upon their deaths, and (2) that it would inflict posthumous harm upon them.

This standard argument in favor of organ taking is persuasive (or, at least, persuasive if one accepts the significant and controversial statist assumption that it is based on)—and so are its proponents' responses to the two main objections that are leveled against it. Clearly, given the arguments in Chapters 1, 2 and 3 the second objection to organ taking can readily be met. And so can the first. As was noted above, one person can respect the autonomy of another by giving her desires due weight in his deliberations. Since this is so, then a State's imposition of a policy of organ taking could be perfectly compatible with it fully respecting the autonomy of all of its citizens, even those that object to the possibility that their organs could be harvested under it. If such persons were given the opportunity to make their objections to such a policy known, and if these objections were given due weight in the deliberations that preceded its implementation (if, for example, they had the opportunity to campaign against it, and then to vote against it in a fair and democratic election) then their autonomy would have been appropriately respected. As such, then, the proponents of organ taking conclude, the implementation of such a policy would not necessarily evince a failure to respect the autonomy of those who objected to the posthumous taking of their organs.

However, this response to this objection moves too fast—although not in a way that undermines its overall legitimacy. As is acknowledged above, simply taking a person's autonomously formed desires into account and giving them due weight in one's deliberations need not be a sufficient ground for the claim that one has thus respected her autonomy. One could not, for example, plausibly provide a defense of the enslavement of a minority on the grounds that their enslavement respected their autonomy, since they were given ample opportunity to campaign and vote against it during the deliberative process that preceded it. Thus, although it will be *necessary* for one person to respect the autonomy of another by giving due weight to her autonomously-formed desires in his deliberations it will not be *sufficient* for this, for a genuine moral concern for the value of her autonomy will also recognize that (to draw on the terminology introduced above) in certain situations absolutist responses to persons' autonomy can be justified. A full account of when such absolutist restrictions would be more legitimate than their proceduralist alternatives is beyond the scope of this Chapter. However, it seems clear that the restrictions placed upon how one person can legitimately treat another while respecting his autonomy would not require that a person should always be protected from the thwarting of his autonomously-formed desires where such thwarting will not benefit him, but only others. It does not, for example, seem contrary to respecting the autonomy of a devoted Humean to prevent him from choosing the destruction of the whole world to prevent the scratching of his finger. However, as the above example of the enslaved minority shows it does seem that a genuine moral concern with respecting a person's autonomy will preclude using him in certain ways for the advantage of others. A complete and defensible account of what respect for autonomy requires will thus have to distinguish between using persons to protect the future exercise of autonomy *simpliciter* by others, and using them to enhance its instrumental value to them, with the former use of persons being more justifiable than the latter. Yet even this distinction would be insufficient on its own, for it would counterintuitively allow that the taking of (at least some of) a person's organs from him while he was alive would be compatible with respecting his autonomy, provided that they could be used to save the lives of others (and hence protect their autonomy *simpliciter*).[47]

These difficulties that will be faced by anyone wishing to develop a defensible account of what is required for one person to respect the autonomy of another in differing contexts need not, however, concern the proponents of organ taking as they defend themselves against the charge that their preferred policy would violate the autonomy of at least some of those subject to it. Part of the difficulty in providing a defensible account of what respect for autonomy requires is that it is not clear how to compare the instrumental value accorded to one person's autonomy with the value *simpliciter* of that of another. (Indeed, it is not even clear that these two ways of valuing personal autonomy are commensurable). Hence, even though on the margins it is clear that respect for autonomy is compatible with compromising the former value of autonomy to protect the latter it is equally clear that this has counterintuitive results when applied as a general principle. Yet this commensurability difficulty is not faced by the proponents of organ taking. This is because it only arises when the instrumental value of one person's autonomy is being assessed against the value *simpliciter* of another's. The removal of a person's organs after she is dead does not have any effect on either the value *simpliciter* of her autonomy or on its instrumental value to her while she is alive. It is clear that the removal of a person's organs postmortem can have no effect on the value *simpliciter* of her autonomy, since, first, corpses are not autonomous beings, and, second, acts performed after a person's death cannot retroactively affect whether her autonomy as respected or not while she was alive. It will also have no effect on the instrumental value of her autonomy to her, either. A person's autonomy has instrumental value to her insofar as its exercise will enable her to achieve some end or goal that she values. The instrumental value of a person's autonomy is thus derivative from the value to her of the goal or end that she uses it to pursue. One might argue that the implementation of a policy of organ taking would compromise the agent-relative instrumental value of the autonomy of those persons who would wish to exercise their autonomy to prevent their organs being removed from their bodies after they are dead. Such an argument would be based on the claim that the non-removal of their organs would have value for the persons who wished to avoid this. Hence, to the extent that this was so a policy of organ taking would compromise the instrumental value of such persons' autonomy to them, since they would no longer be able to exercise it to realize the value (to them) of the non-removal of their organs. But this anti-takings argument is based on the claim that persons can secure value (or be subject to disvalue) through the occurrence of events that occur after they are dead. That is, to put this in more standard terminology, it is based on the claim that persons can be subject to posthumous benefits and harms. But since (as was argued in Chapters 1, 2 and 3) persons cannot be subject to posthumous harms and benefits the instrumental value of their autonomy to them cannot be affected by events that occur after their deaths.[48] Thus, neither the instrumental nor the intrinsic value of a person's autonomy can be affected by the implementation of a policy of organ taking, and so the problems associated with weighing and balancing differing ways of evaluating the autonomy of different persons that were a bar to providing a full account of what respecting a person's autonomy requires dissipate. Since this is so, the only issue that would be germane to the matter of whether the implementation of a given policy of organ taking respected the autonomy of all of those subjected to it would be the question of whether they were able to participate fully in the deliberative measures that preceded it, with the desires that they were autonomous with respect to being given their due consideration.

TWO UNJUSTIFIED ASSUMPTIONS—MOVING TOWARDS MARKETS

Thus far, then, the arguments in favor of organ taking appear strong. Yet they are based on two important and (so far) unjustified assumptions. The first of these is that the above two objections to organ taking should be based on concern for respecting the autonomy of, and avoiding the infliction harm upon, the person whose body the organs are contained in; the second is that the most appropriate body to engage in the taking of organs should be the State.[49]

The Ownership of Organs

Both of these assumptions can be challenged. While it is natural to assume that the taking of bodily organs would be from the person in whose body they are contained (and, hence, if organs are taken from a corpse they are taken from no one, since their original possessor no longer exists) this is not the only possibility. There are no theoretical or practical bars to a person's internal organs being the property of another (either morally or legally) even while the original possessor is still alive. There is, for example, no theoretical or practical bar to one person making a gift of (for example) one of his kidneys to another, where this gift could in principle come complete with the full range of entitlements and duties that A. M. Honore has disaggregated the concept of property into, even if the kidney in question remained within the body of the giver.[50] Were X to, during his life, give his organs to Y (i.e., were he to transfer to Y the full range of duties and entitlements that make up the concept of property) they would be Y's organs even while X was alive, and even if they remained within X's body. As such, if the organs contained within X's body after X had given them to Y were taken upon X's death, then they would be *taken from* Y, and not merely from the dead body of X.[51] But, if this is the case, then both of the above objections to a policy of organ takings could be resurrected. Thus, if the organs contained within X's body were the property of Y then their taking *might* evince a failure to respect Y's autonomy. Taking them might reduce the instrumental value of her autonomy to her, for it would preclude her from exercising it with respect to their disposal in accordance with those of her desires concerning this that she was autonomous with respect to. As such, then, were the organs in question taken for transplant into (e.g.) Z the property of Y, the reduction of the instrumental value of Y's autonomy would, for a person concerned with the moral value of autonomy, have to be justified in terms of the protection of the value *simpliciter* of Z's autonomy (assuming that Z would die without the organs being provided to him). And, as was noted above, it is not clear that such a justification would always be legitimate. It is not, for example, clear that it would be legitimate to claim that the removal of Y's spare kidney against her will did not evince a failure to respect her autonomy simply because it was used to save the life of P (and hence protect P's autonomy *simpliciter*). Thus, once the pro-takings assumption that organs are not being taken from live persons is challenged those who advocate organ taking must abandon their ready response to the autonomy-based challenge to it outlined above, and justify this practice through a general justification of the moral legitimacy of redistribution.[52] Moreover, once it is recognized that even though organs would be removed from postmortem sources they could still be taken from living persons (i.e., those who owned the organs contained within the post-mortem sources) it must also be recognized that even if posthumous harm is impossible the taking of organs could still harm the persons from whom they are taken. Hence, when this recognition is combined with the fact that such taking could possibly be more harmful (as more distressing) to a person, P who owns the organs contained within another's body than could the taking of organs from a *live* source, L, whose "natural" bodily organs were taken from him while he was alive, it must be acknowledged that the taking of organs from a dead source could be *less* justifiable on consequentialist grounds than the taking of organs from living sources. And since this latter type of taking (i.e., from live sources) is generally regarded as being ethically unjustified, so too could the former be also.[53]

However, these objections to organ taking are not decisive. First, arguments might be forthcoming from its proponents that show that acting to compromise the autonomy of the live owners of cadaveric organs is compatible with the Principle of Respect for Autonomy—or if it is not, then it is ethically justifiable to override this Principle in this case.[54] Second, arguments are likely to be forthcoming from the proponents of organ taking that show that even though in certain cases the harm caused to the live owner of the taken organs would outweigh the harm caused by a failure to take them, in general the balance of harm will go the other way. Thus, such persons could conclude, consequentialist considerations would support a policy of organ taking, albeit perhaps with an addendum that allows persons successfully to object in such cases, just as persons can offer conscientious objections to being conscripted into military service.

State or Healthcare Provider Takings?

Yet even if these arguments in defense of organ taking are forthcoming and succesful they would not establish that organs should be taken *by the State*. Instead, all that they would establish is that organs should be taken for the benefit of persons who have medical needs for them. And this conclusion is perfectly compatible with the organs being taken by *non*-State persons or agencies. Moreover, there are good reasons why such takings, if justifiable, should be performed by non-State agencies. Transplantable organs are, even absent a legal market in which they could be sold by their original owners, a valuable resource. Their possession is (obviously) necessary for the performance of lucrative transplants, and this is reflected in the "handling fees" that transplant centers are willing to pay to secure them.[55] Were hospitals and hospices given a mandate to take transplantable organs from those who died within their jurisdiction, then, this would provide them with an incentive to attract persons who are likely to die to do so under their care. Since hospitals and hospices would recognize that others would have a similar incentive this would be likely to lead to a general increase in the quality of end-of-life care afforded to patients as they competed for dying patients.

One might object to such an approach to organ taking on the grounds that providing hospitals and hospices with a mandate to take organs would be to involve them in a clear conflict of interest. But this objection to a healthcare provider (rather than a State) based system of organ taking can be met, for the possible conflict of interest in question would not materialize were healthcare providers to be competing both with each other and with hospices for possible organ sources. Their recognition that this potential conflict of interest would be a concern to the very persons that they are trying to attract would lead them to ensure not only that it would not arise, but that it was clear to both current and prospective patients that it would not.

Takings, Compensation, and Buy-outs

Recognizing that the organ takers could be individual hospices or hospitals rather than the State might appear directly to support the view that allowing such takings would lead directly to hospices and hospitals competing for prospective patients whose organs they could harvest after their deaths, a situation that would appear very similar to an options market in human organs.[56] Yet to draw this conclusion would be overly hasty. Cadaveric organs that are suitable for transplantation are typically secured from persons who have died of trauma, rather than of illness or old age—and persons who die from trauma are not (typically) in a position to choose which medical institution will have jurisdiction over their transplantable organs. Only a very small proportion of transplantable organs, then, would be taken from persons who were in a position to choose which hospital or hospice they would die in. Thus, although in theory allowing hospitals or hospices to take cadaveric organs without consent would lead directly to a situation that appeared very similar to an options market for them, in practice such a market in unlikely to transpire, since these institutions would have little incentive to compete for the small percentage of transplantable organs whose possessors would be in a position to chose where they died.

Yet although the above argument for the view that allowing the taking of cadaveric organs would lead to the development of options markets in them fails, an alternate argument for the related view that such takings would lead to a greater likelihood of organ markets developing can be drawn out of the recognition that the persons whose bodies transplantable organs are located in might not be their owners. Although (as was noted above) recognizing that this could be so need not necessarily block the taking of organs (since consequentialist considerations could still justify this) it is at the very least *prima facie* plausible to hold that persons are morally owed *ex post facto* compensation for the loss of their property that was taken from them.[57] Moreover, if persons are morally owed such *ex post facto* compensation for their organs then a price would have to be placed on them. And if this is so then it would seem plausible to hold (especially within the generally utilitarian framework that this discussion is occurring within) that persons should be allowed the option to buy out of having the organs that they own being removed after the deaths of their possessors (whether this is themselves or another). Allowing persons to have this option to buy out of the removal of the organs that they own would provide some persons with the opportunity to pursue a course of action (buying out) that they believe would be more likely to enhance their well-being.[58] And if the money that they used to buy themselves out of the taking of the organs that they own was then used by the organ takers to purchase organs (in a legal market for them) to replace those that would have been taken allowing persons the option to buy out of having the organs that they own removed would not adversely affect the well-being of potential organ recipients.

There are, however, two objections to allowing such buy-outs, and hence to this move towards the commodification of human organs: (1) that it would reduce the number of organs that would be secured (and hence reduce the well-being of the would-be organ recipients, as a group), and (2) that it would be unjust, for whereas the wealthy could avoid the taking of their organs the poor could not.

The first of these objections is that under a takings system *without* the option of buy-outs all of the transplantable organs would be secured and used, and hence allowing buy-outs would necessarily reduce the number of organs that became available—and hence adversely affect the well-being of those potential organ recipients who would fail to receive organs as a result. There are, however, three responses to this objection to allowing buy-outs. The first is empirical: that it might be the case that a takings system could secure more organs than are needed, and so allowing a limited number of persons to buy out of having their organs taken would not affect the number of organs that would be used at all. Although this response raises issues of its own (how, for example, would one determine who is able to buy out of having their organs taken? Would this be determined by market means, with opt-outs being sold to the highest bidders, or by lottery, or on a first-come-first-excused basis?) the low likelihood that a takings system could secure such an excess of organs renders it moot. The second response begins by noting that the claim that allowing buy-outs from a takings system would reduce the number of organs that become available rests on the assumption that the only sources for organs would be takings or (and to a lesser extent) donations. However, were organs allowed to be purchased from live vendors then the loss of some taken organs from buy-outs could readily be offset by setting their cost at or above the market price of the un-taken organs and using the money thus secured to purchase replacement (i.e., of those lost through buy-outs) organs. Of course, one obvious retort to this second response to this objection to allowing buy-outs is to observe that while this approach might be effective for the procurement of replacement non-essential organs (e.g., kidneys or liver lobes) it would not be effective for the replacement of essential organs (e.g., hearts or whole livers) for these would not be market alienable. There are, however, two replies to this retort. The first of these is simply to note that even essential organs *could* be market alienable. While a full justification of this view is beyond the scope of this volume, it should be noted that since (as was argued in Chapter 5) death is not a harm to the one who dies concern for the well-being of the would be (e.g.) heart vendor should not militate against allowing markets in hearts. Indeed, insofar as such a vendor would benefit either from the knowledge that the *ex post facto* payment for his essential organs would be used in ways that he desired or from the *ex ante* receipt of this payment prior to his death concern for vendor well-being should support allowing such sales.[59] The second reply to this retort is to note that even if essential organs were market inalienable, and so there would be a diminution in the numbers of them procured were buy-outs to be allowed, this does not in itself show that buy-outs would lead to an overall diminution in the well-being of potential organ recipients considered as a group. Persons who wished to buy out of having the organs that they owned taken could be required to provide a sum that would secure enough non-essential organs (i.e., those that could be purchased without the death of the vendor) to save the same (or greater) number of persons who would have been saved had all of the organs that the person who is buying out owned been taken. Thus, although under this system allowing buy-outs would alter who dies among would-be organ recipients (i.e., it would increase the number of persons who die from need of an essential organ, but decrease the number who die for need of a non-essential organ) it need not adversely affect the overall well-being of this population. This leads to the third and final response to this objection. This is that if one is concerned with the well-being of the ill *simpliciter* then it does not matter if buy-outs reduce the number of organs that become available for transplantation *provided that* the money secured from such buy-outs is used to purchase medical supplies that are then used to enhance the well-being of the ill compared to the level that they would enjoy as a group were buy-outs to be disallowed.

The view that allowing buy-outs would reduce the well-being of the would-be organ recipients, as a group, is thus mistaken; what, then, of the objection that this would be unjust? This objection is based on the (correct) view that even with the provision of compensation the taking of organs is (typically) a burden on those from whom the organs are taken. Although the imposition of such a burden might be justified on consequentialist grounds, it would be morally preferable were the same ends to be achieved without it. Thus, if an alternate approach to the procurement of organs would secure as many or as more as a takings system, then, provided that this approach did not have worse moral problems of its own, it would be preferable. But such an alternative system of organ procurement *is* available: to allow markets in human organs, both from neomorts and from living vendors. Rather than merely opposing allowing persons to buy their way out of a takings system, then, this justice-based objection at base opposes such a system altogether, for it would be unjust to impose it upon persons when a morally preferable system is at hand.

Recognizing that the owner of a taken organ might be someone other than the person from whose body it was taken thus lends better support to the view that there should be markets in human organs than does the recognition that institutions other than the State could legitimately take organs. This former recognition could lend support to the view that compensation should be paid for taken organs, a view that begins their commodification.[60] Such commodification of human organs would further be bolstered once it is recognized that (as was argued above) if one is concerned with human well-being then one should both allow persons to buy out of having the organs that they own taken, and also (if one is concerned with the well-being of potential organ recipients) use the money thus secured to purchase organs from live vendors. Thus, even though the recognition that organ takers could be individual hospices or hospitals rather than the State does not directly support the view that allowing such organ takings would lead directly to an options market for cadaveric organs, the recognition that persons other than those in whose bodies transplantable organs are located could be the owners of these organs leads to the view that current markets in human organs should, morally, be allowed. And since such current markets are widely held to be more morally objectionable than their cadaveric cousins, if the former are morally legitimate then the latter are also.

CONCLUSION

Much of the debate concerning the ethical status of policies of presumed consent focuses on the "fewer mistakes" arguments. Persons who are in favor of policies of presumed consent claim they that would lead to fewer mistakes (i.e., fewer mistaken removals of transplantable organs, and fewer mistaken non-removals of such organs) being made than under the current policy of presumed refusal. By contrast, those opposed to such policies claim that fewer mistakes are made under the current policy of presumed refusal—or, if more mistakes are made under the current policy, then they are of lesser moral import than those that would be made under a policy of presumed consent. Both sides to this debate, however, agree that its focus should be on the number of mistakes that would be made under each system of organ procurement. In this Chapter it was argued that this agreed-upon assumption is mistaken.[61] A system of cadaveric organ procurement could fully respect persons' autonomy by taking their expressed wishes concerning the treatment of their bodies seriously. Moreover, neither the mistaken removal nor the mistaken non-removal of a person's transplantable organs would violate her autonomy. This being so, the number of mistaken removals or non-removals of persons' transplantable organs from their postmortem bodies is of no interest to a person concerned with ensuring that personal autonomy is respected and remains inviolate. The autonomy-based versions of the "fewer mistakes" arguments are thus irrelevant to the debate over the ethical status of presumed consent policies. Of course, showing that the autonomy-based versions of the "fewer mistakes" argument are irrelevant to the debate over the ethics of using presumed consent policies (and that the harm-based versions of this argument are unfounded) does not directly address the issue of whether such policies should be adopted. However, the arguments against the usefulness of the "fewer mistakes" arguments within this debate show that antemortem persons will neither necessarily fail to have their autonomy respected nor have it violated if their antemortem wishes are thwarted postmortem. They also show that we have no reason to believe that persons can be harmed by any postmortem mistreatment of their bodies.[62] As such, the arguments offered above against the usefulness of the "fewer mistakes" arguments can be used as *prima facie* evidence to support the introduction of a policy of presumed consent.[63] If persons can neither be harmed by the removal of their organs after their deaths, and if their autonomy will neither fail to be respected nor violated by this even if they did not wish it to occur, there seems to be little reason not to attempt to alleviate the current shortage of transplant organs through instituting a policy of presumed consent. And this line of reasoning can be taken further: that given the need for transplantable organs and the impossibility of posthumous harm, it seems morally justifiable (indeed, perhaps morally required) not just to initiate a policy of presumed consent, but a policy of posthumous organ *taking*. Yet, despite the plausibility of the arguments that have been advanced in favor of this latter position, it was argued above that the two assumptions that they are based on are unwarranted. Once it is recognized that even if organ taking *is* ethically justified this does not entail that the State should act as a taker, it can be seen that allowing organ taking to occur could lead to the commodification of human organs, and hence to the (morally preferable) procurement of organs through market means. And since this is a good thing owing to the recognition of the advantages that typically accrue to voluntary market transactions, the way is paved for the argument to be made that rather than conscripting organs to solve the shortfall, we should allow markets in them.[64]

9   Further Bioethical Applications of Full-blooded Epicureanism

In the last Chapter it was argued that the rejection of the possibility of both posthumous harms and posthumous wrongs would eliminate a set of arguments (the "fewer mistakes" arguments) that have been taken to be central to the contemporary debate over the moral legitimacy of using policies of presumed consent to procure transplant organs. Recognizing the truth of full-blooded Epicureanism is also immediately relevant to other debates in contemporary bioethics, such as the debate over the ethics of assisted posthumous reproduction, the debate over the ethics of medical research on the dead, and the question of posthumous medical confidentiality. For reasons noted in both the Introduction to this volume and the previous Chapter the aim of this Chapter is not, however, to provide a definitive answer to any of these issues. Instead, it is, first, intended to show how a full-blooded Epicurean approach to the metaphysics of death can fruitfully be used to address bioethical issues, and, second, in so doing, to show that this Epicurean approach is not as counterintuitive as it might at first appear.

ASSISTED POSTHUMOUS REPRODUCTION

Assisted posthumous reproduction occurs when the gametes from a dead being are removed and combined with those from another (either living or dead) so that both can reproduce. Such posthumous reproduction is termed *assisted* posthumous reproduction to distinguish it from posthumous reproduction that could occur when one of the procreating agents dies after conception has taken place, but before the birth of his or her offspring.[1] Focusing upon the assisted posthumous reproduction of humans, the question at hand is whether it is morally acceptable to use a person's gametes to create offspring either when she did not consent to this prior to her death, or when she explicitly stated that she did *not* want her gametes to be used in this way. The generally accepted view in both law and bioethics concerning assisted posthumous reproduction is that of presumed *refusal*: that unless a person has explicitly stated that she wishes her gametes to be used for reproductive purposes after her death they should not be so used.[2]

There are three main types of argument offered in support of this view: the arguments from harm, the argument from autonomy, and the arguments from the welfare of those living persons who would affected by the assisted posthumous reproduction in question, including the child (or children) so produced. As will be argued below, however, none of these arguments adequately support the view that policies of presumed refusal are justified.

The Arguments from Harm

The first main argument that is offered in favor of the view that assisted posthumous reproduction is immoral unless persons have explicitly consented to have their gametes used for reproductive purposes after their deaths is the argument from harm. Although the proponents of this argument all focus upon the possibility that assisted posthumous reproduction could harm the antemortem persons who would thus reproduce they differ in their accounts of when the harmful events that they are concerned with would occur. Some hold that persons who did not want to reproduce would be harmed by the state of affairs that would be brought about were they to be the subjects of *successful* assisted posthumous reproduction. Belinda Bennett, for example, holds that "it is clear that there are reproductive interests that can extend after death," and so if a person wished not to reproduce this interest would be thwarted were she to be caused to reproduce posthumously.[3] Similarly, Anne Reichman Schiff argues that "certain acts committed after a person's death can either harm or promote that individual's interest," and so subjecting a person to posthumous reproduction could harm her.[4] Alternatively, rather than basing their arguments on the possibility of posthumous harm some proponents of the argument from harm hold that the possibility that a person might be the subject of posthumous reproduction without her consent would bring about states of affairs during a person's lifetime that she could experience that could harm her. Schiff, for example, has argued that "It is both unfair and undesirable to place the onus upon individuals to state their opposition to posthumous reproduction," on the grounds that since "posthumous reproduction is not the norm in our society, there is no reason to expect people who might be opposed to the practice to make their objection known".[5] Moreover, Schiff contends that the possibility that a person could be caused to reproduce posthumously without her consent "could be a source of apprehension to the living".[6]

Clearly, the arguments from harm that are based on the possibility that persons could be subject to posthumous harm should be set aside, for not only is there no reason to believe that such harm is possible (from Chapters 1 and 2) there is reason to think (from Chapter 3) that it is impossible. What, then, of the claim that the possibility that a person could be caused to reproduce posthumously without her consent could cause harm to the living, either by imposing additional burdens upon them, or by making them apprehensive? The first point to note here is that Schiff's first objection is based on the assumption that "there is no reason to expect people who might be opposed to . . . [having their gametes used for reproductive purposes after their deaths]. . . . To make their objections [to this] known". Schiff justifies this assumption by noting that "posthumous reproduction is not the norm in our society". Yet although Schiff is correct here, whether posthumous reproduction is the norm or not is not the relevant issue. Rather, the relevant issue is whether it would pose an undue burden upon a person who did not want her gametes used for reproductive purposes after her death to require that she express her opposition to this. The answer to this question would depend upon the background assumptions that are in place. If a policy of presumed refusal has been instituted with respect to posthumous reproduction, then it would impose an unwarranted burden upon persons to express their opposition to this, for persons opposed to having their gametes used for reproductive purposes after their deaths should be able to trust that this policy would be adhered to. If, however, a policy of presumed consent is in place, then it would *not* impose an undue burden upon persons who did not want to reproduce posthumously to require them to make their wishes known. Indeed, if such a policy is in place enabling persons to voice their opposition in this way should be viewed not as a burden imposed upon them, but as an opportunity for them to exercise their autonomy to secure states of affairs that they hold to be valuable. Given this, then, Schiff's first objection begs the question, for it is implicitly based on the presupposition that a policy of presumed refusal both is in place, and should be. Schiff's second objection should also be rejected as an argument for presumed refusal. Although it is true that some persons would be apprehensive that their gametes would be used for reproductive purposes without their consent were a policy of presumed refusal not to be in place, this does not in itself support instituting such a policy, even if one is concerned about the well-being of persons who would experience such apprehension. While such apprehension would be alleviated by a policy of presumed refusal, it could *also* be alleviated by a policy of presumed consent, whereby a person's appropriately-expressed desire that her gametes not be used for reproductive purposes after her death would be honored. As such, then, the possibility that persons could be harmed through worrying that their gametes would be used for reproductive purposes that they were opposed to tells only against a policy of gamete *takings*.

The Argument from Autonomy

The second main argument that is offered in favor of instituting a policy of presumed refusal with respect to assisted posthumous reproduction is the argument from autonomy. As with the debate over whether a policy of presumed refusal would be ethically preferable to a policy of presumed consent with respect to the posthumous procurement of transplant organs, some persons who favor a policy of presumed refusal with respect to assisted posthumous reproduction argue that a failure to gain a person's explicit consent to the use of her gametes for reproductive purposes after her death would be a violation of her autonomy. Schiff, for example, argues that "respect for individual autonomy and dignity requires that the deceased's body should not be used in a way that, in all probability, was never contemplated in life".[7]

As Rebecca Collins notes, according to this argument "the main criterion of a disrespectful act is its lack of contemplation by the deceased". However, continues Collins, "it is possible to imagine various situations where such 'disrespect' would not only be appropriate but entirely consistent with the likely wishes of the deceased, had he or she been alive".[8] For example, argues Collins, it would be "unreasonable" to claim that transplanting a man's heart into his daughter who was involved in a car accident within a few hours of his death would exhibit a failure to respect his autonomy simply because he had never contemplated having his heart transplanted to save his daughter's life.[9] More directly, it is simple to imagine cases in which the posthumous removal of gametes for reproductive purposes would have been desired by the antemortem person whose gametes are in question even though he or she never contemplated this possibility while alive.[10]

While these objections to Schiff's argument are sound, let us turn directly to consider the claim that respect for autonomy requires that policies of presumed refusal be instituted. With the arguments from the previous Chapter in hand it is clear that this is not so. Given that autonomy is not the only thing that is valuable, there are various ways in which respect for it could be instantiated, depending upon the way in which it is in competition with other things of value.[11] To recapitulate the taxonomy of the previous Chapter, there are three ways in which respect for autonomy could be instantiated: *Strong absolutism*, *weak absolutism*, and *proceduralism*. As was noted there which of these ways of respecting autonomy would be the appropriate one to adopt would depend upon: (i) the degree of harm that a person P would incur were his autonomous decision not to be adhered to; (ii) the degree to which such a failure to adhere to P's decision would advantage or disadvantage the other persons that it concerned; (iii) whether a failure to adhere to P's decision would serve to prevent harm to others, or provide them with certain benefits; (iv) the issue of whether failing to adhere to P's decision would result in his being required actively to provide some good or service; (v) whether the goods that would be produced by the failure to adhere to P's decision could be produced in another way, and, if so, what the costs of doing so would be. In the previous Chapter it was argued that in the context of the posthumous procurement of human transplant organs a proceduralist approach should be adopted concerning respect for persons' wishes regarding the treatment of their bodies after their deaths. Given the similarities between the posthumous removal of a person's organs for transplant and the posthumous removal of her gametes for reproductive purposes it might seem that the arguments concerning assisted posthumous reproduction should run parallel to those concerning the morality of policies of presumed consent. And, if this is so, then given the arguments in the last Chapter it might seem that the conclusions of both arguments should be that policies of (at least) presumed consent or (possibly and plausibly) takings should be instituted over both persons' organs and gametes. But even though both the posthumous removal of a person's organs and the posthumous removal of her gametes involve the removal of her body parts for the benefit of others there are important differences between such removals that preclude an overly-hasty assimilation of the arguments concerning them.

Considering each of the five questions outlined above in turn, it is clear from the arguments outlined in Chapters 1, 2 and 3 that a person P would not be harmed by either the harvesting of his organs or the harvesting of his gametes.[12] The answer to (i) is thus the same for the harvesting of both organs and gametes. At first sight, the same might appear true of (ii). Since the answer to this question would depend upon the persons involved, it could be the same in the case of the harvesting of organs and the harvesting of gametes. A person who believes that he has little reason to live might believe that his receiving an organ transplant would be of little advantage to him, whereas a bereaved widow who desperately wanted a child with her husband might hold that bearing one would be the greatest benefit that she could ever secure. Conversely, a person who deeply desires to continue to live might consider an organ transplant to be a great benefit to him, whereas a woman who is indifferent towards children might not consider the opportunity to bear those of her deceased husband to be any great benefit at all.[13] However, to claim that the answer to (ii) *could* be the same in the context of deciding which approach to take towards respecting a person's autonomy in the context of posthumous organ procurement and in the context of assisted posthumous reproduction would be to overlook the fact that these questions are asked to decide whether a person's autonomy should be respected absolutely or procedurally within the context of deciding *which public policy concerning this issue is ethically acceptable.* Given that this is why this question is being asked the numbers of persons that are positively or adversely affected by the decision to abide by or override P's autonomy will play a role in determining whether or not to do so, for this datum will serve in this context as a proxy for the amounts of well-being that would result from deciding one way or another.[14] As such, then, it is clear that the answer to (ii) will differ for the questions of whether to harvest organs and of whether to harvest gametes, for the harvesting of organs is in general likely to benefit a greater number of persons than would the harvesting of gametes.[15]

The answer to (iii) will also differ for the harvesting of organs and the harvesting of gametes. As was noted in both Chapter 3 and in the previous Chapter it will be difficult to provide a theoretically defensible account of the appropriate baseline from which to ascertain whether a certain act or event harmed a person. Despite this, however, as noted in the previous Chapter it is intuitively plausible to hold that whereas providing someone with (for example) sperm from a particular individual so that she can reproduce with him is to benefit her, to provide someone with (for example) a functioning kidney is to save her from being harmed by the failure of her organs.[16] As such, then, the harvesting of organs and the harvesting of gametes will differ in that whereas the former saves persons from being harmed the latter confers benefits upon them. By contrast, the answer to (iv) will be the same for both issues, insofar as neither require that (the dead) P actively provide some good or service. Finally, the answers to (v) will differ. The ethical questions that are raised by the issue of assisted posthumous reproduction arise because persons wish to have children with particular individuals who have recently died. The goods that are at issue, then, simply cannot be produced except through their posthumous acquisition from the individuals in question. By contrast, it does not matter to a potential recipient of a transplant organ whose organ it was; all that matters is that it functions properly once transplanted. As such, then, any appropriately functioning organ would be welcome—and such organs could be procured through means other than posthumous procurement from cadavers.

The answers with respect to questions (ii), (iii), and (v) will thus differ with respect to the issues of the posthumous procurement of transplant organs and assisted posthumous reproduction. The question, then, is whether such differences will justify approaching the question of how to respect P's autonomy differently with respect to the issue of posthumous organ procurement and assisted posthumous reproduction. The answers to questions (ii) and (iii) indicate that one should lean more towards a strong absolutist approach to respecting autonomy with respect to assisted posthumous reproduction than with posthumous organ procurement, while the answer to question (v) indicates the opposite. However, the answers to both (ii) and (iii) in the context of the discussion of assisted posthumous reproduction acknowledge that persons could be benefitted through this, and given the arguments of full-blooded Epicureanism, the person P whose autonomy is in question in this context cannot be harmed. As such, then, absent arguments to the contrary it would seem that a proceduralist approach to respecting autonomy would be justified here, just as it would be in the context of posthumous organ procurement.

Before moving to consider the final argument from welfare three related points are worth making. First, it is not the case that any discussion of questions (i) through (v) will lead to a proceduralist approach to respecting autonomy. It is simply likely that, given the truth of full-blooded Epicureanism, such an approach would be justified when considering how to treat persons' remains after they are dead. This point leads to the second: that given this justified lean towards proceduralism with respect to questions of how to respect the desires that persons are autonomous with respect to concerning events that occur after their deaths the truth of full-blooded Epicureanism clearly has practical import for policy making. Finally, even though this discussion of the differences between the answers to the above questions that should be given in the context of posthumous organ procurement and the posthumous retrieval of gametes for assisted posthumous reproduction led to the same policy conclusion, this does *not* mean that this discussion is moot, for the reasons outlined in the Introduction to this volume.

The Argument from Welfare

The final set of arguments that have been offered in favor of the view that policies of presumed refusal should be instituted with respect to assisted posthumous reproduction focus on the effects that having a child through assisted posthumous reproduction would have on the living persons concerned, including the potential child. It is clear that it is likely that the welfare of the living parent of the child conceived through assisted posthumous reproduction could be expected to be enhanced through this, for otherwise he or she would not have requested that the procedure be performed. What, then, of the welfare of the child conceived through this procedure? Although, as Orr and Siegler note, calculating the likely welfare of a potential child is "exceedingly difficult," it is reasonable to assume that, in the absence of clear evidence to the contrary, children who are conceived through assisted posthumous reproduction would be likely to enjoy the same level of well-being as those who grow up in other single-parent families.[17] And since there is no evidence that growing up in such a family itself harms children, it is reasonable to assume that a child so conceived would be likely to enjoy an acceptable level of well-being.[18] No reason to object to assisted posthumous reproduction can thus be developed from the point of the view of the child who would be so conceived.[19]

The surviving would-be parent and the potential child are not, however, the only persons who would be affected by assisted posthumous reproduction: their relatives would be also. This fact has led some to object to assisted posthumous reproduction on the grounds that it would infringe upon the inheritance rights of persons that already exist.[20] On the face of it, this appears to be a weak argument against assisted posthumous reproduction, for, as Jamie Roswell has noted, this argument would also seem to support the view "that second children should not be born because they would detract from the firstborn child's inheritance".[21] However, given that it is possible for assisted posthumous reproduction to take place some years after a person's death one might object to it on the grounds that allowing it would undermine persons' security in his inheritance, for it would render it subject to possible redistribution to a newly-conceived heir. Yet although this would be of real concern, this does not pose an insurmountable problem, for it could be addressed simply by imposing legal restrictions upon the length of time that could elapse between a person's death and the posthumous conception of a legitimate heir.[22] Thus, just as neither the argument from autonomy nor the arguments from harm provide support for adopting a policy of presumed refusal with respect to assisted posthumous reproduction, nor do the arguments from welfare. Indeed, these latter arguments are better marshaled *against* such a policy, rather than for it.

MEDICAL RESEARCH ON THE DEAD

There are many ways in which the dead can be the subjects of research. Biographers attempt to reconstruct the lives of their subjects for public or personal consumption, while genealogists seek to determine the familial relationships of the dead. Archeologists exhume and examine both the possessions and the bodily remains of the dead, while the latter are also of interest to both anthropologists and biologists.[23] And—and more germane to the ethical focus of this volume—the dead are also subject to many different types of medical research, ranging from the relatively common procedures that are performed in autopsies to more esoteric practices, such as those performed on Einstein's brain.[24]

The Argument from the Posthumous Privacy of the Dead

It is now clear that research on the dead cannot be objected to on the grounds that it harms those subject to it.[25] It is also clear that arguments similar to those offered both above and in the previous Chapter could be used to show that persons who are concerned with respecting the autonomy of others should favor a policy of presumed consent (if not outright conscription) with respect to the body parts of the dead that would be useful for medical research. One might, however, offer a further argument in an attempt to show that research on the dead is ethically impermissible, or, at the very least, that it should be ethically restricted: that such research violates persons' interests in having their privacy respected after they are dead. Such an argument has been offered by T.M. Wilkinson, who holds that if persons' interests in privacy are "weighty enough to ground duties while the subjects are alive it is, by symmetry, weighty enough to ground duties while the subjects are dead".[26] Wilkinson rests his argument for the view that respect for the privacy of the dead requires that current research protocols should undergo "major" revision on the claim that persons can be subject to posthumous harm if their interests are violated posthumously.[27] Although this approach is untenable both owing to (as argued in Chapter 1) the failure of this particular approach to grounding the possibility of posthumous harm as well as (as argued in Chapter 3) the impossibility of posthumous harm in general an alternative version of this privacy-based argument could be developed from the distinction between something being a harm *to* a person, and something being a harm *for* her.

If a person values her privacy intrinsically its postmortem violation will be a harm for her, even if it is not a harm to her (i.e., it will not harm her in the usual understanding of what harm is). Since, *ceteris paribus*, persons should avoid bringing about states of affairs that are harms either for or to persons, given that violating a person's privacy could be a harm for her persons have a *prima facie* reason not to violate the privacy of others, whether ante- or postmortem. This *prima facie* reason to respect the privacy of others would thus not apply to the privacy of persons now dead who, while alive, only valued their privacy *instrumentally* for its use in securing or protecting some good whose deprivation would be a harm to them. The violation of such persons' privacy could only be a harm to them, where this harm would accrue from the harm to them that would be inflicted by the deprivation of the good in question. Given the truth of the full-blooded Epicurean's views concerning the impossibility of posthumous harm persons who only valued privacy in this way would be immune from being harmed by its violation after their death. This *prima facie* reason to respect the privacy of persons now dead would also not apply to the privacy of persons who only valued privacy instrumentally for its use in securing some good that they valued for its own sake (i.e., where they valued it even though their deprivation of it would not be a harm to them but only for them) where the good in question is one that could not be affected by events that occur after their death. If, for example, a person valued privacy only for its instrumental value in enabling her to exercise her autonomy as she wished because she held her autonomy to be intrinsically valuable, its posthumous violation would neither be a harm to her nor a harm for her, for this violation would have no effect on her antemortem ability to exercise her autonomy.[28] This *prima facie* reason for respecting privacy *would*, however, apply in the case of a person who valued her privacy instrumentally for the sake of securing some good that she held to be intrinsically valuable, where the existence of the good in question was one that could be affected by events that occur after their death, and whose deprivation would be a harm for her. A much-revered leader might, for example, value keeping private the fact that he had children by one of his slaves, solely because he believed that the disappointment that this revelation would cause among those who revered him would be intrinsically disvaluable.

The relevant question in this context, then, is that of whether or not a person who is a potential subject for research valued her privacy—and, if so, on what grounds she valued it. Neither of these questions will be easy to answer in practice. (Although in some cases the former will be easier to answer than the latter, for persons sometimes take great pains to make it clear that they value their posthumous privacy, by, for example, making this explicit in their wills, or through the inscriptions in their tombs.) However, that persons have a *prima facie* reason not to cause harm for others, and since the violation of a person's privacy could do this, there should be a general presumption against violating the privacy of persons, whether living or dead. Since this is so, it appears that Wilkinson is right, and that recognizing this should "make a major difference to the duties of researchers and the permissibility of research projects".[29]

But this appearance is illusory. This presumption is based upon the view that persons have a *prima facie* reason not to cause harm *for* persons. It is thus only as strong as the *prima facie* reason that it is based upon—and in this case, this reason is not very strong at all. Causing harm for a person is clearly much less bad than causing harm to her. As such, then, it would be better for one person, P, to cause harm *for* another, F, if so doing would prevent harm *to* a third, T. But, if this is the case, then provided that P's act that causes harm for F benefits T in some way, this will override the *prima facie* presumption against its performance that would be based on concern for F's privacy.[30] This argument from privacy, then, would provide a reason only to restrict research on the dead that lacks benefit—and this is a *very* weak proscription indeed. (Indeed, in practice it would proscribe no research, for no one would ever conduct research that was of no benefit to anyone!) However, that the argument from privacy provides only a very weak proscription against performing medical research on the dead, and that there is not only no reason to believe that posthumous harm is possible, but reason to believe that it is not, does not mean that researchers have *carte blanche* to pursue whatever research they wish. Even if the dead cannot be harmed by the research that might be carried out on them, the living that care about them could be (either as it would be a harm to them, or a harm for them), and so consideration of *their* interests could ground restrictions on research. For example, the extreme distress experienced by parents when they discovered that body parts of their small children had been stored and used without their consent at the Alder Hey hospital in Liverpool, in the United Kingdom, would seem sufficient to ground a prohibition against the taking of such parts without parental consent.[31] A full-blooded Epicurean might, however, object that since the dead cannot be harmed there is no basis to be concerned about what happens to a person's body postmortem—and, since this is so, such concerns should be dismissed as irrational. But, for the reasons outlined both in the Introduction to this volume and in the conclusion to Chapter 4, such an Epicurean response would be mistaken, for even a pure hedonist would have a *prima facie* derivative reason to cultivate a social practice whereby persons' preferences for future states of affairs were honored. As such, then, an acceptance of full-blooded Epicureanism, while it cannot itself determine whether or not any given proposed research on the dead would be morally permissible, would serve the useful purpose of re-orientating the debate over this issue in the only philosophically-legitimate direction it can go in. Since the dead cannot be wronged there is no reason to address arguments that focus on the rights of the dead. Similarly, since they cannot be harmed there is no reason to address arguments that focus on the posthumous harms that the proposed research is alleged to bring about. Thus, the only arguments that will be relevant in discussions of the ethics of research on the dead will be those that address the rights of the living regarding the proposed research, or consequentialist arguments that address the effects that it is expected to have on the living.

POSTHUMOUS MEDICAL CONFIDENTIALITY

If a policy of presumed consent is ethically justified for posthumous organ procurement and for assisted posthumous reproduction, and relevantly similar policies could be justified for research on the dead, could similar policies also be justified with respect to the medical records of the dead—especially given the discussion of postmortem privacy, above? That is, could the confidentiality that a person should be able to expect with respect to his medical records during his life be weakened after his death?

As with the discussion of the ethics of research on the dead, a discussion of posthumous medical confidentiality should begin both by noting that given the full-blooded Epicurean arguments of this volume arguments that favor posthumous medical confidentiality that are based on the possibility of posthumous harm should be rejected, while the arguments favoring this out of concern for the autonomy of the dead face the same challenges as those similar autonomy-based arguments that were outlined both above and in the previous Chapter. With these points in hand, it should be noted that, as with the privacy-based discussion of the ethics of research on the dead, concerns about the effects that the breaching of medical confidentiality would have on the *living* are of paramount practical ethical importance. If persons are concerned about people other than their healthcare providers knowing about certain aspects of their medical histories, and are concerned about this even if these others would gain this knowledge after their deaths, it is likely that they would be more reluctant to seek medical advice and treatment if they believed that their medical confidentiality would be likely to be breached posthumously.[32] Thus, if such concern is widespread, concern for the medical well-being of the living would justify imposing rules to restrict even the posthumous breaching of medical confidentiality.[33]

CONCLUSION

Recognizing that not only is there no reason to believe in the possibility of posthumous harm, but that there is good reason to believe that it does not exist, together with a proper understanding of what is involved in respecting autonomy, show that when discussing policies that concern the treatment of the dead there is good reason to move towards those that favor presumed consent, rather than those that favor presumed refusal—with the notable exception of policies pertaining to posthumous medical confidentiality, for the reason outlined above.

With these points in hand it is clear that, as was acknowledged in the Introduction to this volume, adopting a full-blooded Epicurean approach towards the metaphysics of death does not have (many) radical implications for contemporary bioethical debate—although, as was also noted in the Introduction, this does not mean that understanding and accepting this position is not important for contemporary bioethical debate. Even though a full-blooded Epicurean metaphysics of death cannot be used neatly to sever the Gordian knots of many contemporary bioethical issues that concern death, posthumous harm, and the dead, then, this is no reason not to recognize its importance for them, for it will assuredly enable one to become more dexterous in their unpicking.

Conclusion

In David Lodge's academic satire *Changing Places* a mediocre English academic, Philip Swallow, is assigned to teach a course in creative writing at Plotinus University in California, where he is spending a year on exchange. Utterly unfamiliar with this subject Philip writes to Morris Zapp, his high-flying American exchange partner, requesting that he forward to him a copy of a 1927 manual for aspiring novelists (*Let's Write a Novel*, by A. J. Beamish) that Philip kept in his office at his home institution of Rummidge.[1] On finding this book, Zapp opens it and begins reading:

> "Every novel must tell a story," it began. "Oh dear, yes," Morris commented sardonically.
>
> And there are three types of story, the story that ends happily, the story that ends unhappily, and the story that ends neither happily nor unhappily, or, in other words, doesn't really end at all.
>
> Aristotle lives! Morris was intrigued in spite of himself. [. . .] He read on.
>
> The best kind of story is the one with a happy ending; the next best is the one with an unhappy ending, and the worst kind is the story that has no ending at all. The novice is advised to begin with the first kind of story. Indeed, unless you have Genius, you should never attempt any other kind.
>
> "You've got something there, Beamish," Morris murmured.[2]

Judged by Beamish's criteria this volume would resemble both the best kind of story—and the worst. It would resemble the best kind of story because it has a happy ending. Given that, as Epicurus noted, when it comes to death we live in a city without walls, and so will all die, and since it is likely that at least some of our interests will be posthumously thwarted, we can take comfort in knowing that none of these states of affairs can harm us.[3] Furthermore, we can also take comfort in knowing that just as we cannot be harmed after death, so too are we invulnerable to being wronged postmortem. With respect to both their own deaths *qua* deaths, and what comes after, men can be, then, like the Homeric gods, free from care.[4] However,

this volume also resembles Beamish's worst kind of story, for while its arguments support full-blooded Epicureanism they have not done so through a
scorched-earth approach that mutes all opposition.

It was noted in the Introduction to this volume that its starting point was
the claim that an agent's death begins at the first moment of her non-existence. While this is certainly a philosophically respectable way to begin a
discussion such as this, and one that is eminently defensible, such as defense
must be forthcoming, for this account of the timing of death is vulnerable
to criticism.[5] For example, as Kai Draper notes, if one believes that time
is continuous then one "will want to know why we should believe that
there is a first point in time at which [a person] S no longer exists," on the
grounds that "if time is continuous and there is a last point in time at which
S exists, then there is no first point in time at which S no longer exists".[6]
One might also object to this Feinbergian view of death on the grounds
that "events consist in change and a change cannot be contained within
a single moment".[7] Finally, one might argue that it is as yet an open question as to whether or not a person's existence is a matter of degree, and,
if it is, then "there is no determinate first point in time at which someone
who dies no longer exists".[8] And just as one might challenge this starting
point of this volume, so too might one challenge the hedonistic account of
well-being that is developed within it to show that posthumous harm is
impossible. A complete defense of full-blooded Epicureanism, then, would
require establishing both the truth of hedonism, and demonstrating the
falsity of competing accounts of well-being.[9] Finally, just as conclusively
establishing the truth of the Hedonic Variant of the Epicurean argument
for the view that a person's death cannot be a harm to her would require
establishing the truth of hedonism, so too would conclusively establishing
the truth of the Existence Variant of this argument require establishing the
truth of presentism.

Lest one think that these acknowledgements draw the teeth of the conclusions of this volume, one should recall that although the Introduction to
this volume began by noting that its arguments would be ranged against
Aristotelian thanatology this does not imply the rejection of other aspects of
Aristotle's corpus, for his distinction between recklessness and bravery was
a sound one. In this Aristotelian spirit it should be acknowledged that this
volume has not at a stroke definitively overturned the orthodox philosophical opinions of the past two and (almost) a half thousand years on the value
of death and the possibility of posthumous harms and wrongs—although it
can claim to have gone some considerable way towards this. It should also
be reiterated that while the arguments in this volume do not in themselves
always support the drawing of many bold conclusions in those debates in
bioethics in which the thanatological issues that they address play a central
role they *do* support the bold dismissal of many of the prominent arguments that are offered in those areas. Thus, as was argued in this volume,
the truth of full-blooded Epicureanism supports the rejection of many of

the central arguments that occur in the debates over the use of policies of presumed consent for the procurement of transplantable organs, assisted posthumous reproduction, research on the dead, and posthumous patient confidentiality. This Epicurean view is also directly relevant to debates over the morality of suicide, euthanasia, and the *de facto* use of markets to procure cadaveric organs. Despite the above heeding of Aristotle's warnings against hubris, then, one should also recognize, in good Aristotelian fashion, that one should not be overly modest. Thus, one should recognize full-blooded Epicureanism for the drastically revisionary view that it is, in philosophical thanatology, contemporary bioethics—and in all other areas of applied ethics in which the three questions that it answers play a significant role.[10]

Notes

NOTES TO THE INTRODUCTION

1. Aristotle, *Nicomachean Ethics*, 1115a27. In Richard McKeon, trans. and ed., *The Basic Works of Aristotle* (New York, Random House, 1941), 975.
2. Ibid., 1100a17, 946; Aristotle held that "The good or bad fortunes of friends. . . . Seem to have some effect on the dead," although these effects will be "weak and negligible" and will not "make happy those who are not happy nor to take away their blessedness from those who are". Ibid., 1101b2–7, 949. This view is an odd one for Aristotle to endorse—indeed, he himself recognized its apparent incongruity with his account of *eudaimonia*, noting that the Solonic view might seem "quite absurd, especially for us who say that happiness is an activity." 1100a14, 946. Given this, many commentators have, as Kurt Pritzl notes, held that Aristotle does not really believe that persons can be affected by events that occur after their deaths; "Aristotle and Happiness after Death: *Nicomachean Ethics* 1. 10–11," *Classical Philology* 78, no. 2 (1983), 101–111. Pritzl's own reading of this passage treats it as an attempt by Aristotle to harmonize his account of happiness with common views of the possibility of postmortem consciousness. This approach is criticized by Paul W. Gooch, who argues that Aristotle is here showing that while his view of happiness can be harmonized with both possible interpretations of Solon's dictum "look to the end" (i.e., that the virtuous can be called happy in spite of most fortunes, even postmortem ones, and that after a man has died we can assess his life from a third-person viewpoint in light of what follows) he does not endorse either. See "Aristotle and the Happy Dead," *Classical Philology* 78, no. 2 (1983), 112–116. For an alternative reading of this passage in which it is argued that Aristotle is concerned with the possibility that a self might exist postmortem (albeit a self that could not engage in praxis), see Dominic Scott, "Aristotle on Posthumous Fortune," *Oxford Studies in Ancient Philosophy*, XVIII (2000), 211–229.
3. Epicurus, "Letter to Menoeceus," in R.D. Hicks, *Stoic and Epicurean* (New York, Russell & Russell, 1962), 169. Note that although Epicurus' reasoning as to why death is "nothing to us" implies that posthumous harm is impossible, the converse is not true; the view that posthumous harm is impossible does not commit one to holding that death is not a harm to the person who died. For discussions of this point see Christopher Belshaw, *Annihilation: The Sense and Significance of Death* (Stocksfield, England: Acumen, 2009), 78–79, and Ben Bradley, *Well-Being & Death* (Oxford: Oxford University Press, 2009), 43–44. (Of course, one could hold both of these positions, or even view them as being linked, attempting to account for the alleged evil of

death in terms of posthumous harm. See Geoffrey Scarre, "Should we fear Death?" *European Journal of Philosophy* 5, no. 3 (1997), 269–282.) For an account of the role that Epicurean thanatology played in the Epicurean philosophical system see Martha Nussbaum, *The Therapy of Desire: Theory and Practice in Hellenistic Ethics* (Princeton: Princeton University Press, 1994), 195 ff, and Voula Tsouna, *The Ethics of Philodemus* (Oxford: Oxford University Press, 2007), 243 ff.

4. See, for example, Steven Luper, who argues both that death can be a harm to the one who dies, and that posthumous harm is possible, in *The Philosophy of Death* (Cambridge: Cambridge University Press, 2009); these views are also endorsed by Joel Feinberg, in *Harm to Others* (Oxford: Oxford University Press, 1984), 79–95.

5. Steven Luper held that it was "inane" and "absurd" in "Annihilation," in John Martin Fischer, ed., *The Metaphysics of Death* (Stanford: Stanford University Press, 1994), 270; Jack Li held that it was "very odd" in *Can Death be A Harm to The Person Who Dies?* (Dordrecht: Kluwer Academic Publishers, 2002), 19, while Christopher Belshaw notes (fairly) that it would be easier to think of the Epicureans as "freakish" than to prove them wrong. *10 good questions about life and death* (Oxford: Blackwell, 2005), 43.

6. Soren Kierkegaard, "At a Graveside," in Soren Kierkegaard, ed. and trans. Howard V. Hong and Edna H. Hong, *Three Discourses on Imagined Occasions* (Princeton: Princeton University Press, 1993), 73.

7. Mary Mothersill, "Death," in Oswald Hanfling, ed. *Life and Meaning: A Reader* (Oxford: Blackwell, 1987), 88. Richard W. Momeyer held that there is "oddness" in even asking whether death was an evil; see his *Confronting Death* (Bloomington: Indiana University Press, 1988), 15.

8. The Epicurean Philodemus tangentially touched upon the question of whether posthumous harm was possible in his discussion of why one should not be concerned about one's posthumous reputation; see *On Death*, trans. W. Benjamin Henry (Atlanta: Society of Biblical Literature, 2009), XXVIII 32–36, 64. For a brief discussion of this point, see David Armstrong, "All Things To All Men: Philodemus' Model of Therapy and the Audience of *De Morte*," in John Fitzgerald, Dirk Obbink, and Glenn S. Holland, eds., *Philodemus and the New Testament World* (Leiden: Brill, 2004), 43–44.

9. It is thus an "Epicurean" work in Furley's second sense of this term; see David J. Furley, "Lucretius the Epicurean: On the History of Man," in Monica R. Gale, ed., *Lucretius: Oxford Readings in Classical Studies* (Oxford: Oxford University Press, 2007), 158.

10. Joel Feinberg, "Harm to Others," in Fischer, ed., *The Metaphysics of Death*, 172. See also Jeff McMahan, "Death and the Value of Life," in Fischer, ed., *The Metaphysics of Death*, 234. If this view appears to accept too readily presentism (the view that only present objects exist) then one can simply refine it to read that an agent's death begins at the first moment when she does not exist now. However, this possible commitment to presentism is not the only possible problem (if one believes that this is a problem) that the view that a person's death begins at the first moment of her non-existence faces; other (and more serious) difficulties are outlined in the Conclusion to this volume. Naturally, the related questions of what death is and when it occurs are of great importance within bioethics. See, for example, Stephen Holland, "On the Ordinary Concept of Death," *Journal of Applied Philosophy* 27, no. 2 (2010), 109–122.

11. Note that this way of putting things by-passes the question of whether beings can exist *simpliciter* after their deaths. For similar caution see McMahan, "Death and the Value of Life," 384, note 2. For a discussion of this issue

see David Hershenov, "Do Dead Bodies Pose a Problem for Biological Approaches to Personal Identity?" *Mind* 114, no. 453 (2005), 31–59. For an excellent account of how persons could survive their death that lies within the tradition of religious naturalism, see Mark Johnston, *Surviving Death* (Princeton: Princeton University Press, 2010).

12. Although almost all parties to the thanatological debates that are the focus of this volume make this assumption it is by no means a trivial one. (And those persons who do not accept it can still find interest in this volume, taking it as an exercise in how matters would stand in another possible world.) Since there is a non-zero possibility that persons might enter some afterlife after the deaths of their bodies in which they have conscious experiences and retain some or all of what John Davis terms their "investment interests" the assumption that this is not the case is significant—and hence one not to be taken as lightly as it is by A in Cicero's first *Tusculan Disputation*. See John K. Davis, "Surviving Interests and Living Wills," *Public Affairs Quarterly* 20, no. 1 (2006), 18, and the translation of the first *Tusculan Disputation* in James Warren, "The Harm of Death in Cicero's First *Tusculan Disputation*," in James Stacey Taylor, ed., *The Metaphysics and Ethics of Death* (New York: Oxford University Press, forthcoming). See, too, the discussion of the evidence for the existence of an afterlife offered by Russell DiSilvestro, "The Ghost in the Machine is the Elephant in the Room," *Journal of Medicine and Philosophy* (forthcoming). Furthermore, as Belshaw notes, even if one is unpersuaded by the possibility of an afterlife or of the existence of a soul one should not dismiss these views lightly, for there is a "not unrelated position seems often to be thought more philosophically respectable," in which a distinction is drawn between (for example) a person's biological and her biographical life. C. D. Belshaw, "Harm, Change, and Time," *Journal of Medicine and Philosophy*, forthcoming.

13. Even if persons do not immediately exist in some form of afterlife immediately after their deaths there is a non-zero possibility that they might be psychologically reconstructed (e.g., by God) at a later point. If this possibility is combined with the truth of the Wide version of Parfit's Psychological Criterion for personal identity, such reconstructed persons would possibly be the same persons as they were in life. (See Derek Parfit, *Reasons and Persons* [Oxford: Oxford University Press, 1984], 204–209.) If so, then, given that a person's interests will, as Davis has persuasively argued in the context of the debate over the moral authority of living wills, survive from t1 to tn provided that it is nomologically possible that she regain the capacity to care at tn, the possibility of such psychological reconstruction would entail that it is possible that a person's interests could survive her death. (Davis,"Surviving Interests and Living Wills," 23–25.) The question of whether and in what form persons could survive between their physical deaths and Resurrection is a live issue for Christian philosophers. See, for example, Jason T. Eberl, "Do Human Persons Exist between Death and Resurrection?" in Kevin Tempe, ed. *Metaphysics and God: Essays in Honor of Eleonore Stump* (New York: Routledge, 2009), 188–205. See too the essays in Georg Gasser, ed., *Personal Identity and Resurrection: How Do We Survive Our Death?* (Aldershot, England; Ashgate, 2010). Note that these (atheist and theist) claims concerning posthumous existence are much stronger and more controversial than the claim that a human could continue to exist as a corpse after she dies; for an account of the latter, weaker view, see Fred Feldman, *Confrontations with the Reaper* (New York: Oxford University Press, 1992), 105. For a brief account of how Lucretius would object to Davis' reasoning here see Walter Glannon, "Epicureanism and Death," *Monist* 76 (1993), 228.

14. These issues are discussed in (for example) Stuart J. Younger, Robert M. Arnold, and Renie Schapiro, eds., *The Definition of Death: Contemporary Controversies* (Baltimore: The Johns Hopkins University Press, 1999), and in Ana S. Iltis and Mark J. Cherry, eds., *Revisiting Death: Organ Donation and the Dead Donor Rule; The Journal of Medicine and Philosophy* 35, 3 (2010), 223–380. See also R. E. Ewin, *Reasons and the Fear of Death* (Boulder, Co.: Rowman and Littlefield, Inc., 2002), Chapter 6.

15. Note that the arguments above could be put in more positive terms: that it is impossible to confer any posthumous benefits upon agents, and that there is no reason to believe that one can "do right by" the dead through discharging any duties that one believes one owes to them.

16. The relevance of these thanatological issues to suicide and euthanasia will be discussed in Chapter 7; their relevance to the moral status of abortion will be noted in Chapter 2.

17. If death is not a harm to the person who dies, and if one believes that medical resources should be directed at the prevention or alleviation of harm, it would seem that rather than directing resources towards combating mortality one should instead direct them towards the relief of suffering.

18. See, for example, Margaret P. Battin, "Age Rationing and the Just Distribution of Healthcare: Is There a Duty to Die?" *Ethics* 97, no. 2 (1987), 317–340.

19. See James Lenman, "On Becoming Extinct," *Pacific Philosophical Quarterly* 83 (2002), 253–269, John Leslie, "Why Not Let Life Become Extinct?" *Philosophy* 58 (1983), 329–338, and David Benatar, *Better Never to Have Been: The Harm of Coming Into Existence* (Oxford: Clarendon Press, 2006), 194–200.

20. This will be discussed in Chapter 8.

21. See, for example, Hazel Biggs, "Speaking for the Dead—Life in Perpetuity," *Res Publica* 8 (2002), 93–104, Dorothy Nelkin and Lori Andrews, "Do the Dead have Interests? Policy Issues for Research After Life," *American Journal of Law and Medicine* XXIV, nos. 2&3 (1998), 261–291, and Mark R. Wicclair and Michael deVita, "Oversight of Research Involving the Dead," *Kennedy Institute of Ethics Journal* 14, no. 2 (2004), 143–164. For a discussion of this issue in the light of the Alder Hey scandal in Britain—in which parts of childrens' bodies were taken postmortem and used for research without parental consent—see T. M. Wilkinson, "Parental Consent and the Use of Dead Children's Bodies," *Kennedy Institute for Ethics Journal* 11, no. 4 (2001), 337–358.

22. See, for example, M. Masterton, M. G. Hansson, A. T. Hoglund, G. Helgesson, "Can the Dead be Brought into Disrepute?" *Theoretical Medicine and Bioethics* 28, no. 2 (2007), 137–149, and "Queen Christina's moral claim on the living: justification of a tenacious moral intuition," *Medicine, Health Care, and Philosophy* 10, no. 3 (2007), 321–327.

23. See, for example, Jessica Berg, "Grave Secrets: Legal and Ethical Analysis of Postmortem Confidentiality," *Connecticut Law Review* 34, no. 1 (2001), pp. 81–122. This issue will be discussed in Chapter 9.

24. This will be discussed in Chapter 9.

25. See, for example, Daniel Sperling, *Management of Post-Mortem Pregnancy: Legal and Philosophical Aspects* (Aldershot: Ashgate, 2006), 78–82.

26. See, for example, Davis, "Surviving Interests and Living Wills".

27. See Porphyry's account of the Epicurean view of philosophy: "Every disturbance and unprofitable desire is removed by the love of true philosophy. Vain is the word of that philosopher who can ease no mortal trouble. As there is no profit in the physician's art unless it cure the diseases of the body, so there

is none in philosophy, unless it expel the troubles of the soul." *Porphyry the Philosopher to Marcella*, 31. Available at http://www.tertullian.org/fathers/porphyry_marcella_03_revised_text.htm (Accessed June 16th, 2010.) That this is an Epicurean view was noted by Nussbaum, in "Therapeutic arguments: Epicurus and Aristotle," in Malcolm Schofield and Gisela Striker, eds., *The Norms of Natures: Studies in Hellenistic Ethics* (Cambridge: Cambridge University Press, 1986), 31. For discussions of the therapeutic use of Epicurean thanatology see Margaret Graver, "Managing Mental Pain: Epicurus vs. Aristippus on the Pre-Rehearsal of Future Ills," *Proceedings of the Boston Area Colloquium in Ancient Philosophy*, 17 (2002), 155–177, Mikel Burley, "Anticipating Annihilation," *Inquiry* 49, no. 2 (2006), 172 ff, and William James Earle, "Epicurus: 'Live Hidden!'," *Philosophy* 63, no. 243 (1988), 97–100.

28. See, for example, David D. Friedman, *Law's Order: What economics has to do with law and why it matters* (Princeton: Princeton University Press, 2000), 96.

29. See, for example, Stephen E. Rosenbaum, "Death as a Punishment: A Consequence of Epicurean Thanatology," in Dane R. Gordon, David B. Suits, eds., *Epicurus: His continuing influence and contemporary relevance* (Rochester, NY.: RIT Cary Graphic Arts Press, 2003), 195–207.

30. See, for example, Stephen E. Rosenbaum, "The Harm of Killing: An Epicurean Perspective," in Robert M. Baird, William F. Cooper, Elmer H. Duncan, Stuart E. Rosenbaum, eds., *Contemporary Essays on Greek Ideas: The Kilgore Festschrift* (Waco, TX: Baylor University Press, 1987), 207–226, Peter Carruthers, *The Animals Issue: Moral theory in practice* (Cambridge: Cambridge University Press, 1992), Chapter 4, and Samantha Brennan, "The Badness of Death, the Wrongness of Killing, and the Moral Importance of Autonomy," *Dialogue* XL (2001), 723–737.

31. See Craig Howes, "Afterword," in John Paul Eakin, ed., *The Ethics of Life Writing* (Ithaca, NY: Cornell University Press, 2004), 245.

32. See Peter Kivy, *The Fine Art of Repetition: Essays in the Philosophy of Music* (Cambridge: Cambridge University Press, 1993), Chapter 5.

33. See, for example, Geoffrey Scarre, "Can archaeology harm the dead?", and Sarah Tarlow, "Archeological ethics and the people of the past," both in Chris Scarre and Geoffrey Scarre, eds., *The Ethics of Archeology: Philosophical perspectives on archaeological practice* (Cambridge: Cambridge University Press, 2006), 181–198; 199–216. See, too, Geoffrey Scarre "Archeology and Respect for the Dead," *Journal of Applied Philosophy* 20, no. 3 (2003), 237–249, Robert Pogue Harrison, *The Dominion of the Dead* (Chicago: The University of Chicago Press, 2003), 24, Joe Watkins, "Archaeological Ethics and American Indians," in Larry J. Zimmerman, Karen D. Vitelli, and Julie Hollowell-Zimmer, eds., *Ethical Issues in Archeology* (Lanham, Md.: AltaMira Press, 2003), 131, and Paul Bahn, "Do Not Disturb? Archaeology and the Rights of the Dead," *Journal of Applied Philosophy* 1, no. 2 (1984), 213–225. Bahn's views concerning the putative rights of the dead fall prey to the criticisms of the rationality of ascribing rights to dead persons that are developed in Chapter 4.

34. On the first of these issues see D. W. Haslett, "Is Inheritance Justified?" *Philosophy and Public Affairs* 15, no. 2 (1986), 122–155, and S. Stewart Braun, "Historical Entitlement and the Practice of Bequest: Is there a moral right of bequest?" *Law and Philosophy* 29, no. 6 (2010), 695–715; on the second see James Warren, *Facing Death: Epicurus and his Critics* (Oxford: Clarendon Press, 2004), 162–199. For an account of the ways in which American law recognizes persons' (legal) rights to exert control of property beyond

the scope of their own lives (in a manner that Thomas Paine would consider tyrannical!) see Ray D. Madoff, *Immortality and the Law: The rising power of the American dead* (New Haven: Yale University Press, 2010). For Paine's views, see his *Rights of Man* (Harmondsworth, UK: Penguin, 1969), 63–64.

35. See, for example, Axel Gosseries, "Intergenerational Justice," in Hugh LaFollette, ed., *The Oxford Handbook of Practical Ethics* (New York: Oxford University Press, 2003), 459–484, Bob Brecher, "Our Obligation to the Dead," *Journal of Applied Philosophy* 19, no. 2 (2002), 109–119, Janna Thompson, "Intergenerational Responsibilities and the Interests of the Dead," in H. Dyke, ed., *Time and Ethics: Essays at the Intersection* (Dordrecht: Kluwer Academic Publishers, 2003), 71–83, and Edward A. Page, *Climate Change, Justice and Future Generations* (Cheltenham, UK: Edward Elgar, 2006), 124–129.

36. See Lukas H. Meyer, "Reparations and Symbolic Restitution," *Journal of Social Philosophy* 37, no. 3 (2006), 406–422, and Michael Ridge, "Giving the Dead Their Due," *Ethics* 114 (2003), 38–59.

37. For accounts of attempted posthumous punishments, see Chapter 1, n. 1. For an example of an attempted posthumous reward, see Linda R. Rabieh, *Plato and the Virtue of Courage* (Baltimore, Md.: The Johns Hopkins University Press, 2006), 2.

38. See, for example, John Harris, "Doing Posthumous Harm," in James Stacey Taylor, ed., *The Metaphysics and Ethics of Death* (New York: Oxford University Press, forthcoming.)

39. See, for example, Tim Mulgan, "The Place of the Dead in Liberal Political Philosophy," *The Journal of Political Philosophy* 7, no. 1 (1999), 52–70.

40. Note that the claim here is just that such a general antipathy *could* justify the retention of P, not that it *would*. This leaves open the possibility that, as Jeremy Bentham held (surprisingly, given his hedonistic and utilitarian commitments), desires that persons have for a practice P that imposes significant costs upon others and which are acknowledged even by those who possess them to have no rational basis should not be used to justify P. (Bentham was here writing in the context of laws against homosexuality; see his *Offences Against One's Self*, available at: http://www.columbia.edu/cu/lweb/eresources/exhibitions/sw25/bentham/index.html. Accessed January 7th, 2010.)

41. In particular, it might have practical import for persons who were previously afraid of their own future non-existence. For a persuasive set of examples that show that such a fear exists, see Kathy Behrendt, "A Special Way of Being Afraid," *Philosophical Psychology* 23, no. 5 (2010), 669–682.

42. It might be tempting here also to refer to Mill's claim that one is better off being Socrates dissatisfied than a pig satisfied. (J. S. Mill, *Utilitarianism* [Indianapolis, Ind.: Hackett Publishing Company, 1979], 10.) However, recognizing the truth of full-blooded Epicureanism would make one better off than Mill's dissatisfied Socrates, for once one grasps that one cannot be harmed by one's own death a possible source of fear will be removed from one's life!

43. See, for example, R. Cummins, "Reflection on Reflective Equilibrium," in M. DePaul and W. Ramsey, eds., *Rethinking Intuition: The Psychology of Intuition and Its Role in Philosophical Inquiry* (Lanham, MD: Rowman & Littlefield, 1998), 113–128; Michael Devitt, "The Methodology of Naturalistic Semantics," *Journal of Philosophy* 91 (1994), 545–572, and J. Weinberg, S. Nichols, and S. Stich, "Normativity and Epistemic Intuitions," *Philosophical Topics* 29, nos. 1–2 (2001), 429–460.

44. I thank Griffin Trotter for a very helpful discussion of this issue.

45. These different ways of understanding the subject of philosophical analysis are outlined in Alvin Goldman, "Philosophical Intuitions: Their Target, Their Source, and Their Epistemic Status," *Grazer Philosophische Studien* 74 (2007), 1–26. This identification of harm as the primary subject of the philosophical analysis of this volume endorses Stephen Rosenbaum's perspicacious claim that much of the debates in the metaphysics of death are really debates over standard philosophical concepts—for Rosenbaum, that of value—and so their import is not philosophically provincial. See Rosenbaum's "Concepts of Value and Our Thinking about Death," in Taylor, ed., *The Metaphysics and Ethics of Death*, forthcoming.

46. Goldman, "Philosophical Intuitions," 13.

47. Note that this could be true even if one adopts a constitutive approach to the relationship between concepts (as this term is understood above) and evidencehood (such that "possessing a concept tends to give rise to beliefs and intuitions that accord with the contents of the concept" [ibid., 15]), for one engaged in philosophical analysis could have external reasons for re-evaluating her own intuitions (for example, were she to jettison some after re-evaluation she would need to bite fewer bullets, and this is a value for her).

48. To describe a policy whereby a person's organs are available for harvest independently of whether she consented to this or not as a policy of organ conscription is mistaken, because the term "conscription" implies that the goods being conscribed could be taken from the person from whom they are conscribed without her consent. At the time at which a person's organs would be conscribed from her under those "conscription" policies that are the cousins of policies of presumed consent (i.e., after her death), however, the issue of consent is moot, since the person is now a corpse. Rather than being policies of conscription, then, which carries with it connotations of involuntariness, such policies are more accurately termed policies of organ taking. I thank Larry White and Lloyd Cohen for pressing me on this point.

NOTES TO CHAPTER 1

1. Christian D. von Dehsen, *Philosophers and Religious Leaders: An Encyclopedia of People Who Changed the World* (Phoenix, AZ: Oryx Press, 1999), 199. Imposing posthumous punishments on persons used to be a not uncommon practice. It is, for example, in this context common to observe that certain (non-State-sanctioned) suicides in Athens would be punished by having the hand that killed them cut off postmortem; see, for example, Alan Warren Friedman, *Fictional Death and the Modernist Enterprise* (Cambridge: Cambridge University Press, 1995), 52. Although Friedman gives no source for this claim it is from Aeschines, trans. C.D. Adams, *Against Ctesiphon* (London: William Heinemann, 1919), 244. However, as Elise P. Garrison argues, not only is this the only Greek reference to such a treatment of a suicide, it also occurs in the context of an attempt to discredit Demosthenes for his role in instigating the battle of Chaeronea. It is thus not unreasonable to read this reference to the treatment of suicides as being a normative rather than a descriptive one, with Demosthenes, the slayer of his own soldiers, being implicitly compared to the hand that kills its own supporting body. (See Elise P. Garrison, *Groaning Tears: Ethical & Dramatic Aspects of Suicide in Greek Tragedy* [Leiden: Brill Academic Publishers, 1995], 19). However, even though claims concerning this allegedly ancient form of punishing suicides might have suspect legitimacy, it is clear that attempts were

made to punish suicides in ancient Greek society by "certain marks of dishonor," as Aristotle notes in the *Nicomachean Ethics*, trans. H. Rackham (Cambridge, Mass.: The Harvard University Press, 1934), V, xi, 3–4, 360–365. Rome, too, attempted to inflict posthumous punishment on persons; see Katariina Mustakallio, *Death and Disgrace: Capital Penalties with Post Mortem Sanctions in Early Roman Historiography* (Helsinki: Suomalainen Tiedeakatemia, 1994), and Eric R. Varner, "Punishment after death: mutilation of images and corpse abuse in ancient Rome," *Mortality* 6, no. 1 (2010), 46–64. For an account of attempts made to punish suicides in late medieval France, see Esther Cohen, *The Crossroads of Justice: Law and Culture in Late Medieval France* (Leiden: E. J. Brill, 1993), 141–143. In England John Bradshaw, Henry Ireton, and Oliver Cromwell were all posthumously hung, drawn, and quartered at Tyburn for their roles in the regicide of Charles I. See *Journal of the House of Commons, Vol. 8, 1660–1667* (London: House of Commons, 1802), 26–27. Similarly, the English Murder Act of 1752 provided for the possibility of dissecting the bodies of persons executed for murder as an alternative to gibbeting; see Alastair V. Campbell, *The Body in Bioethics* (London: Routledge, 2009), 108.

2. Lest this be construed as a smug sideswipe against the Catholic Church it should be noted that belief in posthumous harms is perfectly rational against the background of a religious belief in an afterlife; as will be argued in this volume it does not make sense *absent* such a belief. And yet the contemporary proponents of the view that posthumous harm is possible attempt to support it without these religious underpinnings—an approach that no doubt would have been considered odd indeed by the historical Epicurus. The contemporary proponents of the view that the dead can be harmed include Robert C. Solomon "Is There Happiness After Death?" *Philosophy* 51 (1976), 189–193, Barbara Baum Levenbook, "Harming Someone after His Death," *Ethics*, 94 (1984), 407–419, Dorothy Grover, "Posthumous Harm," *The Philosophical Quarterly*, 39 (1989), 334–353, Steven Luper, "Posthumous Harm," *American Philosophical Quarterly*, 41 (2004), 70–71, "Past Desires and the Dead," *Philosophical Studies* 126 (2005), 331–345, "Mortal Harm," *The Philosophical Quarterly* 57, no. 227 (2007), 239–251, Anthony Serafini, "Callahan on Harming the Dead," *Journal of Philosophical Research* XV (1989–1990), 329–339, F. M. Kamm, *Morality, Mortality Volume I: Death and Whom to Save from It* (New York: Oxford University Press, 1993), 63, and H. E. Barber, "Ex Ante Desire and Post Hoc Satisfaction," in Keim Campbell, J., M. O'Rourke, and H. Silverstein, eds. *Time and Identity: Topics in Contemporary Philosophy* (Cambridge, Mass.: The MIT Press, 2010), 249–267. That the view that posthumous harm is possible is (pretheoretically) held by some persons was noted by Robert M. Gordon, *The Structure of Emotions: Investigations in cognitive philosophy* (Cambridge: Cambridge University Press, 1987), 7. But (obviously) not everyone has endorsed the possibility of posthumous harm: Shakespeare's Macbeth, for example, held that "Duncan is in his grave;/After life's fitful fever he sleepes well;/Not steel, nor posion,/Malice domestic, foreign levy, nothing/Can touch him further". William Shakespeare, *Macbeth* (New York: Longman's, Green, & Co., 1896), Act III, Scene II.; see too Psalms 49: 10–12, 17. Similarly, Stephen Darwall notes (albeit, like Macbeth, without argument) that "it is hard to see how things entirely beyond the boundaries of a person's life *can* benefit or harm that person intrinsically, how they can make an intrinsic difference in the value of life *for that person*." "Self-Interest and Self-Concern," in Ellen Frankel Paul, Fred D. Miller, Jr., and Jeffrey Paul, eds., *Self-Interest* (New York: Cambridge University Press, 1997), 164. See also Adam Smith, *The Theory*

of Moral Sentiments, ed. D. D. Raphael and A. L. Macfie, vol. 1 of the Glasgow Edition of *The Works and Correspondence of Adam Smith* (Indianapolis, IN: Liberty Fund, 1982), Chapter 1, Of Sympathy. Accessed from http://oll.libertyfund.org/title/192/200058/3301252 on April 17, 2012.

3. Joan C. Callahan noted the first of these phenomena in "On Harming the Dead," *Ethics* 97 (1987), 341; the second is discussed in Masterton, et al., "Queen Christina's moral claim on the living," 321–327, and "Can the Dead be Brought into Disrepute?" 137–149.

4. George Pitcher, "The Misfortunes of the Dead," in Fischer, ed. *The Metaphysics of Death*, 157–168.

5. Feinberg, "Harm to Others," 171–190. Although Feinberg simply adopted this account of posthumous harm from Pitcher, since the discussions of it are typically addressed together it would not be inaccurate to say that it is now known as the "Feinberg-Pitcher" account of posthumous harm.

6. W. Glannon, "Do the sick have a right to cadaveric organs?" *Journal of Medical Ethics*, 29 (2003), 153–154, and C.L. Hamer and M.M. Rivlin, "A stronger policy of organ retrieval from cadaveric donors: some ethical considerations," *Journal of Medical Ethics*, 29 (2003), 197–199.

7. See, for example, Aaron Spital and James Stacey Taylor, "In Defense of Routine Recovery of Cadaveric Organs: A Response to Walter Glannon," *Cambridge Quarterly of Healthcare Ethics* 17, no. 3 (2008), 337–343, "Routine Recovery of Cadaveric Organs for Transplantation: Consistent, Fair, and Life Saving," *Clinical Journal of the American Society of Nephrology* 2 (2007), 300–303, and Cecile Fabre, *Whose Body is it Anyway?* (New York: Oxford University Press, 2006), Chapter 4. For criticisms of Fabre's views on organ taking see James Stacey Taylor, "Liberalism, the Duty to Rescue, and Organ Procurement," *Political Studies Review* 6, 3 (2008), 314–326; for a revised version of Taylor's view on organ taking see Chapter 8.

8. See, for example, Masterton et al., "Queen Christina's moral claim on the living," 323–325.

9. See, for example, A.R. Schiff, "Arising from the dead: challenges of posthumous procreation," *North Carolina Law Review* 75, 3 (1997), 901–965.

10. See, for example, Sperling, *Management of Post-Mortem Pregnancy*, 79.

11. T.M. Wilkinson, "Last Rights: the Ethics of Research on the Dead," *Journal of Applied Philosophy* 19 (2002), 31–41.

12. The title of my "The Myth of Posthumous Harm," *American Philosophical Quarterly* 42, no. 4 (2005), 311–322, is thus hubristic, for even though this paper shows that the Feinberg-Pitcher account of posthumous harm is mistaken it does not thereby show that posthumous harm is impossible. This point is made independently in Benjamin S. Yost, "The Irrevocability of Capital Punishment," *Journal of Social Philosophy* 42, no. 3 (2011), 330.

13. As do, for example, the arguments of Callahan, "On Harming the Dead," 341–342, W. J. Waluchow, "Feinberg's Theory of "Preposthumous" Harm," *Dialogue* 25 (1986), 727—734, and Julian Lamont, "A Solution to the Puzzle of When Death Harms Its Victims," *Australasian Journal of Philosophy* 76 (1988), 203–205. The objections in these papers are outlined and rebutted in James Stacey Taylor, "Harming the Dead," *Journal of Philosophical Research* 33 (2008), 185–202.

14. The change in focus from harming the dead to wronging them is not merely terminological for it carries with it some considerable theoretical baggage. The proponents of some moral theories (such as act utilitarianism) hold that it is impossible to wrong someone without harming them. Since this is so, those participants in the bioethical debates in which posthumous harm plays a role whose moral views preclude the possibility of harmless wrongdoing

would not simply switch the focus of their arguments from harms to wrongs if it is shown that posthumous harm is impossible. Instead, they would abandon their concerns with the putative interests of the dead altogether. (Or, at least, would abandon any concern that they had with these putative interests for the sake of the dead themselves; they could still retain an indirect concern for them as a result of being directly concerned about the interests of living people who were concerned about the dead; see the discussion of this point in Chapter 4.) On a related note, even were it to be shown that the dead could be wronged but not harmed, this would, given the dominance of *harm*-based consequentialist approaches within contemporary Western bioethics, undercut the concern that many of the participants within the debates in which the question of posthumous harm plays a role have for the putative interests of the dead. Shifting the focus of discussion in certain debates in bioethics from posthumous harms to posthumous wrongs would thus serve (at best) to marginalize the putative interests of the dead in the debate in which they now play a central role, even though they would still be items of direct concern for some.

15. Note that this modified Epicurean argument is compatible with the truth of the belief that *all* persons possess everlasting life through God—although if this claim were true the Epicurean argument that were persons not to possess this they would be immune from posthumous harm would not be a very interesting one!

16. Jens Johansson notes that the problem of the subject is a misnomer in the context of the Epicurean argument for the view that death is not a harm to the person who dies, for it is clear that the subject of such harm must be the antemortem person whose death is at issue. As such, claims Johannseen, the proper response to the Epicurean challenge is to provide an account of when the antemortem person is harmed by her own death. Jens Johansson, "The Time of Death's Badness," *Journal of Medicine and Philosophy*, forthcoming. The currently-competing accounts of when a person is harmed by her own death include priorism (whose proponents hold that death can be bad for the one who dies prior to her death), eternalism (whose proponents hold that death can be eternally bad for the one who dies), concurrentism (whose proponents hold that death can be bad for its victims at the times of their deaths), and subsequentism (whose proponents hold that death can be bad for its victims after they die). For an outline of these competing positions see Bradley, *Well-Being & Death*, 84 (The analogue in the debate over posthumous harm would be to provide an account of how the antemortem person is harmed, although it should be noted here that not all who believe in the possibility of posthumous harm believe that it would befall the antemortem person whose interested were thwarted; see here the discussion of Sperling's views on posthumous harm in the next Chapter.) Should one wish to reformulate the debate in this way, the arguments offered in Chapter 5 should be read as providing reasons to believe that no such account of when the antemortem person is harmed by her own death could be forthcoming.

17. Epicurus, "Letter to Menoeceus," in Hicks, *Stoic and Epicurean*, 169.

18. Oddly, John Broome fails to recognize the problems involved in endorsing the possibility of backwards causation of when he endorses the possibility of posthumous harms; see his *Weighing Lives* (Oxford: Oxford University Press, 2004), 47. For a précis of a complex argument against the possibility of backwards causation, see Michael Tooley, *Time, Tense, and Causation* (Oxford: Clarendon Press, 1997), 118–119; see also D. H. Mellor, *Real Time* (Cambridge: Cambridge University Press, 1981), Chapter 10. In Chapter 5 it will be argued in the context of defending one version of the Epicurean

argument that death is not a harm to the person who dies that presentism is defensible. Since presentists have, as Craig Bourne argues, an "explanatory advantage on why backwards causation does not occur" the truth of presentism would provide significant support for a full-blooded Epicurean thanatology, as it could be used to ground both objections to the possibility of posthumous harm and the view that death is not a harm to the person who dies. (See Craig Bourne, *A Future for Presentism*, [New York: Oxford University Press, 2007], 134–135.) However, as will be argued in Chapter 5, the full-blooded Epicurean thanatology that will be defended in this volume does not depend on presentism.

19. The force of this argument was recognized by Aristotle: "For both good and evil are thought to exist for a dead man, as much as for one who is alive but not aware of them." *Nicomachean Ethics* 1100a, 19–20. See McKeon, *The Basic Works of Aristotle*, 946–947.
20. Parfit, *Reasons and Persons*, 495. Feinberg, "Harm to Others," 181–182.
21. Feinberg, "Harm to Others," 181–182.
22. Feinberg acknowledges that there might be a difference between these cases insofar as in Case B "there might seem to be no subject of the harm, the woman being dead at the specific moment when the harm occurred." ("Harm to Others," 182). He argues, however, that this problem is defused by Pitcher's arguments (outlined below) for the possibility of posthumous harm.
23. Parfit, *Reasons and Persons*, 495. Parfit does not explicitly endorse the view that the dead can be harmed.
24. Feinberg, "Harm to Others," 182
25. Note that Feinberg merely assumes that these conspirators posthumously betray this woman's trust; he does not argue for this. This assumption should be challenged, for, a betrayal is a form of wrong, and, as will be argued in Chapter 4, not only is there no reason to believe that the dead can be wronged there is reason to believe that they cannot. See also Chapter 2, note 30.
26. Feinberg, "Harm to Others," 182–183.
27. Ibid., 183
28. It will be argued that the dead cannot be wronged in Chapter 4.
29. Feinberg, "Harm to Others," 171–190, Pitcher, "The Misfortunes of the Dead". Since Feinberg's account of how the dead can be harmed is a reiteration of Pitcher's, the arguments in this section focus on Pitcher's views.
30. Pitcher, "The Misfortunes of the Dead," 161.
31. Ibid., 161.
32. Ibid., 168.
33. Ibid., 168.
34. This counterfactual view of harm has been outlined and defended by Thomas Nagel, "Death," in Fischer, ed., *The Metaphysics of Death*, 65–66. It will be discussed more fully in the context of hedonism in Chapter 3.
35. A similar point has been made independently by Mark H. Bernstein, *On Moral Considerability* (Oxford: Oxford University Press, 1998), 65.
36. Dorothy Grover, "Posthumous Harm," 336–337.
37. Solomon, "Is There Happiness After Death?" 189–193, Luper, "Posthumous Harm," 69.
38. Some proponents of the view that posthumous harm is possible argue that since a person's posthumous reputation can wax or wane without backwards causation, attributing posthumous harm to a person need not require it either. (See Levenbook, "Harming Someone After His Death," 408, 416, and Luper. "Posthumous Harm," 69.) However, as Callahan has argued, this argument fails, for saying that (e.g.) Einstein's posthumous reputation waxes

or wanes "is not a description of something *Einstein* has or has not got; it is a description of us—that is, it is a description of what some in the existing community of believers believe." Callahan, "On Harming the Dead," 342–343.

39. The arguments in this section are effective not only against the Feinberg-Pitcher account of posthumous harm, but those accounts of how posthumous harm is possible that are variants of this view. See, for example, Steven Luper, "Posthumous Harm," 69–71, Dorothy Grover, "Posthumous Harm," 336–339, 352–353, and Paul Griseri, "Can a Dead Man Be Harmed?" *Philosophical Investigations* 10 (1987), 317–329.

40. The major alternative accounts that have been developed will be discussed in the next Chapter.

41. For further discussion of this way in which a person's autonomy can be usurped see James Stacey Taylor, *Practical Autonomy and Bioethics* (New York: Routledge, 2009), Chapter 1.

42. To accept this possibility is to accept that a person can be said to be harmed as a result of undergoing a Cambridge change, that is, it is to accept that a person can be harmed by an event even though she herself undergoes no change as a result of it. This is important, for denying that harm could be the result of Cambridge changes in a person's properties would preclude the possibility that the dead could be harmed. See Lamont, "A Solution," 198, n.5, William Grey, "Epicurus and the Harm of Death," *Australasian Journal of Philosophy* 77 (1999), 361, and Geoffrey Scarre, *Death* (Montreal: McGill-Queen's University Press, 2007), 105–110, and "The Invulnerability of the Dead," in Taylor, ed., *The Metaphysics and Ethics of Death* (Oxford University Press, forthcoming). The distinction between real changes in the properties of objects and changes in the properties of objects that occur as a result of changes in their relations to other objects (phoney, or "Cambridge" changes) was first outlined by Peter Geach, *God and the Soul* (New York: Schocken Books, 1969), 71–72.

43. While this certainly accommodates the intuition that the woman in Case A has been harmed, a more robust response to Feinberg—and one that is better supported by the arguments in this volume—would hold that this woman was *not* harmed by the collapse of her enterprise as this had no negative effects upon her experiences. This response to Feinberg could be defended by drawing on the arguments in Chapter 4.

44. Note that this is a weaker claim than that made in Taylor, "The Myth of Posthumous Harm"

45. Note that this observation does not commit one to holding that the woman in Case A was harmed.

46. See Callahan, "On Harming the Dead," 36.

47. Feinberg, "Harm to Others," 183.

48. I owe this example to Paul Tudico. An example making the same point has been developed by Steven Luper, *The Philosophy of Death*, 149.

49. For further discussion of this point see Taylor, *Practical Autonomy*, Chapter 1, and the discussion of Dorothy Grover's account of how posthumous harm is possible in Chapter 2 of this volume.

50. That one can refer to dead persons does not imply that one can predicate properties of them. See David-Hillel Ruben "A Puzzle About Posthumous Predication," *The Philosophical Review* 98 (1988), 213.

51. Douglas Portmore, "Desire Fulfillment and Posthumous Harm," *American Philosophical Quarterly* 44, 1 (2007), 27–38. Portmore's rejection of accounts of posthumous harm that are based on the desire theory of welfare does not commit him to rejecting the possibility of posthumous harm

simpliciter. Indeed, an alternative version of how such harm is possible can be drawn from his "Welfare, Achievement, and Self-Sacrifice," *Journal of Ethics & Social Philosophy* 2, no. 2 (2007). Available at: http://www.jesp.org/PDF/DouglasPortmore.pdf, Accessed January 8, 2010. Note that although Portmore writes of desires and Feinberg and Pitcher wrote primarily about interests nothing in these arguments turns on this distinction.

52. Portmore, "Desire Fulfillment and Posthumous Harm," 27.
53. Ibid., 27.
54. Ibid., 28.
55. Parfit, *Reasons and Persons*, 494. Quoted by Portmore, "Desire Fulfillment and Posthumous Harm," 28.
56. Ibid., 28.
57. Mark Overvold, "Self-Interest and Getting What You Want," in H. B. Miller and W. H. Williams, eds., *The Limits of Utilitarianism* (Minneapolis: University of Minnesota Press, 1982), 190.
58. Portmore, "Desire Fulfillment and Posthumous Harm," 28. As Portmore notes, it is for this reason that Gregory Kavka and Brad Hooker have objected to Overvold's version of the desire theory of welfare. See G. Kavka, *Hobbesian Moral and Political Theory* (Princeton, NJ: Princeton University Press, 1986), 41, and Brad Hooker, "A Breakthrough in the Desire Theory of Welfare," in J. Heil, ed., *Rationality, Morality and Self-Interest: Essays Honoring Mark Carl Overold* (Lanham, Md.: Rowan and Littlefield, 1993), 205–213.
59. Hooker, "A Breakthrough in the Desire Theory of Welfare," 212, quoted by Portmore, "Desire Fulfillment and Posthumous Harm," 28–29.
60. Ibid., 29.
61. Ibid., 29.
62. Ibid., 30.
63. Ibid., 30, note 14. Note that this account of what it is voluntarily to abandon a desire is similar to Christman's account of what it is to be autonomous with respect to one's effective first-order desires. See John Christman, "Defending Historical Autonomy: A Reply to Professor Mele," *Canadian Journal of Philosophy* 23, 2 (1993), 288. For a criticism of such a negative approach to analyzing autonomy, and, hence, to analyzing what it is voluntarily to abandon a desire, see James Stacey Taylor, *Practical Autonomy and Bioethics*, 13.
64. Portmore, "Desire Fulfillment and Posthumous Harm," 31. Portmore also holds that this View has a second counterintuitive implication: that if one dies when one desired A, then the postmortem occurrence of ~A would be a harm to one no matter how fleeting one's desire for A was, and no matter how longstanding one's desire for ~A was. But, granting the acceptability of the desire theory of welfare (a provision that is in line with the general thrust of Portmore's arguments) this does not seem to be as "absurd" as Portmore believes. Assuming for the sake of argument that the possibility of posthumous harm is a live one, it does not seem odd to say that one would have harmed an elderly billionaire by refusing to honor his recent will in which he left his fortune to his recently-acquired trophy wife, instead giving his estate to the foundation that he had worked for all his life.
65. Ibid., 32.
66. Although Portmore here assumes that a person's desires would be extinguished after her death (and so, presumably, would her interests) it is possible that they would not be; see Davis' discussion of the way in which a person's investment interests could survive her death in "Surviving Interests and Living Wills," 23–27.

67. Portmore, "Desire Fulfillment and Posthumous Harm," 33.
68. Ibid., 33.

NOTES TO CHAPTER 2

1. Silverstein's complex 4D argument for the possibility of posthumous harm will be discussed in the next Chapter, in the context of defending the view that the correct connection between an A-relative evil x and A's negative experiences is that x is the cause of these experiences. Levenbook has recently developed a new argument supporting her view that posthumous harm is possible that is based attempting to establish that persons can be degraded by bodily mistreatment after they no longer exist. While this is certainly a novel and complex argument it will not be addressed here, simply because the scope of the concept of "degradation" is extremely unclear, and so absent its clear delineation any argument that is based upon it will be fraught with difficulties. See Barbara Baum Levenbook, "Welfare and Harm After Death," in Taylor, ed., *The Metaphysics and Ethics of Death*, forthcoming.
2. Levenbook, "Harming Someone after His Death"; Levenbook's criticisms of the Feinberg-Pitcher account of how posthumous harm is possible occur on 408–412.
3. Ibid., 412.
4. Ibid., 412. Levenbook notes that these are not the only necessary conditions for a person to be harmed by a loss, nor are they jointly sufficient. However, she sets to one side the question of what other conditions might be required as being "relatively minor to the present concerns". Ibid., 413.
5. Ibid., 413.
6. Ibid., 413.
7. Ibid., 416.
8. Ibid., 416.
9. Ibid., 416.
10. Harry S. Silverstein, "The Evil of Death," *Journal of Philosophy* 77 (1980), 404–405, ff; this exegetical account of his view is given by Levenbook, "Harming Someone after His Death," 417.
11. Ibid., 418.
12. Ibid., 418.
13. Joan C. Callahan, "On Harming the Dead," *Ethics* 97, no. 2 (1987), 343. A similar point is made by Don Marquis, "Harming the Dead," *Ethics* 96 (1985), 159. Oddly, Marquis fails to recognize the implications that this point has for his view of the morality of abortion; see Walter Sinnott-Armstrong, "You Can't Lose What You Ain't Never Had: A Reply to Marquis on Abortion," *Philosophical Studies* 96 (1997), 59–72.
14. Ibid., 343. This point has also been made by Don Marquis, "Harming the Dead," 159–160.
15. Callahan, "On Harming the Dead," 342–343. Levenbook is thus mistaken to claim in a later paper that "The linguistic evidence suggests that the ordinary concept of loss does not demand an existing loser . . . ," on the basis of noting that "we . . . ordinarily speak of people losing the respect of others, or their own good reputations, when the same thing occurs after their death that would justify saying that they have lost these things if it occurred before their death". Barbara Baum Levenbook, "Harming the Dead, Once Again," *Ethics* 96 (1985), 163. Callahan's point is also telling against Waluchow's support for his claim (offered in support of the possibility of posthumous harm), that it is not true that "A person can acquire or lose properties only

during those times when he is in existence," which is based on the view that a person's literary reputation could wax or wane after her death. Waluchow, "Feinberg's Theory of 'Preposthumous' Harm," 734.

16. Feinberg, "Harm to Others," 178; Dorothy Grover, "Posthumous Harm," 339.
17. Ibid., 344.
18. Ibid., 343.
19. Ibid., 347.
20. Ibid., 347, 348.
21. Ibid., 351
22. Ibid., 351,
23. Ibid., 351. The question of whether the dead can be wronged will be taken up in Chapter 4.
24. Ibid., 352.
25. Ibid., 353.
26. An argument similar to the "Knowledge and Autonomy View" is used by Grover to argue that death can be a harm to the person who dies; see her "Death, and Life," *Canadian Journal of Philosophy* 17, no. 4 (1987), 721 ff.
27. See, for example, his classic poem "Railway Bridge of The Silvery Tay," in Robert Crawford and Mick Imlah, eds., *The Penguin Book of Scottish Verse* (London: Penguin, 2006), 349–350.
28. Note that this counterexample to Grover does not depend on posthumous harms and benefits being possible—the possibility of the former is only mentioned in this context to emphasize that Grover's account of how posthumous harm is possible must be mistaken even in the eyes of one who believes that persons can be affected by events that occur after their deaths.
29. Grover recognizes that her account of how posthumous harm is possible would be subject to the objection that it requires the possibility of backwards causation, and attempts to meet this by noting that some properties of ante-mortem persons can be affected by events that occur after their deaths. The property that she draws upon to exemplify this possibility (that of being a killer) however, is, as was argued in the previous Chapter, disanalogous to the property of harm, and so cannot support her (and Feinberg's and Pitcher's) claim that posthumous harm does not require backwards causation. See Grover, "Posthumous Harm," 336–337.
30. Ibid., 351. Although Grover believes that it is possible posthumously to betray someone, this assumption is not obviously correct, for a betrayal is a type of wrong, and (as will be argued in Chapter 4) not only is there no reason to think that the dead can be wronged, there is reason to believe that such wronging is impossible. I thank Barbara Baum Levenbook for bringing to my attention the need to clarify my views on the possibility of posthumous betrayal; see her "The Retroactivity Problem," in Joseph Keim Campbell, Michael O'Rourke, and Harry S. Silverstein, eds., *Time and Identity* (Cambridge, Mass.: MIT Press, 2010), 307, n. 3. However, since nothing in this argument against Grover's view turns on the issue of whether or not it is possible to betray the dead, the discussion of why this is so can be left until Chapter 4.
31. This account of the relationship between deception, betrayal, and autonomy is outlined more fully in Taylor, *Practical Autonomy and Bioethics*, Chapter 1.
32. This example is relevant to the discussion of the autonomy-based "fewer mistakes" arguments discussed in Chapter 8.
33. This was case of the woman in Feinberg's Case A that was discussed in the previous Chapter.

34. For a discussion of this see Taylor, *Practical Autonomy and Bioethics*, 6–7.
35. Ibid., 84–85.
36. Daniel Sperling, *Posthumous Interests: Legal and Ethical Perspectives* (Cambridge: Cambridge University Press, 2008), 34.
37. Ibid., 34–35.
38. Ibid., 35.
39. Ibid., 36
40. The moral implications of loving persons who are dead will be discussed in Chapter 4, in the context of Jeffrey Blustein's "Rescue from Insignificance" argument for the view that we owe duties to the dead.
41. Sperling, *Posthumous Interests*, 39
42. Naturally, these phenomena lead to interesting philosophical puzzles. For a discussion of the puzzles associated with referring to and predicating properties of things that do not exist, see Chapter 5. For a classic discussions of our putative emotional attitudes towards things that we believe do not exist (such as fictional entities), see Kendall L. Walton, "Fearing Fictions," *The Journal of Philosophy* 75, no. 1 (1978), 5–27.
43. It is possible that a Human Subject might be harmed symbolically, as we might hold that a person is symbolically harmed were something that is a harm for him to occur, as will be discussed in Chapter 3. But to refer to *symbolic* harm in this way would be to tacitly acknowledge the absence of any *actual* harm, just as Rex Mottram's claim in Evelyn Waugh's *Brideshead Revisited* that it would be "raining spiritually" when it did not rain despite the Pope's prediction that it would acknowledges that it would not really be raining at all. Evelyn Waugh, *Brideshead Revisited* (New York: Alfred A. Knopf, 1993), 174–175.
44. Paul Griseri, "Can a Dead Man be Harmed?" 317. Griseri motivates his discussion by quoting a claim by Raimond Gaita, that " . . . those murdered suffer not only the evil of death but also that of being murdered. So, for example, an unjust act e.g. a lynching 'for the sake' of the murdered dead makes matters worse for them, for they are then not only the murdered but also the unjustly avenged dead and so are forced even deeper into a quagmire of evil". Raimond Gaita, "Better one than ten," *Philosophical Investigations* 5, no. 2 (1982), 103, n.1. Griseri's account of how posthumous harm is possible it is directly relevant to bioethical issues, insofar as, for some persons, it is an open question as to whether certain medical procedures that might be performed on cadavers (e.g., the posthumous taking of human organs for transplant) are intrinsically unjust.
45. Griseri, "Can a Dead Man be Harmed?" 318.
46. Ibid., 321. A person is harmed "morally" for Griseri when the harm inflicted upon her "is connected with their moral concerns". (Ibid., 319.)
47. Ibid., 319
48. Ibid., 327. The idea of inherited guilt is, of course, a recurring feature of Attic tragedy. For an excellent discussion of it in this context see N. J. Sewell-Rutter, *Guilt by Descent: Moral Inheritance and Decision Making in Greek Tragedy* (Oxford: Oxford University Press, 2007), Chapter 2. See also E. R. Dodds, *The Greeks and the Irrational* (Berkeley: University of California Press, 1951), 31 ff., and R. Parker, *Miasma: Pollution and Purification in Early Greek Religion* (Oxford: Clarendon Press, 1983), 198 ff.
49. Griseri, "Can a Dead Man be Harmed?" 328.
50. Larry May, "Metaphysical Guilt and Moral Taint," in Larry May and Stacey Hoffman, eds., *Collective Responsibility: Five Decades of Debate in Theoretical and Applied Ethics* (Savage, Md.: Rowman and Littlefield, 1991), 240. Quoted by Marina A.L. Oshana, "Moral Taint," *Metaphilosophy* 37, nos. 3–4 (2006), 359–360.

51. Ibid., 370–371.
52. Ibid., 371–382.
53. This claim will be defended more fully in Chapter 5.
54. And so the title of Taylor, "The Myth of Posthumous Harm," is vindicated.

NOTES TO CHAPTER 3

1. Note that the account of hedonism developed above differs from pure hedonism. Pure hedonism is the view that the only bearers of intrinsic value are states of affairs (in the Chisholmian sense) and that a person's well-being depends on her "taking pleasure or pain to some degree in some proposition". See Bradley, *Well-Being & Death*, 9. This account of hedonism follows that of Roderick Chisholm, *Person and Object* (LaSalle, Ill.: Open Court Publishing Co., 1976), Chapter 4, and Fred Feldman, *Pleasure and the Good Life: Concerning the Nature, Varieties, and Plausibility of Hedonism* (New York: Oxford University Press, 2004). Here, the question of whether hedonic value atoms are the only ones possible is left open.
2. Luper, "Posthumous Harm," *American Philosophical Quarterly* 41, no. 1 (2004), 67.
3. Ibid., 67.
4. Ibid., 67. For Luper, a desire is thwarted "if it is never either satisfied or voluntarily given up before satisfaction becomes impossible". (Ibid., 67; see also Steven Luper, *Invulnerability: On Securing Happiness* [Chicago: Open Court Publishing Co., 1996], 30.) This is an odd account of what it is to thwart a desire, for it precludes by definition a person's having a desire that is neither thwarted nor satisfied. As such, it leads Luper to claim that a desire has been thwarted when it would be more accurate to claim that it had been eliminated, as when he claims that "what (permanently) removes a desire thwarts it, by ruling out the possibility of its being satisfied". (See Luper, "Posthumous Harm," p. 68; see also Luper, "Annihilation," 271.) Worse yet, since there are clear cases of desires that are intuitively neither thwarted nor satisfied (consider, for example, the "perpetual and restless desire of power after power, that ceaseth only in death"; Thomas Hobbes, *Leviathan* (Indianapolis: Hackett Publishing Co., Inc., 1994), 58) Luper's account of thwarting is mistaken. A better account of what it is to thwart a desire is that a desire D is thwarted by an event E that precludes D from being satisfied although D still exists. It should also be noted that Luper uses the term "satisfaction" broadly, to cover both instances of desire satisfaction (in Ross's sense) and instances of desire fulfillment. (See W.D. Ross, *Foundations of Ethics* [Oxford; Oxford University Press, 1939], 300.) Nothing substantive, however, turns on either of these terminological differences.
5. On this view death will be a harm to the person who dies insofar as it thwarts some of her desires. This account of death's badness will be challenged below.
6. Luper, "Posthumous Harm," 69.
7. Ibid., 69.
8. The first two examples of personally defined projects that are held to render a person vulnerable to posthumous harms are from Luper, ibid., 69.
9. Ibid., 69. Luper recognizes that this argument in defense of the possibility of posthumous harm is faced by what he terms the timing puzzle; the difficulty of dating when a person is harmed by the events that occur after her death. Luper argues that Pitcher's response to this puzzle is "the best," and "it is persuasive". (Ibid., 70). Unfortunately, as was argued in Chapter 1, although

Pitcher's account of how posthumous harm is possible, and hence his solution to this puzzle, might be the best available, it is not persuasive.

10. Although see note 4, on Luper's odd account of "thwarting".

11. Parfit, *Reasons and Persons*, 157. Cited by Luper, "Posthumous Harm," 70.

12. Parfit, *Reasons and Persons*, 151, Cited by Luper, "Posthumous Harm," 70.

13. Ibid., 71. Luper again draws on Pitcher's arguments to explain when such posthumous harm would occur.

14. Ibid., 67.

15. This section will thus offer a positive argument in favor of hedonism, rather than lending support to it by undermining its competitors. The latter strategy has been adopted by Bradley, whose work should thus be seen as complementary to this section. See Bradley, *Well-Being & Death*, Chapter 1.

16. Robert Nozick, *Anarchy, State, and Utopia* (Oxford: Blackwell, 1974), 42–45. It is not clear whether Nozick intended this thought experiment to support this conclusion, for his example of the experience machine was directed at the claim that all that matters to us are our experiences. It is, however, compatible with the account of hedonism that is developed here to hold that something, S, other than a person's experiences can matter to her; S would just not play in role in determining the degree of her well-being.

17. Nozick, *Anarchy, State, and Utopia*, 42.

18. It is interesting to note that the this thought experiment is posed in terms of a person's having the opportunity to plug into the experience machine, rather than being told that she is already in it, and having the opportunity to unplug, with the knowledge of her status as being within the machine being erased from her memory should she chose to remain within it. Given this, it is an open question as to whether persons would choose to unplug from their currently-experienced lives (and hence from their currently-experienced families, friends, pets, and jobs), or stay in them if they were informed that they were living in the experience machine. And if persons tended to chose to remain within the machine, it might be that a simple preference for the *status quo*, rather than for experiences generated from without the machine, underlies persons' reluctance to plug in.

19. For an innovative defense of hedonism against this understanding of the source of this reluctance see Eduardo Rivera-Lopez, "Are Mental State Welfarism and Our Concern for Non-experiential Goals Incompatible?" *Pacific Philosophical Quarterly* 88 (2007), 74–91.

20. Joseph Mendola, "Intuitive Hedonism," *Philosophical Studies* 128 (2006), 455. Although Mendola does not recognize this, this Berkeleyian approach to defending hedonism would, strictly speaking, only be possible within a theistic framework. (I owe this point to James Worth.) As such, given the plausible assumption that this framework would countenance some form of afterlife, this approach to defending hedonism would be in tension with the thanatological concerns of the historical Epicurus.

21. This was noted by Geoffrey Scarre, "On Caring About One's Posthumous Reputation," *American Philosophical Quarterly* 38, no. 2 (2001), 209. Note that holding that a person could value the well-being of her children for its own sake, independently of any effect that this might have on her own well-being, is not directly to reject the possibility that only hedonic value matters; rather, it is only to reject egoistic hedonism.

22. This move is thus not open to Bradley, for he endorses pure hedonism. However, one could hold that whereas persons' beliefs that things other than their experiences are intrinsically valuable could motivate them not to enter the experience machine, these beliefs are mistaken, and so one could provide

a descriptive account of persons' reluctance to enter while still holding that they should do so.

23. A similar distinction is made by Josie Fisher, "Harming and Benefiting the Dead," *Death Studies* 25 (2001), 563–564. The importance of this distinction is implicitly recognized by Alan E. Fuchs, in defending Overvold's view that posthumous harm is impossible; "Posthumous Satisfactions and the Concept of Individual Welfare," in John Heil, ed., *Rationality, Morality, and Self-Interest: Essays Honoring Carl Overvold* (Lanham, Md.: Rowman & Littlefield Publishers, 1993), 220.

24. This objection might arise if one accepts Stephen Darwall's rational care theory of well-being, on which "what it is for something to be good for someone is for it to be something that is rational (makes sense, is warranted, or justified) to desire for him insofar as one cares about him". Stephen Darwall, *Welfare and Rational Care* (Princeton, NJ: Princeton University Press, 2002), 8–9. However, accepting Darwall's theory of well-being need not commit one to rejecting the distinction between something being a harm to a person and its being a harm for her. (And, of course, if one believes that it *does* commit one to denying this distinction then one could try to preserve it by arguing that Darwall's theory should be rejected.) One might, for example, hold that Darwall's theory of well-being is only a theory of what would be good to a person, not what would be good for her. I thank David Shoemaker for pressing me on these points.

25. This distinction is also compatible with the claim that posthumous events could be harms to a person, and thus could harm her *simpliciter*, for it does not rule out the possibility that a person could be harmed by events that do not affect her experience.

26. Although an event that causes a bad experience might be just one part of a larger event that would lead him to have a good experience, or a better experience that he might have otherwise done. If so, the person's overall experience (i.e., of the larger event in question) would not be a harm to him.

27. Robert S. Olick is thus wrong to hold that this cliché captures the view of those who believe setbacks to interests must be known about to be harmful. See his *Taking Advance Directives Seriously: Prospective Autonomy and Decisions near the End of Life* (Washington, D.C.: Georgetown University Press, 2001), 64.

28. This point is discussed more fully in Chapter 5, in the context of discussing the Existence Variant of the Epicurean argument that death is not a harm to the one who dies.

29. See Parfit, *Reasons and Persons*, 499.

30. As such, these versions of this hedonistic account of well-being will be immune to the objection to hedonism that James Griffin developed from the example of Freud's preference for thinking in torment rather than being unable to think clearly without pain. See James Griffin, *Well-Being* (Oxford: Clarendon Press, 1986), 8.

31. For a discussion of this and related issues, see Kai Draper, "Disappointment, Sadness, and Death," *The Philosophical Review* 108, no. 3 (1999), 390–394.

32. As such, then, the objections that were leveled in Chapter 1 against the Feinberg-Pitcher account of how posthumous harm is possible were too meek. First, instead of holding that the woman in Feinberg's Case A was harmed by the deceptive actions of her friends because by deceiving her they thwarted her interest in exercising her autonomy, it should instead have been held that she was *benefited* by them, in that they made her experiences better than they otherwise would have been, although this does not preclude one from

regretting on her behalf that she was subject to deception. Second, and more tellingly, since on this account of what it is for an event to cause harm to a person the harm is *caused* by the event in question, and not merely *made true* by it, events that cause harm to persons must occur prior to the harm that they cause, and so persons cannot be harmed by events that occur after their deaths.

33. The view that an event or state of affairs harms someone through *causing* harm to her is often taken to be axiomatic; see, for example, Matthew Hanser, "The Metaphysics of Harm," *Philosophy and Phenomenological Research* 77 no. 2 (2008), 421, and Elizabeth Harman, "Harming as Causing Harm," in Melinda A. Roberts and David T. Wasserstrom, eds., *Harming Future Persons: Ethics, Genetics, and the Nonidentity Problem* (Dordrecht: Springer,2009), 139. However, given that this volume is arguing against thanatological views that are similarly often taken to be axiomatic, a defense of the view of harm as being caused is needed.

34. Harry S. Silverstein, "The Evil of Death Revisited," in Peter A. French and Howard K. Wettstein, eds., *Midwest Studies in Philosophy Volume XXIV, Life and Death: Metaphysics and Ethics* (Boston, Mass.: Blackwell, 2000), 122.

35. Ibid., 122. Note that Silverstein does not distinguish between x being a harm *to* A and x being a harm *for* A. Silverstein's view is based on a four-dimensional framework in which time and space are treated equivalently. For an earlier exposition of this view, see Harry S. Silverstein, "The Evil of Death," in Fischer, ed., *The Metaphysics of Death*, 93–116. For recent elaborations and clarifications of this view, see Harry S. Silverstein, "The Time of the Evil of Death," in Joseph Keim Campbell, Michael O'Rourke and Harry S. Silverstein, eds., *Time and Identity* (Cambridge, Mass.: The MIT Press, 2010), 283–295, and Harry S. Silverstein, "The Evil of Death One More Time: Parallels Between Time and Space," in Taylor, ed., *The Metaphysics and Ethics of Death*, forthcoming.

36. Stephen Rosenbaum, "How to Be Dead and Not Care: A Defense of Epicurus," in Fischer, ed., *The Metaphysics of Death*, 129–131.

37. Ibid., 130.

38. Silverstein, "The Evil of Death Revisited," 123.

39. Ibid., 123.

40. Ibid., 124.

41. Ibid., 124.

42. Although in Case 2 they might have been sustained by Ann's affair, if Jim confronted her about it and found out the truth.

NOTES TO CHAPTER 4

1. Alexander McCall Smith, *Friends, Lovers, Chocolate* (New York: Pantheon Books, 2005), 209.

2. Isabel is not alone in thinking that the question of whether the dead can be harmed and the question of whether they can be wronged go hand in hand. J. Jeremy Wisnewski explicitly conflates them in "What We Owe the Dead," writing "I cannot help but accept that the dead can be wronged, *and hence harmed . . .*" (emphasis added), *Journal of Applied Philosophy* 27, no. 1 (2009), 57. These questions are also conflated by P. E. Digeser in *Political Forgiveness* (Ithaca: Cornell University Press, 2001), 88–92, while Charles C. Hinkley conflates them throughout Chapter 5 ("Can We Wrong the Dead?") of his *Moral Conflicts of Organ Retrieval: A case for constructive pluralism*

(Amsterdam: Editions Rodophi, BV, 2005). Similarly, Raymond A. Bellotti, in arguing that dead humans have both interests and rights, conflates these questions in outlining a possible argument that could be leveled against his view and a (one line!) response to it:

1) Suffering negative sensations is a necessary condition for having one's interests harmed.

2) The dead lack the capacity for experiencing sensations and for cognitive awareness.

Therefore, the dead cannot be harmed.

But this argument confuses (i) being wronged with (ii) knowing that one has been wronged.

(Raymond A. Belliotti, "Do Dead Human Beings Have Rights?" *The Personalist* 60 (1979), 202.) It is clear that Bellotti here understands the claim that a person's interests have been harmed to be synonymous with the claim that the person whose interests they are has been wronged. Note that Bellioti's response to what he terms "the argument from cognitive awareness" goes awry, for the proponents of the version of it that he considers could simply respond by noting that a person need not know that his interests have been thwarted for him to be harmed by this, provided that such thwarting adversely affects his experiences in some way. For the same reason Bellioti's objection would fail as an objection against the account of what it is for an event to cause harm to a person that was developed in the preceding Chapter. Furthermore, just as the question of whether one can harm the dead is separate from the question of whether one can wrong them, so too is the question of whether one can wrong the dead entirely distinct from the question of whether one can forgive them for wrongs that they did to one during their lives. This latter question is more concerned with what mode of forgiveness is available to the injured party than to questions concerning the possible relational properties of the dead themselves. For a discussion of this, see Charles L. Griswold, *Forgiveness: A Philosophical Exploration* (New York: Cambridge University Press, 2007), 120–121.

3. Note again that this observation does not commit one to endorsing the view that it is possible to wrong someone without thereby harming her.

4. Just as the question of posthumous harm is a question concerning whether antemortem persons can be harmed by events after their deaths, so too the question of posthumous wrong is a question of whether antemortem persons can be wronged by events that occur after their deaths—it is not the question of whether one can wrong a corpse. This observation is not, however, as trivial as one might assume, for some persons confusedly believe that corpses do have rights. See, for example, John Sutton Baglow, "The rights of the corpse," *Mortality* 12, 3 (2007), 223–239. For a decisive rejection of this view see James Stacey Taylor and Aaron Spital, "Corpses do not have rights: A response to Baglow," *Mortality* 13, 3 (2008), 282–286. See also Norman L. Cantor, *After We Die: The Life and Times of the Human Cadaver* (Washington, D.C.: Georgetown University Press, 2010), 64, who holds that corpses have legal rights to "decent sepulture" and "quiet repose". It is clear that Cantor is unaware of the possibility that antemortem persons could be held to have rights whose objects extend beyond the scope of their lives, and hence in ignorance assigns the rights that he believes are held by the dead to corpses. (Lest this comment be considered too harsh, consider how Lucretius would have treated his view that the dead have a right to "quiet repose"!) In this regard John Chipman Gray observes that corpses lack legal rights; see John Chipman Gray, *The Nature and Sources of the Law* (New York: Columbia University Press, 1916), 38. More recently—and

again *contra* Cantor—Alison Dundes Renteln notes that the view that the dead have the legal right not to have their corpses mistreated has gained little currency in Anglo-American jurisprudence; *The Cultural Defense* (Oxford: Oxford University Press, 2004), 179.

5. T. M. Wilkinson develops an argument for the claim that one "has a right to control what happens to one's body after death" "in the context of organ retrieval from the dead". Wilkinson's argument is essentially that one has such a right because the body in question is one's own. (*Ethics and the Acquisition of Organs* [New York: Oxford University Press, 2011], 44.) But there is a problem with this argument as an argument for the possibility that one might wrong the dead through violating their property rights: once one is dead one cannot own anything, for one does not exist, and hence there can be no property rights to violate.

6. Stephen Winter argues that the dead do not have rights, and, hence, that they cannot be wronged by rights-violations. Stephen Winter, "Against Posthumous Rights," *Journal of Applied Philosophy* 27, no. 2 (2010), 186–199. Yet Winter's focus is on showing that the dead cannot be wronged in the sense of having their claims violated, where a claim "is equivalent to a justifying reason for constraint that is relative to an entity" (188), where these claims are grounded on interests (189). As such, then, Winter's argument against the existence of posthumous rights should properly be understood as an argument against the view that one can thwart a person's interests after her death—that is, as an argument against the view that a person could be posthumously harmed, on the Feinberg-Pitcher understanding of what this involves—rather than as an argument against the view that one can wrong the dead *per se* (i.e., *independently* of thwarting their interests).

7. For example, in the Midrash (a collection of stories that arose in the Jewish tradition, elaborating on biblical tales and adding others) it is simply taken for granted that the posthumous slander of Nadab and Abihu wrongs them; see Carol Ochs, *Women and Spirituality* (Lanham, Md.: Rowman and Littlefield, Inc., second edition, 1997), 85. Similarly, both Nick Smith and Raymond Gaita accept without argument the possibility that the living could wrong the dead. Smith accepts that Kantian view that we could wrong the dead by failing to give them the apologies we owe them in *I Was Wrong: The Meanings of Apologies* (New York: Cambridge University Press, 2008), 130); Gaita discusses the possibility of wronging the dead by dishonoring them through mistreating their corpses in *The Philosopher's Dog: Friendships with Animals* (New York: Random House, 2002), Chapter 6. (For Kant's view see Immanuel Kant, Mary J. Gregor, ed., *The Metaphysics of Morals* (Cambridge: Cambridge University Press, 1996), 76.) Yet while the view that the dead can be wronged is widespread, it is not universally held; John Harris, for example, holds that it is "doubtful" whether the dead have any posthumous rights, basing his arguments for this on the view that such rights would not be supported on either the choice or the benefit theories of rights. See his "Mark Anthony or Macbeth: Some Problems Concerning the Dead and the Incompetent when it Comes to Consent," in Sheila A.M. Maclean, ed., *First Do No Harm: Law, Ethics, and Healthcare* (Aldershot: Ashgate, 2006), 289–290. (But see Wilkinson, *Ethics and the Acquisition of Organs*, 56–59.) And, despite his mistaken views on the possibility of both posthumous harms and wrongs, Feinberg at least recognized that it might not be meaningful or conceptually possible to ascribe rights to the dead. Joel Feinberg, "The Rights of Animals and Unborn Generations," in Ernest Partridge, *Responsibilities to Future Generations: Environmental Ethics* (Buffalo, NY: Prometheus Books, 1981), 140.

8. Annette Baier, for example, uses the claim that we "already accept" that the dead have rights as one of the starting points for her argument that future persons have rights. "The Rights of Past and Future Persons," in Partridge, *Responsibilities to Future Generations*, 172. Similarly, there is a long-standing but often unargued-for tradition that the dead have at least a right to burial; Grotius, for example, devotes an entire chapter of his magnum opus *The Rights of War and Peace* to this subject. See Hugo Grotius, *The Rights of War and Peace, including the Law of Nature and of Nations*, trans. A. C. Campbell (New York: M. Walter Dunne, 1901), Chapter XIX. The existence of such a natural right is criticized by Catalin Avramescu on the grounds that were it to exist it "must be common to the majority of nations," but "not all nations adhere to the same funerary standards." (Catalin Avramescu, trans. Alistair Ian Blyth, *An Intellectual History of Cannibalism* [Princeton: Princeton University Press, 2009], 54–55.) But this objection is erroneous in two respects. First, the fact that funerary rights vary does not in itself show that the right to burial is not common to the "majority" of nations, for some variance is still compatible with this claim. Second, and more damning, what actual practices persons engage in does not by itself indicate what natural rights there are, for they could simply be unrecognized or ignored. That death's apparent companion in certainty, taxation, is widespread does not show that there is no natural right to be free from having one's property extorted from one, but (perhaps) only that such a right is widely violated.
9. Feinberg, "Harm to Others," 182–183. As Belshaw notes, however, Feinberg is too sanguine to assume that there is a victim of posthumous wrongdoing—and, moreover, even if he is correct here "it needs to be recognized that a route in [i.e., to establishing the possibility of posthumous harm] can only work in a subset of cases," for "Most putative examples of posthumous harms involve accidental misfortune rather than malicious, thoughtless, or selfish human agency." *Annihilation*, 138.
10. Loren Lomasky attempts to establish that the dead have rights on the basis of arguing that they can be harmed through having their projects thwarted after death, drawing on a modified version of Feinberg's account of how posthumous harm is possible to establish the latter claim. See *Persons, Rights, and the Moral Community* (New York: Oxford University Press, 1987), 218–220. A similar argument is also offered by Meyer, "Reparations and Symbolic Restitution," 414. However, since (as has been argued in Chapters 1, 2 and 3) posthumous harm is impossible, Lomasky's and Meyer's attempts to establish that the dead have rights are also mistaken.
11. Nelson P. Lande, "Posthumous Rehabilitation and the Dust-Bin of History," *Public Affairs Quarterly* 4, no. 3 (1990), 271. Lande continues his argument to the conclusion that rectificatory justice requires that a person who has been unjustly saddled with a bad name should have this removed from him by the entity that affixed it to him, or that if a person's good name was taken from him, or that he was prevented from having a good name, by another, that other should rehabilitate his good name by restoring it to him.
12. Ibid., 271. Lande's argument continues after (e) to establish the conclusion outlined above.
13. Ibid., 285, n. 9.
14. Ibid., 285, n. 9.
15. Ibid., 285, n. 9.
16. For a discussion of the duties concerning the treatment of the bodies of one's enemies and of enemy prisoners that were generally accepted in Homeric times, see Samuel Eliot Basset, "Achilles' Treatment of Hector's Body,"

Transactions and Proceedings of the American Philological Association 64 (1933), 41–65.

17. Indeed, so simple, elegant, and persuasive is it that the reason for the paucity of arguments in favor of the view that the dead can be wronged might be that it is widely believed that establishing this possibility is as simple a matter as this. Indeed, as was noted above, this appears to be Feinberg's view.

18. Jeffrey Blustein, *The Moral Demands of Memory* (Cambridge: Cambridge University Press, 2008), 245. Blustein states that we have a *moral* obligation to remember the dear departed (Ibid., 269). Thus, since our obligation to remember is a moral one, and assuming that it is owed to the dead, were we not to fulfill it we would wrong the dead. Since the arguments below rest on the assumption that Blustein holds that the obligation to remember the dead is owed to the dead, it should in fairness to Blustein be noted that if this is not his view, then to the extent that they rest on it these arguments would not be criticisms of his position. In this case, then, these arguments should be understood as being criticisms of any possible attempt to use Blustein's arguments to establish that the dead can be wronged. The view that we have an obligation to remember the dead is also expressed by David Cockburn, in his *Other Times: Philosophical perspectives on past, present and future* (Cambridge: Cambridge University Press, 1997), 154–160, by Soren Kierkegaard, *Works of Love*, ed. and trans. Howard V. Hong , Edna H. Hong (Princeton: Princeton University Press, 1995), 347, and by Malin Masterton, Matts G. Hansson, Anna T. Hoglund, "In search of the missing subject: narrative identity and posthumous wronging," *Studies in the History and Philosophy of Biological and Biomedical Sciences* 41 (2010), 340-346. A rather confused account of why justice imposes upon us a duty to remember the dead victims of past crimes that appears to vacillate between holding that this is duty owed to no-one, and that this is a duty owed to the dead, is outlined in W. James Booth, *Communities of Memory: On Witness, Identity, and Justice* (Ithaca: Cornell University Press, 2006), 128–133.

19. All three of these arguments employ an expressive justificatory strategy, rather than a consequentialist one; that is, they focus on the attitudes that persons are required to adopt towards those who have died, rather than focusing on the good to be promoted by remembering them. This distinction between consequentialist and expressive approaches to arguing for the moral imperative to remember is outlined by Blustein, Ibid., 261–269. It should also be noted that these three arguments for the view that we have a moral obligation to remember the dead are not mutually exclusive; see Blustein, Ibid., 281.

20. Ibid., 270.

21. Ibid., 272. Blustein here quotes James Hartley, *Suffering Witness* (Albany, NY: State University of New York, 2000), 24; italics added by Blustein. Blustein notes that there are various ways in which the possession of dignity can be grounded, ranging from the Kantian approach of grounding it in persons being ends-in-themselves, to other rationality or autonomy-based accounts, to those that ground it in the "irreplaceability of the individual or the relationships of care that we have with each other" (*The Moral Demands of Memory*, 272). The dignity-based "rescue from insignificance" approach to grounding the obligation to remember the dead is not, however, based on any one account of the grounding of dignity, but is compatible with them all. This is because even though Blustein recognizes that "Different accounts of the basis of dignity will be associated with different ways of appropriately responding to it" they all share the view that respect is the appropriate way to respond to persons as possessors of dignity (Ibid., 272).

22. See, for example, R.S. Downie's comments on the Alder Hey scandal in "Research on Dead Infants," *Theoretical Medicine* 24 (2003), 166.
23. Blustein, *The Moral Demands of Memory*, 273.
24. Ibid., 273.
25. Ibid., 274.
26. Ibid., 274.
27. Ibid., 275.
28. Ibid., 278; quoting Janna Thompson, "Inherited Obligations and Generational Continuity," *Canadian Journal of Philosophy* 29, no. 4 (1999), 503.
29. Blustein, *The Moral Demands of Memory*, 279.
30. Ibid., 258. A similar point is made by Sperling, *Posthumous Interests*, p. 39.
31. Note that these actions need not be overt; private, internal rituals or acts of remembrance that are not socially expressive would satisfy this expressive account of evaluation.
32. See, for example, Christine M. Korsgaard, *The Sources of Normativity* (Cambridge: Cambridge University Press, 1996), Lecture 4, and Thomas E. Hill, Jr., *Autonomy and Self-respect* (Cambridge: Cambridge University Press 1991), Chapter 1.
33. Especially as there is an equally voluminous literature showing that humans do not have this special moral status; see, for example, Peter Singer, *Animal Liberation* (New York: New York Review, 1975), 1–23, and R.G. Frey, "Autonomy, Diminished Life, and the Threshold for Use," in James Stacey Taylor, ed., *Personal Autonomy: New Essays on Personal Autonomy and Its Role in Contemporary Moral Philosophy* (Cambridge; Cambridge University Press, 2005), 330–346.
34. Note that this would not merely be a theoretical nicety, for it would commit us to pursuing justice in response to the wrongs that were done to persons during their lives even after they had died to acknowledge that the wrongs done to them then were genuine wrongs. This does not commit us to claiming that if we failed to do so we would wrong the dead victims, for to fail to secure justice is not necessarily to wrong the victim.
35. See Blustein, *The Moral Demands of Memory*, 270–271.
36. Ibid., 270–271. Blustein notes that there might be cases in which there is an overriding reason not to acknowledge that someone existed, and so in these cases it would not be obviously imperative for the living to remember the dead.
37. See, for example, Harry G. Frankfurt, "On the Usefulness of Final Ends," in Harry G. Frankfurt, ed., *Necessity, Volition, and Love* (Cambridge; Cambridge University Press, 1999), 82–94.
38. Blustein, *The Moral Demands of Memory*, 274.
39. Ibid., 274.
40. In fairness to Blustein he does not seem to be convinced by the reasoning that he offers either, for immediately after his outline of this purported relationship between love, honor, and duty he writes that "It is uncontroversial that we can be faulted for not fulfilling duties of love and honor, *assuming there are such. . . .*" Ibid., 274; italics added.
41. Ibid., 275
42. For a discussion of this point in the context of bequests see Hillel Steiner, *An Essay on Rights* (Oxford: Blackwell, 1994), 249–258.
43. Blustein, *The Moral Demands of Memory*, 279.
44. It is important to note that this argument does not show that one could never establish that there are positive duties. The Rescue from Insignificance view, outlined above, for example, is an attempt to establish that persons have a positive duty to remember the dead in a non-question-begging manner.

Note, too, that although Blustein has failed to show here that persons have a moral obligation to the dead to remember them the Reciprocity View could be used to support the view that if they have posterity-directed desires of the appropriate sort then persons have a prudential obligation (to themselves) to remember their predecessors, to maintain (or perhaps establish) a tradition of remembering from which they would benefit. This possibility is further discussed at the end of this Chapter.

45. Note that this argument does not show that the dead cannot be wronged *simpliciter*, it only shows that they cannot be wronged through violation of their alleged rights. The scope of this argument against the possibility of the dead being wronged will be expanded below.

46. A defense of this claim will be offered in the next Chapter, in the context of discussing the Existence Variant of the Epicurean argument for the view that the dead cannot be harmed.

47. Lande, "Posthumous Reputation and the Dust-Bin of History," 273–274. Lande continues this argument to the conclusion that no argument for the posthumous rehabilitation of a person's good name can be based on her possession of rights, and so no arguments for such rehabilitation can be based on considerations of justice. The sense in which the dead no longer exist here is the sense in which they no longer exist as interest bearers. As such, this argument avoids Feldman's arguments in favor of the view that the dead do exist in some form; see the second caveat concerning the scope of this volume outlined in the Introduction.

48. Ibid., 274.

49. Ibid., 275. The example of the improper execution of a person's will being a violation of his right to dispose of his property as he wished is from Feinberg, "Harm to Others," 189.

50. This is fortunate, for, as Steiner has argued, it is not at all natural or intuitive to ascribe rights to the dead in this way. Steiner, *An Essay on Rights*, 249–258—although see Wilkinson, *Ethics and the Acquisition of Organs*, 58–59.

51. Luper, "Posthumous Harm," 69.

52. Lande, "Posthumous Reputation and the Dust-Bin of History," 275. Lande notes that the fulfillment of certain desires can only occur after a person's death, "such as the desire to found a dynasty, or . . . to possess a good name posthumously".

53. Ibid., 275.

54. Ibid., 275.

55. Not all accept that a person's interests will continue to exist after her death. The denial of this claim had led some to argue against the moral authority of living wills and other forms of advance directives, on the grounds that since a person's investment interests will not survive the loss of her capacity to care about their objects they should not be privileged over her surviving welfare interests—and since advance directives do typically support such privilege they illegitimately privilege non-existent interests over existing ones. See, for example, Rebecca Dresser, "Autonomy Revisited: The Limits of Anticipatory Choices," in Robert H. Binstock, Stephen G. Post, and Peter J. Whitehouse, *Dementia and Aging: Ethics, Values, and Policy Choices* (Baltimore, Md.; The Johns Hopkins University Press, 1992), 75–76, and by John A. Robertson, "Second Thoughts on Living Wills," *The Hastings Center Report* 21, no. 6 (1991), 7. For a response, see Davis, "Surviving Interests and Living Wills," 17–30. For a discussion of the relevance for this issue to the assumptions that underlie this volume, see note 12 in the Introduction.

56. Note that one could accept that a person's desires and interests could be thwarted by an event that occurs at time t even if one does not believe that

the desires and interests in question exist at t. It is possible for an entity or state to undergo (mere Cambridge) changes in its properties after it ceases to exist, and so the non-existence of an interest at t is no bar to its acquiring the property of "being thwarted" at an earlier time (t-n) when it did exist as a result of its being subject to a Cambridge change at t-n. The existence of an entity (or state) E at time t, then, is not necessary for an event A at time t to make it true that property Q can be correctly attributed to E. For a further discussion of posthumous predication see Ruben, "A Puzzle about Posthumous Predication," 211–236.

57. This argument against Lande's views concerning posthumous wrongs is parallel to the argument offered in Chapter 1 against the Feinberg-Pitcher account of how posthumous harm is possible.

58. The ways in which it is possible to accommodate the intuitions that appear to support the view that the dead can be wronged that these arguments have orphaned without endorsing this view were outlined in Chapter 1.

59. One final, brief, argument in favor of the view that the dead can be wronged deserves mention here. J. Jeremy Wisnewski argues that the view that there are no obligations to the dead leads to paradox, and so should be rejected. He begins by noting that making a promise creates a *prima facie* obligation on the promiser. Promises have both legitimacy conditions (conditions that must be met for the promise to be legitimate), and satisfaction conditions (actions that must be performed for the promise to be fulfilled). If A promises to B to perfom an act P after B's death the obligation created seems to be to B, and the satisfaction conditions (do P) are transparent to both A and B. But if there are no obligations to the dead there are no satisfaction conditions for the promise, since one cannot fulfill an obligation to one who is dead. As such, then, while the initial promise had satisfaction conditions when made, it lacked satisfaction conditions when the time came for it to be performed. As such, holds Wisnewski, this promise would both have and lack satisfaction conditions—and this is absurd. And since this absurdity is generated by the assumption there are no obligations to the dead, this assumption should be rejected. (J. Jeremy Wisnewski, "What We Owe the Dead," *Journal of Applied Philosophy* 27, no. 1 (2009), 58–60.) Unfortunately for Wisnewski, as the above outline of the argument makes clear the absurd result that he believes is generated does not hold. Wisnewski fails to recognize that the promise's having satisfaction conditions and its lacking them do not temporally co-exist; the former exists when it is made, and when B is alive, the latter exists after B is dead. And since it would be absurd only were a promise both to have and to lack satisfaction conditions *at the same time* the assumption that there are no obligations owed to the dead does not lead to absurdity, and so the *reductio* that Wisnewski believes he has identified does not exist.

60. For a discussion of this possibility see Jesse M. Bering and Katrina McLeod, "Reasoning about Dead Agents Reveals Possible Adaptive Trends," *Human Nature* 16, no. 4 (2005), 360–381. Less strikingly, it might be that (as discussed in Chapter 1, in the context of accommodating the orphaned intuitions concerning this matter) persons believe that the dead can be wronged because they do not pay enough attention to the underlying justifications for the claims that they make that appear to support this view.

61. Alternatively, one could provide a sociobiological account of how persons *could* (derivatively) be harmed after their deaths by focusing on a person's inclusive genetic fitness through his genetic relatedness to his kin, rather than on the individual phenotype. Here, a person could be harmed after his death if events occurred that adversely affected his inclusive genetic fitness

by adversely affecting the likely reproductive success of his kin. Since such harm would befall the person's genotype, however, this would not be a case of posthumous harm *per se* since the genotype that is harmed (if it is coherent to say that a genotype is harmed) would still exist. I thank Neil Tennant and Paul Bentley for independently suggesting this line of argument to me.

62. Note that this line of reasoning does not establish that one would wrong the dead were one not to respect their wishes; see the responses to Blustein in the context of the Argument from Reciprocity, above. Moreover, not all wishes will be so honored; we might not, as Callahan observes, euthanize a perfectly heathy and contented dog as the death-bed request of his owner; "On Harming the Dead," 350. The line of argument that is offered here is further developed by Ernest Partridge, "Posthumous Interests and Posthumous Respect," *Ethics* 91 (1981), 259–264.

63. It is thus not odd that Epicurus left a will. For a discussion of Epicurus' will in the light of the criticisms leveled against his leaving it by Cicero, see James Warren, *Facing Death*, 162–199. Given these remarks, something other than a general "love of humanity" could motivate persons to respect the wishes of the dead; a love for one's children, for example, or for one's own projects. See D. Goldstick, "The Welfare of the Dead," *Philosophy* 63 (1988), 113.

NOTES TO CHAPTER 5

1. Feinberg, "Harm to Others," 174. This view is also held by Walter Glannon, "Persons, Lives, and Posthumous Harms," *Journal of Social Philosophy* 32 (2001),132. As Bradley observes, Glannon seems to endorse this position because he believes that hedonists must deny that death is a harm to the one who dies, because he believes that "death is bad because it deprives its victim of extrinsic goods". However, as Bradley notes, no deprivation theorist believes this. Bradley, *Well-Being & Death*, 43, n. 78.

2. Ibid., 111

3. Ibid., 44. Bradley notes that a similar point is made by Jens Johansson, *Mortal Beings: On the Metaphysics and Value of Death* (Stockholm: Almquist & Wiksell International, 2005), 98–99. The possibility of separating the view that death is a harm to the person who dies from the view that she might be harmed by events that occur after her death was also noted by Ivan Soll, "On the Purported Insignificance of Death: Whistling before the dark?" in Jeff Malpas and Robert C. Solomon, eds., *Death and Philosophy* (London: Routledge, 1998), 30

4. For reconstructions of Epicurus' argument see Warren, *Facing Death*, 18–19, 23.

5. Epicurus, *Kyriai Doxai*. In Graziano Arrighetti, *Opere* (Turin: Einaudi, 2nd edition, 1973), 123. It is thus important for Epicureans to reject the Democritean doctrine that corpses can experience some residual sensations; see Cicero, *Tusculan Disputations*, trans. J. E. King (Cambridge, MA.: Harvard University Press, 1960), I, xxxiv, 82; 97. For a discussion of this issue see C. C. W. Taylor, *Pleasure, Mind, and Soul: Selected Papers in Ancient Philosophy* (Oxford: Clarendon Press, 2008), Chapter 18.

6. Epicurus, *Letter to Menoeceus*. This translation of this key passage is from David Furley, "Nothing to us?" in Malcolm Schofield and Gisela Striker, eds. *The Norms of Nature: Studies in Hellenistic Ethics* (Cambridge: Cambridge University Press, 1986), 75. For a note on this translation, see Furley, "Nothing to Us?", 75, n. 2 and 3. Note that adopting the proper Epicurean view towards death is compatible with both a desire for immortality and a

desire to lengthen one's life (see Rosenbaum, "Epicurus and Annihilation," in Fischer, ed., *The Metaphysics of Death*, 295)—a point that has obvious implications for bioethical discussions of life-extension technologies. For such a discussion, see Margaret Pabst Battin, *Ending Life: Ethics and the way we die* (New York: Oxford, 2005), 269–276 and Christine Overall, *Aging, Death, and Human Longevity: A Philosophical Inquiry* (Berkeley: University of California Press, 2003). For discussions of whether immortality is actually desirable, see Bernard Williams, "The Makropulos Case: Reflections on the Tedium of Immortality," in Fischer, ed. *The Metaphysics of Death*, 71–92, J. Jeremy Wisnewski, "Is the immortal life worth living?" *International Journal for the Philosophy of Religion* 58 (2005), 27–36, James Lenman, "Immortality: A Letter," *Cogito* 9 (1995), 164–169, John Martin Fischer, "Why Immortality Is Not So Bad," *International Journal of Philosophical Studies* 2, no. 2 (1994), 257–270, "Epicureanism about Death and Immortality," *The Journal of Ethics* 10 (2006), 355–381, John Martin Fischer and Ruth Carl, "Appendix: Philosophical Models of Immortality in Science Fiction," in John Martin Fischer, ed., *Our Stories: Essays on Life, Death, and Free Will* (New York: Oxford University Press, 2009), 93–101, Timothy Chappell, "Infinity Goes Up on Trial: Must Immortality Be Meaningless?" *European Journal of Philosophy* 17, no. 1 (2007), 30–44, and Todd May, *Death* (Stocksfield: Acumen, 2009), Chapter 2.

7. There are many different versions of each of these two primary interpretations. See, for example, Feldman, *Confrontations with the Reaper*, Chapter 8; Kai Draper, "Epicurean Equanimity Towards Death," *Philosophy and Phenomenological Research* 69, no. 1 (2004), 92–114, Stephen Rosenbaum, "How to be Dead and Not Care," 121–122; McMahan, "Death and the Value of Life," 233–242, and Li, *Can Death be a Harm to The Person Who Dies?*, 11–19.

8. Note that this Epicurean argument could be modified so that it is compatible with the truth of a belief in the afterlife; see both the Introduction, and note 15, Chapter 1.

9. This account of harm is drawn from Chapter 3, and will be defended more fully below. Note that on this account of harm an event or a state of affairs must occur for it to cause harm to a person. Thus, even though this account of harm will, as will be argued below, support the claim that a person could be harmed by an event that caused him to have worse experiences than he would have had had it not occurred (even if the experiences that he does have are still positive ones) it will not support the claim that the non-occurrence of an event could harm a person whose life would have gone better than it actually did had that event occurred. This account of harm is thus not subject to the criticism (offered by Kai Draper against Feldman's similarly comparative account of the value that a state of affairs P could hold for a person S, on which "the extrinsic value for S of P = the difference between the intrinsic value for S of the life S would lead if p is true and the intrinsic value for S of the life S would lead if P is false". [*Confrontations With the Reaper*, 150]) that it "expands the notion of a misfortune well beyond its ordinary boundaries". Draper, "Disappointment, Sadness, and Death," 389. For further criticisms of Feldman's comparative account of the value that S has for P, see Earl Conee, "Dispositions Towards Counterfactuals in Ethics" in Kris McDaniel, Jason R. Raibley, Richard Feldman, and Michael J. Zimmerman, eds., *The Good, the Right, Life and Death* (Aldershot, England: Ashgate, 2006), 181–183, and David B. Suits, "Why Death is Not Bad for the One Who Dies," *American Philosophical Quarterly* 38, no. 1 (2001), 73–75.

10. This version of the Hedonic Variant of the Epicurean argument that death cannot be a harm to the person who dies is similar to that developed by Stephen E. Rosenbaum:

   (A) A state of affairs is bad for person P only if P can experience it at some time.

   Therefore,

   (B) P's being dead is bad for P only if it is a state of affairs that P can experience at some time.

   (C) P can experience a state of affairs at some time only if it begins before P's death.

   (D) P's being dead is not a state of affairs that begins before P's death.

   Therefore,

   (E) P's being dead is not a state of affairs that P can experience at some time.

   THEREFORE, P's being dead is not bad for P.

   Stephen Rosenbaum, "How to be Dead and Not Care: A Defense of Epicurus," 121–122. Rosenbaum's neo-Epicurean argument has been criticized by Jack Li. Li argues that premise (A) is based on four assumptions: "(1) 'P exists when a state of affairs (or event) occurs' is a necessary condition for the state of affairs (or event) being a harm . . . for P"; "(2) 'P can (logically or metaphysically) experience a state of affairs (or event)' is a. . . . necessary condition for the state of affairs (or event) being a harm (or bad thing) for P"; "(3) 'P experiences a state of affairs (or event) when the state of affairs (or event) occurs' is a . . . necessary condition for the state of affairs (or event) being a harm (or bad thing) for P"; "(4) 'P experiences and feels a state of affairs (or event) as bad when the state of affairs (or event) occurs' is a *sufficient* condition for the state of affairs or event being a harm (or bad thing) for P. 'P experiences and feels a state of affairs (or event) as good when the state of affairs (or event) occurs' is a *sufficient* condition for the state of affairs (or event) being a good thing for P." *Can Death be a Harm to the Person Who Dies?*, 26. Li then argues that since (1), (3), and (4) of these assumptions are mistaken, Rosenbaum's Epicurean argument should be rejected. There are two points to make in response to this criticism. First, if Rosenbaum accepts a hedonic account of harm similar to that outlined in this volume, and hence distinguishes between extrinsic and intrinsic harms, he need not accept assumptions (1) or (4). (Accepting such a view of harm is compatible with Rosenbaum's neo-Epicurean position.) If he adopts such a view of harm he could accept that an event that occurs prior to a person's existence could cause harm to him (thus rejecting assumption 1), and also that an event that is experienced as intrinsically good or bad by P could still be an extrinsic harm to him (thus rejecting assumption 4). Second, although Rosenbaum (and other neo-Epicureans who offer a hedonically-based version of the Epicurean argument that death is not a harm to the person who dies) must accept assumption (3) (although not necessarily the temporality claim that Li included within it), Li's argument against this assumption is flawed in two respects. To argue that (3) should be rejected Li offers a case in which a man in unaware that his wife is unfaithful to him and that her partner in infidelity has damaged his reputation with false rumors. Li claims that this case shows that (3) (and hence Rosenbaum's argument) should be rejected, for "although . . . [the man in question] . . . does not actually experience this misfortune, we would judge that he was severely harmed by this event" (29). In holding that this man is harmed by the events that *ex hypothesi* have no effect on his experience Li is begging the question against the Epicurean accepter of (3).

11. As such, they will not engage with the debate as to whether Epicurus was concerned with allaying fears about a possible afterlife, rather than with allaying fears about annihilation; see Richard Sorabji, *Self: Ancient and Modern Insights about Individuality, Life, and Death* (Chicago: The University of Chicago Press, 2006), 96, 301.
12. For an argument that it this that we are afraid of, and not death itself (and hence that Epicurus' arguments miss the point), see C. G. Prado, *Coping with Choices to Die* (Cambridge: Cambridge University Press, 2010), Chapter 7.
13. Grieving pet owners, then, can take comfort from the Epicurean view. However, one need not be an Epicurean to hold that an animal's death is not a harm to it; see Ruth Cigman, "Death, Misfortune, and Species Inequality," *Philosophy and Public Affairs* 10, no. 1 (1981), 47–64, and John Harris, "Four Legs Good, Personhood Better!" *Res Publica* 4, no. 1 (1998), 57–58.
14. The phrase "appears to" is included here so as not to beg the question against those who hold that persons do exist prior to their births. For an argument that leads to this (counterintuitive) conclusion, see Silverstein, "The Evil of Death," 109–116. Note that persons who hold that the unborn exist are not thereby committed to the view that they can be harmed, for they might exist in a state in which they are invulnerable to this.
15. Fred Feldman, "Some Puzzles About the Evil of Death," in Fischer, ed., *The Metaphysics of Death*, 314.
16. Ibid., 319.
17. Ibid., 319.
18. This is the approach taken by Warren in response to examples such as Feldman's. See Warren, *Facing Death*, 43. Its implausibility rests on the fact that events can harm persons not only through their occurrence, but also by their effects. See Grey, "Epicurus and the Harm of Death," 359.
19. Ronald Wright, *A Scientific Romance: A Novel* (New York: Picador, 1999).
20. The view that a person's death can be a harm to her by depriving her of the goods is life is extremely common, and is often regarded as a "simple", common-sense point; see, for example, John Broome, *Ethics out of Economics* (Cambridge: Cambridge University Press, 1999), 173.
21. Jeff McMahan terms this the *Wide Experience Requirement*, distinguishing it from what he terms the *Narrow Experience Requirement*; "that an event can be bad for a person only if he experiences it as bad". "Death and the Value of Life," 234.
22. This objection to Epicurean arguments has been offered by McMahan, ibid., 234.
23. See, for example, Feldman, *Confrontations with the Reaper*, Chapters 8 and 9; Thomas Nagel, "Death," in Fischer, ed., *The Metaphysics of Death*, 59–69; L. W. Sumner, "A Matter of Life and Death," *Nous* 10 (1976), 162, 165–166. McMahan also has a deprivation view of death's badness, but does not claim that death is bad for the person who dies; instead, he claims that the harm of death is a "quasi-impersonal" harm. "Death and the Value of Life," 240.
24. Nagel, "Death," 62, 64. See also Thomas Nagel, *The View from Nowhere* (New York: Oxford University Press, 1986), 230.
25. Nagel, "Death," 65.
26. The phrase "misfortune to" has been used instead of the more usual "misfortune for" to avoid confusion, given the distinction between "harm to" and "harm for" that is used in this volume.
27. As Stephan Blatti notes, the consensus among those who believe that death can be a harm to those who die is that it is so in virtue of its depriving them

of the goods of life. But, in addition to this putative harm of death, Blatti also holds that there is another distinctive harm that death visits upon an autonomous agent: that "no exercise of her autonomy fails to be possibly limited, and this limitation is intrinsically harmful". "Death's Distinctive Harm," *American Philosophical Quarterly*, forthcoming. Blatti acknowledges that this view is based on the assumption that autonomy is intrinsically valuable. As such, while novel, this account of how death can harm its autonomous victims is subject to the criticism that autonomy is not intrinsically valuable. See, for example, Taylor, *Practical Autonomy and Bioethics*, Chapter 10.

28. Feldman, *Confrontations with the Reaper*, 137–140; Bradley, *Well-Being & Death*, chapter 2.
29. Feldman, *Confrontations with the Reaper*, 138.
30. Ibid., 138.
31. Ibid., 139.
32. Bradley, *Well-Being & Death*, 48. Here, something is instrumentally good for a person in virtue of its leading to other things that are good for her, while something is intrinsically good for a person if it is good for her even if it does not lead to any other good things. These characterizations of something's being instrumentally (extrinsically) good for a person and something's being intrinsically good for her are outlined in Bradley, ibid., 3.
33. Ibid., 49. See also David Lewis, *Counterfactuals* (New York, Blackwell, 1973); Robert Stalnaker, *Inquiry* (Cambridge, Mass.: MIT Press, 1984).
34. Bradley, *Well-Being & Death*, 49. Bradley follows Lewis in analyzing closeness in terms of similarity. (See David Lewis, *On the Plurality of Worlds* (New York: Blackwell, 1986), 20–27.) Bradley notes that which world is closest is not always determinate, since this "depends on which features of actual world we want to keep fixed, or on what similarity relation we are employing." *Well-Being & Death*, 49.
35. Ibid., 50.
36. Ibid., 50
37. Williams, "The Makropulos Case: Reflections on the Tedium of Immortality," 76.
38. Ibid., 76–77.
39. Glenn Braddock, "Epicureanism, Death, and the Good Life", *Philosophical Inquiry* 22 (2000), 55.
40. See also Martha Nussbaum, "The Damage of Death: Incomplete Arguments and False Consolations," in Taylor, ed., *The Metaphysics and Ethics of Death*, forthcoming. Note that this does not commit one to claiming that the intelligent man ceases to exist *simpliciter*, and so it does not beg the question against those who believe that the dead continue to exist. This response to Nagel is rejected by Brian Sayers on the grounds that it "threatens to overpopulate us with subjects," supporting this claim by noting that if it is accepted "we would have to posit hundreds of subjects, one having existed for perhaps sixty years, subsequent ones merely a week or two" in cases of humans who suffer from Alzheimer's disease. "Death as a Loss," 153. As an objection to this response to Nagel, however, this is weak, for it is not implausible to believe that several subjects do exist in such cases. For an illuminating discussion of whether persons can be said to survive brain injuries, see Walter Glannon, "Brain Injury and Survival," in Taylor, ed., *The Metaphysics and Ethics of Death*, forthcoming.
41. This man would thus be relevantly similar to a person who was harmed by a slander that she never suspects, even though its effects adversely affect her experiences.

42. O.H. Green further argues that Nagel's objection to the Epicurean position should be rejected on the basis that the state of the intelligent man when reduced to the position of a contented infant is not a subjective evil for him, for "Consciousness of a state or event which is a subjective good or evil is necessary for its being so," and this man is not conscious of his reduced condition. "Fear of Death," *Philosophy and Phenomenological Research* XLIII, no. 1 (1982), 100–101.

43. Objections to Feldman's arguments here have been offered in James S. Taylor, "Nothing in the Dark: Deprivation, Death, and the Good Life," in Noel Carroll and Lester H. Hunt, eds., *Philosophy in the Twilight Zone* (Oxford: Blackwell, 2009), 178–181.

44. A similar objection to deprivation arguments of the sort that Feldman employs has been offered by Silverstein, who notes that the "life-life" comparisons of the sort that Feldman employs in his two examples are irrelevant to addressing the Epicurean claim that "life-death" comparisons of the form "*A*'s death is worse for *A* than *A*'s (continued) life is (bad) for *A*" are incoherent. See "The Evil of Death," 96–100; the quotation is from 97. For further criticisms of Feldman's arguments here see John M. Collins, "Feldman's Account of Death's Badness, and Life-Death Comparatives," *Southwest Philosophy Review* 21, no. 2 (2005), 90–95.

45. Bradley develops this example to object to the first premise of the version of the Existence Variant of the Epicurean argument that he considers: "(1) Anything that is bad for someone must be bad for that person at a particular time. (2) There is no time at which death is bad for the one who dies. (Death is not bad for someone before she dies, since it has not occurred yet; it is not bad for her once she dies, because from that point on she no longer exists.) Therefore, (3) death is not bad for the one who dies." *Well-Being & Death*, 73.

46. Ibid., 76

47. Ibid., 76

48. Ibid., 77

49. Hence, Bradley holds that the version of the Existence Variant of this Epicurean argument that he considers should be rejected, for its first premise is mistaken. Bradley offers other examples of apparently timeless evils, such as "the evil of never seeing one's beloved again," and the evil of never getting what one deserves. Ibid., 77–78.

50. Ibid., 78; Aristotle, *Nicomachean Ethics*, 1115a27, in McKeon, trans. and ed., *The Basic Works of Aristotle*, 975.

51. Bradley acknowledges this in the context of discussing subsequentism, when discussing the Difference-Making Principle for Times: "The overall value of event E for subject S at world w and time t = the intrinsic value of t for S at w minus the intrinsic value of t for S at the nearest possible world to w at which E does not occur". (Note that Bradley here suppresses the relativization to similarity conditions for ease of exposition.) *Well-Being & Death*, 90, and 90, n. 32.

52. Grey, "Epicurus and the Harm of Death," 364; quoted by Bradley, *Well-Being & Death*, 92. Bradley notes that this strategy could work for the other examples of apparently timeless evil that he mentioned, such as the evil of not getting what one deserves.

53. This is how Williams's argument is (plausibly) construed by Silverstein; see "The Evil of Death," 100–102. On this understanding Williams's argument is, as Silverstein notes, subject to the criticisms that beset that of other deprivation-based arguments (such as Feldman's) that move from claims concerning life-life comparisons to claims concerning life-death comparisons.

54. Williams, "The Makropulos Case," 77.
55. Bradley has developed these arguments for use against the version of the Existence Variant of Epicurean argument that is outlined in note 45, above.
56. Ibid., 80
57. Ibid., 81.
58. As Bradley neatly puts it, "The eternalist thinks of existence-at-a-time in the same way as existence-at-a-place". Ibid., 81.
59. Ibid., 82.
60. Ruben, "A Puzzle about Posthumous Predication," 213. Sperling attributes this to Ruben as his view ("For, as David Hillel-Ruben [sic] himself argues, 'if a property is true of some object at t, then surely the object of which the property is true at t must itself exist at t, just in order to display or exemplify that property at that time'.") [David-Hillel Ruben, *Action and its Explanation* (Oxford: Clarendon Press, 2003), 11–12] and then criticizes him for it. (Sperling, *Posthumous Interests*, 31.) However, as Ruben makes clear, this is a view that he *rejects*—the sentence from Ruben quoted by Sperling, above, is introduced with the sentence "The thought that generates the puzzle of posthumous predication seems to me to be deep and initially compelling, *even though finally wrong*." (Ruben, *Action and Its Explanation*, 11, emphasis added.) That Ruben rejects this view (rather than endorsing it, as Sperling holds) is not surprising, since the article in which it first appears is an article in which Ruben offers an account of how posthumous predication (the predication of properties to objects that no longer exist) is possible. See Ruben, "A Puzzle about Posthumous Predication," 214.
61. Ibid., 224. For an argument that this solves the puzzle of posthumous predication see ibid., 224–236.
62. However, even the standard view that for a relation to hold at t between two relata they must both exist at t need not pose any problems for presentism. As Bourne argues, presentists should claim that any genuine relations that might exist between spatio-temporal objects "are all either (a) spatio-temporal or (b) causal relations". (*A Future for Presentism*, 95). Arguing that presentists can account for temporal relations using just "conjunction, the notion of truth *simpliciter* for *u*-propositions, and the *greater than* relation defined over real numbers," Bourne then holds that they should then deny that *cause*s is a genuine relation. (Ibid., 97). Those relations that seem to hold between relata at different times which fall into neither category (a) nor category (b) (e.g., such as *taller than*) are determinables, which the presentist could deny are genuine relations. (Ibid., 96).
63. As Mark Hinchliff notes, "on the description theory, reference is determined by a cluster of properties associated with the name. All that the presentist requires is that the properties be suitably tensed so as not to imply that past objects exist. On the causal theory, reference is determined by a causal chain linking name to referent. All that the presentist requires is that the chain be specified in suitably tensed terms so as not to imply that past objects exist." "The Puzzle of Change," *Noûs* 30, *Supplement: Philosophical Perspectives 10, Metaphysics* (1996), 125. See also Bourne's account of how presentists can avoid committing themselves to holding that statements involving the proper names of past objects (such as "Socrates") are meaningless, which is based on elucidating A.N. Prior as holding that general statements can be made about past individuals, even if singular statements cannot be, as "proper names (at least for past objects) should be treated not as referring expressions, but as quantifier phrases, in the style of Russell's theory of ordinary proper names . . . which utilizes his theory of descriptions . . ." (*A Future for Presentism*, 99–101, esp. 101; the quotation is from 100; Bourne refers to A.N. Prior,

"Now," in A. N. Prior, *Papers on Time and Tense* [Oxford: Clarendon Press, 2003], 171–193). Russell's theory of ordinary proper names can be found in his "Knowledge by Acquaintance and Knowledge by Description," *Proceedings of the Aristotelian Society* 11 (1911), 108–128, and his "Lectures of the Philosophy of Logical Atomism," in Bertrand Russell, ed. R.C. Marsh, *Logic and Knowledge. (Essays 1901–1950)* (London: Routledge, 1956), 175–281. For Bourne's arguments that a version of the causal theory of reference is available to presentists, see *A Future for Presentism*, 103–108, and chapter 4. For an interesting discussion of how it is possible to refer to objects that do not exist "right now" see Palle Yourgrau, "Kripke's Moses," in Taylor, ed., *The Metaphysics and Ethics of Death*, forthcoming.

64. Note, though, that presentists differ on the possibility of the predicating properties to non-existent entities. Unrestricted Presentism holds that objects can have properties and stand in relations even when they do not exist, while Serious Presentism holds that existence is a necessary condition for both the possession of properties and standing in relations. See Ned Markosian, "A Defense of Presentism," in Dean W. Zimmerman, ed., *Oxford Studies in Metaphysics, volume 1* (Oxford: Clarendon Press, 2004), 51–52.

65. See Ruben, "A Puzzle about Posthumous Predication," 214.

66. See James Warren, *Epicurus and Democritean Ethics: An Archaeology of Ataraxia* (Cambridge: Cambridge University Press, 2002), 3–4. See also Julia Annas, *The Morality of Happiness* (New York: Oxford University Press, 1993), chapters 7 and 16, David Konstan, *Some Aspects of Epicurean Psychology* (Leiden: E.J. Brill, 1973), 10 ff, Raphael Woolf, "Pleasure and Desire," in James Warren, ed., *The Cambridge Companion to Epicureanism* (New York: Cambridge University Press, 2009), 158–178, and "What Kind of Hedonist was Epicurus?" *Phronesis* X:IX, no. 4 (2004), 303–322, Philip Mitsis, *Epicurus' Ethical Theory: The Pleasures of Invulnerability* (Ithaca: Cornell University Press, 1988), Chapter 1, Martha Nussbaum, *The Therapy of Desire*, 212 ff, Michael Trapp, *Philosophy in the Roman Empire: Ethics, Politics, and Society* (Aldershot: Ashgate, 2007), 40–41, John M. Cooper, *Reason and Emotion: Essays on ancient moral psychology and ethical theory* (Princeton: Princeton University Press, 1999), Chapter 22, Mitsis, *Epicurus' Ethical Theory*, Chapter 1, Boris Nikolsky, "Epicurus on Pleasure," *Phronesis* XLVI, no. 4 (2001), 440–465, Stephen E. Rosenbaum, "Epicurus on Pleasure and the Complete Life," *Monist* 73, no. 1 (1990), 21–41, Gisela Striker, "Epicurean hedonism," in Jacques Brunschwig and Martha C. Nussbaum, eds., *Passions and Perceptions: Studies in Hellenistic Philosophy of Mind Proceedings of the Fifth Symposium Hellenisticum* (Cambridge: Cambridge University Press, 1993), 1–17, Clay Spawn, "Updating Epicurus's Concept of *Katastematic* Pleasure," *The Journal of Value Inquiry* 36 (2002), 473–482, James Warren, "Epicurus and the Pleasures of the Future," in David Sedley, ed., *Oxford Studies in Ancient Philosophy XXI* (Oxford: Clarendon Press, 2001), 135–179, and Malte Hossenfelder, "Epicurus—hedonist malgre lui," in Schofield and Striker, eds. *The Norms of Nature*, 245–263.

67. A point made by Philodemus, *On Death*, III 30–36; 8. For a discussion of this see Braddock, "Epicureanism, Death, and the Good Life," 58, and Tsouna, *The Ethics of Philodemus*, 255. Draper, however, argues that "it is quite likely that Epicurus himself was a deprivationist and so rejected the 'Epicurean view' that death cannot be to the advantage or disadvantage of its subject". Draper, "Epicurean Equanimity Towards Death," 104. Draper holds this view since he believes that were Epicurus to reject it "he would have been committed to the proposition that even if one would be showered with blessings should one's life continue, one would have no good egoistic

reason to make the slightest effort to avoid death . . . But there is no suggestion of such an extreme position in the surviving works of Epicurus." Ibid., 104. Draper's attribution of this deprivationist position to Epicurus is thus based on the view that if life is a good for one, and so one has reason to pursue its continuance, then the cessation of life will be a harm. But the apodosis clause does not follow from the protasis. It is not analytic to hold that the absence of something that is a good for one is thereby a harm to one, *especially* if the absence occurs as a result of one's nonexistence, and so without further argument there is no reason to accept the attribution to this deprivationist position to Epicurus.

68. Note that while the Epicurean arguments considered here will be supported by those offered by Lucretius, they are independent of it; the converse is not, however, true of the Lucretian arguments vis a vis their Epicurean predecessors, as will be observed in the next Chapter.

NOTES TO CHAPTER 6

1. Lucretius is not the only ancient philosopher to have offered such an argument; as Stephen Rosenbaum has noted, versions of it have also appeared in Pseudo-Plato, Cicero, Seneca, and Plutarch. See his "The Symmetry Argument: Lucretius Against the Fear of Death," *Philosophy and Phenomenological Research* 50, no. 2 (1989), 354.

2. Although, according to James Boswell, David Hume was convinced by a version of it, and drew comfort from it as he was dying. See Charles McC. Weis and Frederick A. Pottle, eds., *Boswell in Extremes 1776–1778* (New York: McGraw-Hill Book Company, Inc., 1970), 12. For an interesting account of what Hume was reading on his deathbed, see Annette C. Baier, *Death and Character: Further reflections on Hume* (Cambridge, Mass.: Harvard University Press, 2008), Chapter 6.

3. For a wonderful discussion of *De Rerum Natura* see Charles Segal's monumental *Lucretius on Death and Anxiety: Poetry and philosophy in De Rerum Natura* (Princeton: Princeton University Press, 1990). For an excellent discussion of *De Rerum Natura* III 830–1094 see Barbara Price Wallach, *Lucretius and the Diatribe Against the Fear of Death: De Rerum Natura* III 830–1094 (Leiden: E. J. Brill, 1976).

4. Lucretius, *De Rerum Natura* , trans. W. H. D. Rouse, revised by Martin Ferguson Smith (Cambridge, Mass.: Harvard University Press, 2006), 3.830–43; 253.

5. Ibid., 3.972–6; 265.

6. Nussbaum identifies two further arguments thanatological arguments in Lucretius; the "banquet" argument, in which he holds that, like a banquet, life has a structure which has a natural end point, and the "population" argument, that there is a need for the old to die to avoid overpopulation. Nussbaum discusses these in *The Therapy of Desire*, Chapter 6. For a discussion of Nussbaum's views on the banquet argument, see John Martin Fischer, "Contribution to Symposium on Nussbaum's *The Therapy of Desire*," *Philosophy and Phenomenological Research* 59 (1999), 787–792, and "Epicureanism About Death and Immortaility," in Fischer, ed., *Our Stories*, 121–124, and Tim O'Keefe, "Lucretius on the Cycle of Life and the Fear of Death," *Apeiron* 36, no. 1 (2003), 43–65. See also Nussbaum's initial reply to Fischer, "Reply to Papers in Symposium on Nussbaum, *The Therapy of Desire*," *Philosophy and Phenomenological Research* 59 (1999), 811–812. For further discussion of the view that persons' lives can have a narrative

structure in the context of a discussion of whether death can be a harm to the person who dies (albeit one without reference to Lucretius' banquet argument) see James Lindemann Nelson, "Death's Gender," in Margaret Urban Walker, ed., *Mother Time: Women, Aging, and Ethics* (Lanham, Md.: Rowman & Littlefield Publishers, Inc., 1999), 121–124, and Warren, *Facing Death*, Chapter 4. An alternative (and highly unusual) way of understanding Lucretius' symmetry argument has been developed by Joseph Raz in the context of a discussion of whether life is intrinsically valuable. Raz distinguishes between "longevity preferences" (i.e., to live for as long as possible) and "time-location preferences" (to live at a particular time). Raz holds that Lucretius' symmetry argument is designed to show that persons should not hold a longevity preference. As understood by Raz, Lucretius' argument is based on the claim that persons cannot both hold a longevity preference and an asymmetrical time-location preference, for if one holds an asymmetrical time-location preference one will not prefer a *longer* life, but only that one now receive *more* life. Thus, since persons' time-location preferences are always asymmetrical, persons do not have a longevity preference. Joseph Raz, *Value, Respect, and Attachment* (Cambridge: Cambridge University Press, 2001), 88–99. Raz's understanding of Lucretius argument has been trenchantly criticized by Warren on both exegetical and philosophical grounds. See Warren, *Facing Death*, 93–100.

7. This is not always true; consider, for example, the person described by Nabokov in his autobiographical work *Speak, Memory* who was horrified to see a home movie produced a few weeks before he was born, where his perambulator was waiting for him. Quoted by Sorabji, *Self*, 338–339. But such cases at least border on the pathological.

8. Warren argues persuasively that only the ontological version of this argument is supported by Lucretius' text; see James Warren, "Lucretius, Symmetry arguments, and fearing death," *Phronesis* LXVI, no. 4 (2001), 466–480. See also Furley, "Nothing to Us?", 76. However, since the focus of this volume is on establishing the truth of the claim that death cannot be a harm to the person who dies, rather than on providing an accurate exegesis of the ancient arguments for this conclusion, any exegetical support that can be drawn for the focus on the ontological version of this Lucretian argument will be eschewed.

9. The possibility that this lack of rational responsiveness to arguments concerning death and posthumous harms and wrongs might be the result of evolutionary adaptation was briefly discussed at the end of Chapter 4.

10. Even if a person's distress at the prospect of his own death originates from his belief that it will be a harm to him the removal of this belief will not itself guarantee the extinction of his distress, for a person's emotions towards particular objects can survive the removal of their rational basis. For a discussion of why this might be so (albeit with respect to a person's actions, rather than emotions, although the argument is readily generalized) see Robert Noggle, "Autonomy, Value, and Conditioned Desire," *American Philosophical Quarterly* 32, no. 1 (1995), 57–69. Of course, noting this is not intended to undercut Jeffrie Murphy's correct observation that "rational thinking sometimes provides solace for some people—e.g., witness the lives and deaths of Spinoza, Hume, and Freud". "Rationality and the Fear of Death," *The Monist* 59 (1976), 188. See also Rosenbaum, "The Symmetry Argument," 355.

11. The reasonableness of such distress is not disputed by Epicureans, and so the proponents of the Lucretian argument outlined above do not intend it to ameliorate it.

12. Note that it is important here that such a person feels *distress* while contemplating his own death, rather than *fearing* it, for while distress at the thought of the occurrence of an event or a state of affairs that one holds to be intrinsically bad might be warranted, it is not clear that persons should fear the occurrence of such events or states of affairs unless they are directly related to them (e.g., they cause them pain).

13. Mill, *Utilitarianism*, 35. Note, too, that such a person might be especially susceptible to endorsing the Backfire Problem that will be outlined below, if he believes that it is not just his death but his nonexistence as an experiencing being that is the intrinsic bad that is the object of his distress.

14. Nagel, "Death," 67–68. Nagel does not here distinguish clearly between the ontological and the attitudinal versions of the Lucretian argument, but it is clear that his objection, if sound, will undermine the ontological version.

15. Rosenbaum, "The Symmetry Argument," 368. A version of this argument has also been developed by Fred Feldman, "Some Puzzles about the Evil of Death," in Fischer, 323.

16. This was noted, although not endorsed, by Richard Sorabji, *Time, Creation, and the Continuum: Theories in antiquity and the early middle ages* (Ithaca: Cornell University Press, 1983), 179.

17. Feldman, "Some Puzzles about the Evil of Death," 323.

18. Noted by Rosenbaum, "The Symmetry Argument," 368.

19. Feldman, *Confrontations with the Reaper*, 154–155.

20. Derek Parfit, *Reasons and Persons*, 165–166.

21. Ibid., 167.

22. Seneca, *Epistulae Morales*, 77.12. Trans. R. M. Gummere. Available at: http://www.molloy.edu/sophia/seneca/epistles/ep77.htm Accessed July 20th, 2010. The symmetry argument that Seneca discusses in these passages is similar to the Lucretian argument, although it draws its symmetry between the foolishness exhibited by two different persons, rather than between the equivalence of the time that exists prior to, and following after, one person's life. This argument occurs in Seneca at 77.11.

23. Note that on the Stoic account of fate neither the period of time prior to a person's birth, nor the period of time after his death, could ever be correctly said to belong to him, for it is fated that he will never exist contemporaneously with them. (These periods of time are *aliena*.) If this is correct, then counterfactual accounts of how death can be a harm to the person who dies (such as Feldman's) which trade on the idea that a person could have lived longer than he did, and thus is deprived by death of the goods of life that he could have had, are mistaken, for the time of a person's death is *necessarily* fixed. For a discussion of this point see D. N. Sedley. "Chrysippus on psychophysical causality," in J. Brunschwig and M. Nussbaum, eds., *Passions and Perceptions: studies in Hellenistic philosophy of mind* (Cambridge: Cambridge University Press, 1993), 316–318.

24. Although Seneca's point would still hold even if one rejected the Stoic account of fate, provided that one accepted the truth of metaphysical determinism.

25. Stephen Hetherington, "Lucretian Death: Asymmetries and Agency," *American Philosophical Quarterly* 42, no. 3 (2005), 212. Hetherington uses the term "almost" to accommodate what Nagel calls "the brief margin permitted by premature labor". Quoted by Hetherington,"Lucretian Death," 217, n. 6. Hetherington's argument is here dubbed an *anti*-Stoic argument because it is based on counterfactual claims concerning a person's earlier birth and later death that would be rejected by the Stoics.

26. Ibid., 212.

27. Ibid., 212.

28. Ibid., 212.
29. Rosenbaum, "The Symmetry Argument," 362. Rosenbaum notes that Nagel claims that a person could not have been born earlier than she was, but notes that the issue is really about whether one could have been *conceived* earlier, rather than *born* earlier, since the Lucretian argument concerns the symmetry between pre-natal and postmortem non-existence, and it seems that persons cease to be non-existent once they are conceived. Two points should be noted here. First, Rosenbaum's argument (and that of Lucretius) can accommodate the claim that the unborn exist, for if this is true the arguments could simply be modified to the claim that persons do not exist pre-natally as experiencing beings, and it is the existence of persons *qua* such beings that is at issue. Second—and importantly, given the arguments below—Rosenbaum's assumption that persons come into existence at the moment of conception is mistaken, for two reasons. First, it is possible that a zygote could split after conception to form monozygotic twins, and so the point at which a person could be said to have come into existence should occur after such splitting is possible. Second, since it is plausible to hold that persons are not identical with their organisms, but, instead, with (at least) certain mental states, persons will only come into existence once these mental states appear. As such, then, persons are never identical with embryos, although they owe their origins to them. See Jeff McMahan, "The Lucretian Argument," in Kris McDaniel, Jason R. Raibley, Richard Feldman, and Michael J. Zimmerman, eds., *The Good, the Right, Life and Death: Essays in Honor of Fred Feldman* (Aldershot, England: Ashgate Publishing Co., 2006), 214.
30. Nagel, "Death," 68.
31. See S. Kripke, "Naming and Necessity," in D. Davidson and G. Harman, eds., *Semantics of Natural Language* (Dordrecht: Reidel, 1972), 314. That Nagel seems to be relying on this Kripkean point has also been noted by Rosenbaum, "The Symmetry Argument," 362–363, n.31, and Philip Mitsis, "Epicurus on Death and the Duration of Life" in *Proceedings of the Boston Area Colloquium in Ancient Philosophy* 4 (1989), 309.
32. Rosenbaum, "The Symmetry Argument," 363. Accepting that a person's genetic origin is essential to her identity is not the same as accepting that she must owe her origins to a particular set of gametes, for there is no (conceptual) bar to there being numerically distinct but qualitatively identical gametes.
33. Ibid., 363.
34. Frederik Kaufman, "Death and Deprivation; Or, Why Lucretius' Symmetry Argument Fails," *Australasian Journal of Philosophy* 74, no. 2 (1996), 307.
35. Ibid., 307.
36. Ibid., 307. Kaufman notes that Lucretius was also concerned about psychological personhood, quoting him as claiming that " . . . if time should gather together our substance after our decease and bring it back again as it is now placed, if once more the light of life should be vouchsafed to us, yet, even were that done, it would not concern us at all, when once the remembrance of our former selves were snapped in twain." *DRN*, III, 854; quoted by Kaufman, "Death and Deprivation," 308.
37. Ibid., 308.
38. Ibid., 309. A similar point is made by Peter C. Dalton, "Death and Evil," *The Philosophical Forum* XI, no. 2 (1979–1980), 209, and Christopher Belshaw, "Death, Pain, and Time," *Philosophical Studies* 97, no. 3 (2000), 337.
39. Kaufman, "Death and Deprivation," 309.
40. Ibid., 309.
41. Nagel, "Death," 68.

42. Versions of this argument also appear in Frederik Kaufman, "An answer to Lucretius' symmetry argument against the fear of death," *Journal of Value Inquiry* 29, no. 1 (1995), 57–64, and "Pre-Vital and Post-Mortem Non-Existence," *American Philosophical Quarterly* 36, no. 1 (1999), 1–19.
43. This objection is developed by McMahan, "The Lucretian Argument," 215, and, more elaborately, by Anthony Brueckner and John Martin Fischer, "Being born earlier," *Australasian Journal of Philosophy* 76, no. 1 (1998), 110–114.
44. Brueckner and Fischer, "Being born earlier," 111. Note that Brueckner and Fischer do not believe that our pre-vital times are symmetrical with our post-mortem times, for they agree with Parfit that we have a natural bias towards the future. See their "Why is Death Bad?" *Philosophical Studies* 50 (1986), 213–221. For trenchant criticisms of their view see Ishtiyaque Haji, "Pre-vital and Post-Vital Times," *Pacific Philosophical Quarterly* 72 (1991), 171–180.
45. Ibid., 111.
46. Ibid., 113.
47. Kaufman, "Pre-Vital and Post-Mortem Non-Existence," 11–13; John Martin Fischer and Daniel Speak, "Death and the Psychological Conception of Personal Identity," in John Martin Fischer, ed., *Our Stories: Essays on Life, Death, and Free Will* (New York: Oxford University Press, 2009), 52–54.
48. Kaufman, "Pre-Vital and Post-Mortem Non-Existence," 12.
49. Fischer and Speak, "Death and the Psychological Conception of Personal Identity," 54. Like Nagel and Kaufman, Fischer and Speak accept the mistaken view that a person's death could be bad for her if it deprives her of the goods of life that she would have otherwise had. It is not clear, however, why Fischer and Speak concede to Kaufman that a person's thick self could not have existed earlier, given the arguments offered in Anthony L. Brueckner and John Martin Fischer, "Why is Death Bad?" in Fischer, ed., *Our Stories*, 27–35. (This latter paper was first published in 1986; the paper by Fischer and Speak was first published in 2000.) Fischer, however, retracts this concession in his "Earlier Birth and Later Death: Symmetry through Thick and Thin," in McDaniel et al., eds., *The Good, the Right, Life and Death*, 195.
50. Fischer and Speak, "Death and the Psychological Conception of Personal Identity," 55.
51. Ibid., 56.
52. Frederik Kaufman, "Thick and Thin Selves: A Reply to Fischer and Speak," in French and Wettstein, eds., *Midwest Studies in Philosophy Volume XXIV*, 96–97.
53. Fischer, "Earlier Birth and Later Death," 195.
54. Ibid., 195.
55. Such a self is a person in Frankfurt's sense, in that it could form second-order volitions. See Harry G. Frankfurt, "Freedom of the Will and the Concept of a Person," in Harry G. Frankfurt, ed., *The Importance of What We Care About* (New York: Cambridge University Press, 1988), 12–16.
56. Fischer, "Earlier Birth and Later Death," 195.
57. Kaufman, "Thick and Thin Selves," 96.
58. The reason why "conception" is used here rather than birth will become clear below.
59. The focus of this argument is on a person's conception rather than her birth to allow for the fact that a fetus can feel pain, and thus can be harmed.
60. Note that this is distinct from the claim that no event that occurs prior to a person's conception could harm her. Note, too, that if one wishes both to retain the structure of the Hedonic Variant of the Epicurean argument developed in Chapter 5, and remain neutral on the question of whether persons

exist pre-natally, one could add in a further premise: (5) A person's pre-natal existence does not occur after her conception, which, together with premise (4), will support the conclusion: Therefore, a person's pre-natal existence is not a harm to her.

61. Rosenbaum correctly argues that the proponents of the attitudinal version of this Lucretian argument can meet the Backfire Problem without drawing on additional Epicurean support in this way. See Rosenbaum, "The Symmetry Argument," 369–373

62. That the proponent of this Lucretian argument should respond in this way to the Backfire Problem shows that this argument should not be taken to provide an argument that operates independently of the original Epicurean argument for the view that death is not a harm to the person who dies. Instead, as was noted at the end of the previous Chapter, it should be understood as an argument that is designed simply to reinforce the original Epicurean conclusion.

63. Feldman, *Confrontations with the Reaper*, 154 (italics added).

64. It also has no direct bearing on the attitudinal version of this argument, for to undermine that argument Feldman must undermine the intuitive force of premise (3), which is ignored by his *explanation* of why persons have the attitudes that they do (rather than a *justification* of why they should have them).

65. Kaufman, "Pre-Vital and Post-Mortem Non-Existence," 7–8. It is not at all clear that Kaufman's latter claim is true!

66. Ibid., 8.

67. Parfit claims that persons' bias towards the future is simply a contingent matter, and that persons could have temporal attitudes that are different than they currently are. To support this claim he develops the example of Timeless, who is distressed to discover that he experienced past pains, and pleased to hear that he will experience future enjoyment. Parfit, *Reasons and Persons*, 174. Having noted that were persons to be like Timeless it would be easier for them to appreciate Symmetry Arguments (at least in their attitudinal form), Kaufman argues that Timeless is not conceivable, for if he were a person Prior who is "biased toward the past and indifferent toward the future" would also be conceivable. ("Pre-Vital and Post-Mortem Non-Existence," 8). However, argues Kaufman, Prior is not conceivable as an agent, for his indifference towards the future makes it "hard to see how he can intend anything, make choices, or have a will," and so it seems that Parfit's optimism about the fungibility of persons' temporal attitudes is misplaced. (Ibid., 9.) Kaufman is mistaken here; for Prior is not conceivable because he is indifferent towards the future. Timeless, however, is not so indifferent, and so that Prior is, is of no relevance to the conceivability of Timeless.

68. Kaufman, "Pre-Vital and Post-Mortem Non-Existence, 9.

69. Similar objections can be leveled against F.M. Kamm's arguments that death is bad to the person who dies whereas pre-natal non-existence is not on the grounds that death, but not pre-natal non-existence, is an "Insult" to persons (in that it "takes away what we think of as already ours and . . . emphasizes our vulnerability), and inspires "Terror" in them. See F.M. Kamm, "Why is Death Bad and Worse than Pre-natal Non-existence?" *Pacific Philosophical Quarterly* 69 (1988), 162–163. For a response to Kamm that is similar to that developed above in response to the possible use of Parfit's hospital example to undermine this Lucretian argument, see Fred Feldman, "F.M. Kamm and the Mirror of Time," *Pacific Philosophical Quarterly* 71 (1990), 23–27.

70. Walter Glannon, "Temporal Asymmetry, Life, and Death," *American Philosophical Quarterly* 31, no. 3 (1994), 240. Glannon cites E. O'Callaghan, et

al., "Schizophrenia after Prenatal Exposure to 1957 A2 Influenza Epidemic," *The Lancet* 337 (1991), 1248–1250.

71. For literary examples of this point see Edwin Brock's pessimism about the middle of the twentieth century in his "Five Ways to Kill a Man," (available at: http://www.davidpbrown.co.uk/poetry/edwin-brock.html ; accessed January 18th, 2010), or the relative levels of danger assigned to traveling to different periods of history in Connie Willis, *Doomsday Book* (New York: Spectra, 1993).

NOTES TO CHAPTER 7

1. See, for example, Barry R. Schaller, *Understanding Bioethics and the Law: The promises and perils of the brave new world of biotechnology* (Westport, Conn.: Praeger, 2008), chapter 4, Jonathan Glover, *Causing Death and Saving Lives* (Harmondsworth: Penguin Books, 1977), 201, and John Bigelow, John Campbell, and Robert Pargetter, "Death and Well-Being," *Pacific Philosophical Quarterly* 71 (1990), 119–140. Strangely, this view was endorsed by the Epicurean Philodemus—although in fairness to him it should be noted that he endorsed the view that "the foolish" would be better off dying young in the context of sneering at those (non-Epicureans) who thought that it is pitiable to die young. Philodemus, *On Death* XII.26-XIII.17, 28, 30. The view that *everyone* would be comparatively better off dead was allegedly argued for by Hegesias; see Wallace I. Matson, "Hegesias the Death-Persuader: or, the Gloominess of Hedonism," *Philosophy* 73 (1998), 553–557. For a defense of Epicurus' response to this view, see Fred D. Milller, Jr., "Epicurus on the Art of Dying," *The Southern Journal of Philosophy* 14, no. 2 (1976), 171.
2. William Shakespeare, *Hamlet*, III.1. In William Shakespeare, *The Complete Works of William Shakespeare* (New York: Avenel Books, 1975), 1088. For examples of arguments in favor of suicide see Mary Rose Barrington, "Apologia for Suicide," in M. Pabst Battin and David J. Majo, eds., *Suicide: The Philosophical Issues* (New York: St. Martin's Press, 1980), 90–103; M. Pabst Battin, "Suicide: A Fundamental Human Right?" in Battin and Majo, eds., *Suicide*, 268; Richard B. Brandt, *Morality, utilitarianism, and rights* (Cambridge: Cambridge University Press, 1992), 320–323, and C.G. Prado, *Choosing to Die: Elective death and multiculturalism* (Cambridge: Cambridge University Press, 2008). An alternative justification of suicide that is nevertheless compatible with (although not committed to) the view that a person might be "better off dead" is offered by Christine M. Korsgaard, who holds that suicide could be justifiable if it is the only way to preserve one's identity against the ravages of "severe illness, disability, and pain". Korsgaard, *The Sources of Normativity*, 162. For examples of such arguments in favor of euthanasia see Glover, *Causing Death and Saving Lives*, chapter 14; Margaret Pabst Battin, *The Least Worst Death: Essays in bioethics on the end of life* (New York: Oxford University Press, 1994), chapter 5; Gerald Dworkin, R.G. Frey, Sissela Bok, *Euthanasia and Physician-Assisted Suicide: For and Against* (Cambridge; Cambridge University Press, 1998), Part One, and Robert Young, *Medically Assisted Death* (Cambridge: Cambridge University Press, 2007), chapter 2.
3. Torquatus, for example, held that "we might leave life calmly if it please us not"; see Cicero, *De Finibus Bonorum et Malorum* I. 49; available at http://www.thelatinlibrary.com/cicero/fin1.shtml#49 (Accessed July 17th, 2010). Epicurus allegedly sustained his last few days by recollecting his past philosophical conversations, even though he was in extreme pain from the kidney stones that led to his death. See Diogenes Laertius, "Life of Epicurus,"

in Cyril Bailey, trans. and ed., *Epicurus: The Extant Remains with short critical apparatus* (New York: Georg Olms Verlag, 1970), 150. Cicero was understandably skeptical of this; see Cicero, trans. J. E. King, *Tusculan Disputations*, 515–516, V. xxxi. 86–88. For a discussion of the Epicurean view of suicide, see Walter Englert, "Stoics and Epicureans on the Nature of Suicide," in John J. Cleary and William Wians, eds., *Proceedings of the Boston Area Colloquium in Ancient Philosophy: Volume X 1994* (Lanham, Md.: University Press of America, 1994), 86–95.

4. The Epicurean thus seems to be precluded from holding that suicide could be choice-worthy on the hedonistic grounds that it could be used to avoid harm, especially since such a pro-suicide argument appears to be the mirror image of the deprivationist argument for the view that death is a harm to the one who dies. See Margaret P. Battin, "Can Suicide be Rational? Yes, Sometimes," in James L. Werth, Jr., *Contemporary Perspectives on Rational Suicide* (Philadelphia, Pa.: Brunner/Mazel, 1999), 18–20. Note that the phrase "commit suicide" is not used here, for the reasons outlined by Benatar. See David Benatar, "Suicide: A Qualified Defense," in Taylor, ed., *The Metaphysics and Ethics of Death*, forthcoming.

5. From now on this will be referred to simply as "euthanasia" for the sake of simplicity.

6. McMahan, "Death and the Value of Life," 235.

7. Ibid., 236. As written, this claim seems to imply that coming into existence would be good for the person before he exists. But it is clear that McMahan does not intend to locate the beneficiary of such an existence in his pre-vital time, for he later writes that such a beneficiary "is here before us, enjoying the goods of life". (Ibid., 237.) As such, then, it would be more accurate for this claim to be understood as being temporally indexed, such that if a person's life goes well then he was benefited by his coming into existence.

8. Draper holds that for this reason the Epicurean should not deny that death would be a comparative harm to the person who dies; see Kai Draper, "Epicurus and the Anticipation of Death," in Taylor, ed., *The Metaphysics and Ethics of Death*, forthcoming. However, Draper's arguments rests on accepting the Comparative View, which (as will be outlined below) McMahan correctly rejects; see McMahan, "Death and the Value of Life," 239.

9. Note that the claim that continuing to live is good is here understood as being good because of its being a precondition for the goods of life, rather than good in itself. This claim is thus in accord with those made in the context of discussing the views of Levenbook and Silverstein in Chapter 2.

10. Note that McMahan does not refer to Perverse Epicureanism, but only to "the Epicurean"—although it is clear that not all Epicureans (but only perverse ones) would reject the reconciliation strategy.

11. Ibid., 237.

12. Ibid., 236.

13. Ibid., 239.

14. Ibid., 239.

15. Ibid., 235.

16. Further Epicurean responses to the concern that Epicureanism cannot morally condemn killing are outlined below, in the context of showing how the moral issue of euthanasia could be no more straightforward for an Epicurean than for a non-Epicurean.

17. As Stephen Rosenbaum notes, there is no inconsistency in an Epicurean preferring to continue to live. See "Epicurus and Annihilation," in Fischer, ed. *The Metaphysics of Death*, 295.

18. Moreover, if the person contemplating suicide held suffering to be intrinsically disvaluable then a world in which there was less suffering rather than more would also be one that was good *for* her (and hence one that she had a reason to bring about).
19. For a defense of reasoning without comparing, see David K. Chan, "Reasoning Without Comparing," *American Philosophical Quarterly* 47, no. 2 (2010), 149–160.
20. Note that this Epicurean way of explaining why it might be rational for a person to perform an action that she knows would bring about her death does not commit the Epicurean to denying that she could be morally responsible for her death, even if she did not directly intend to bring about her death but only relieve her suffering. This Epicurean analysis of the rationality of suicide is thus orthogonal to the question of the legitimacy or otherwise of the Doctrine of Double Effect.
21. Although he does not couch his argument in terms of noncomparative reasons, it seems that this is a view endorsed by Warren, *Facing Death*, 199–201.
22. That the Epicurean's prudential justification for suicide will typically rest on noncomparative reasons obviates the need to respond to arguments that are based on the claim that suicide could not be rational owing to the fact that one's own death is "an unknown quantity," and so one cannot even begin to decide whether one should kill oneself. See Philip E. Devine, *The Ethics of Homicide* (Ithaca, NY: Cornell University Press, 1978), 25. For a discussion of Devine's argument, see Feldman, *Confrontations With the Reaper*, 219–223. Note that while the Epicurean could hold that a person's suicide was *rational* this does not commit her to claiming that it would therefore be *moral*.
23. See John Donnelly, "Suicide and Rationality," in John Donnelly, ed., *Language, Metaphysics, and Death* (New York: Fordham University Press, 1978), 96.
24. Similar points with respect to the view that accepting the Epicurean view that death is not a harm to the person who dies would lead to a removal of the proscriptions on killing are made by Stephen Rosenbaum, "The Harm of Killing," 207–226.

NOTES TO CHAPTER 8

1. Lucretius, *De Rerum Natura* 5.177–80, p. 393. Warren argues that this Lucretian view is unsatisfactory, for "The Epicureans appear to offer no significant positive reason for wishing to continue to live, beyond a mere inertia". Warren, *Facing Death*, 210. A similar concern is expressed by Luper-Foy, who argues that "Epicureans have sabotaged their motivation for living". Luper-Foy, "Annihilation," 278, and in Steven Luper, "Adaptation," in Taylor, ed., *The Metaphysics and Ethics of Death*, forthcoming. A compelling response to such concerns is developed by Stephen Rosenbaum, in "Epicurus and Annihilation," in Fischer, ed., *The Metaphysics of Death*, 293–304; see also McMahan's arguments for the reconciliation strategy outlined in the previous Chapter, and in his "Death and the Value of Life," 235–240.
2. Lisa Bortolotti convincingly argues that there is no reason to believe that life extension would be undesirable for individuals. See her "Agency, Life Extension, and the Meaning of Life," unpublished mss., and (with Y. Nagasawa), "Immortality without Boredom," *Ratio* 22 (2009), 261–277. In the former paper Bortolotti argues against the views of (among others) Bernard Williams, "The Makopoulos Case," 73–92, and L. James, "Shape and the

meaningfulness of life," in L. Bortolotti, ed., *Philosophy and Happiness* (Basingstoke: Palgrave, 2009), Chapter 4. Bortolotti also notes the ethical issues that successful life-extension technology might raise, "such as widespread longevity generating overpopulation, disincentives to reproduce, or stagnation of ideas, and concerns about fairness in the distribution of this newly acquired resource" mss., 9. These issues were also raised by John Wyndham, in his novel *Trouble with Lichen* (New York: Walker and Company, 1960). Williams' views are also criticized in Ben Bradley and Kris McDaniel, "Death and Desires," in Taylor, ed., *The Metaphysics and Ethics of Death*, forthcoming.

3. See, for example, Richard H. Thaler, Cass R. Sunstein, *Nudge: Improving Decisions about Health, Wealth, and Happiness* (New Haven, Conn.: Yale University Press, 2008). Thaler's and Sunstein's earlier work on "libertarian paternalism" is trenchantly criticized by Gregory Mitchell, "Libertarian Paternalism is an Oxymoron," *Northwest University Law Review* 99 (2005), 1245–1277.

4. The question of whether policies of presumed consent, or their more radical cousins, policies of posthumous organ takings, are morally legitimate will be the subject of this chapter. A more ethically sound system of organ procurement—namely, the use of markets—is defended in Mark J. Cherry, *Kidney for Sale by Owner: Human Organs, Transplantation, and the Market* (Georgetown: Georgetown University Press, 2005), James Stacey Taylor, *Stakes and Kidneys: Why markets in human body parts are morally imperative* (Aldershot: Ashgate Publishing, 2005), and Benjamin E. Hippen, "In Defense of a Regulated Market in Kidneys from Living Vendors," *Journal of Medicine and Philosophy* 30, no. 6 (2005), 593–626.

5. For the reasons outlined in the Introduction to this volume "organ taking" will be used here instead of the more common but less accurate "organ conscription". The former term is also used by David Price, apparently for the same reason, although he does not make this explicit; see his *Legal and Ethical Aspects of Organ Transplantation* (Cambridge: Cambridge University Press, 2000), 84.

6. According to the United Network for Organ Sharing there were 105, 357 waiting list candidates in the United States as of 11.23pm on January 23rd, 2010, while from January to October 2009 only 23, 846 transplants had been performed. See http://www.unos.org/ . Accessed January 23rd, 2010.

7. Although it is intuitively plausible that the introduction of a system of presumed consent would lead to an increase in the availability of transplantable organs it is difficult to support this view by comparing the procurement rates of countries which have such a system and those that do not, for other differences besides their procurement policies prevent easy comparisons. For example, the different rates of organ procurement that exist between countries that have presumed consent policies in place and those that do not might be owed to the number of transplant centers they have, the number of fatal road accidents that each has that generate transplantable organs, and what sort of organs are required by persons on their waiting lists.

8. Debates over other proposed means of alleviating the shortage of transplantable organs typically focus on several independent issues. For example, the debate over whether markets could be used to procure additional transplantable organs has several foci, such as whether such markets would enhance or compromise the autonomy of the potential vendors, whether they would illegitimately commodify the human body, and whether they would lead to a diminution in the number of organs procured. For discussion of these arguments see Taylor, *Stakes and Kidneys*, Cherry, *Kidney for Sale by Owner*,

and Hippen, "In Defense of a Regulated Market in Kidneys from Living Vendors," 593–626. See also James Stacey Taylor, "Autonomy and Organ Sales, Revisited," *Journal of Medicine and Philosophy* 34 (2009), 632–648, and Mark J. Cherry, "Why Should We Compensate Organ Donors When We Can Continue to Take Organs for Free? A Response to Some of My Critics," *Journal of Medicine and Philosophy* 34 (2009), 649–673.

9. That this is the issue that the debate over the ethical status of presumed consent policies focus on has been explicitly recognized in a White Paper published by the Organ Procurement and Transplantation Network. See J. Michael Dennis, Patricia Hanson, Ernest E. Hodge, Ridd A.F. Krom, Robert M. Veatch, "An Evaluation of the Ethics of Presumed Consent and a Policy Based on Required Response," *UNOS Update* 1, no. 2 (1994), 16–21. This issue is of interest to a full-blooded Epicurean not because she would endorse this approach, but because, as will be argued below, she will reject it.

10. See, for example, Michael B. Gill, "Presumed Consent, Autonomy, and Organ Donation," *Journal of Medicine and Philosophy* 29, 1 (2004), 37–59.

11. See, for example, R.M. Veatch and J.B. Pitt, "The myth of presumed consent: Ethical problems in organ procurement strategies," *Transplantation Proceedings* 27 (1995), 1888–1892. The view that treating persons' postmortem remains as they would wish them to be treated is required by respect for autonomy, and that this restricts the postmortem procurement of organs is expressed by B. Farsides, "Respecting wishes and avoiding conflict: understanding the ethical basis for organ donation and retrieval," *British Journal of Anaesthesia* 108 (2012), 73–79.

12. This latter view was expressed by Hamer and Rivlin, "A stronger policy of organ retrieval from cadaveric donors," 197, 198, and Glannon, "Do the sick have a right to cadaveric organs?" 154.

13. Organs takings (under the guise of "routine recovery" or "organ conscription,") have been defended by Aaron Spital, "Conscription of Cadaveric Organs for Transplantation: Neglected Again," *Kennedy Institute of Ethics Journal* 13, no. 2 (2003), 169–174, Spital and Taylor, "In Defense of Routine Recovery of Cadaveric Organs: A Response to Walter Glannon," 337–343, and "Routine Recovery of Cadaveric Organs for Transplantation: Consistent, Fair, and Life Saving," 300–303; Cecile Fabre, *Whose Body is it Anyway?*, Chapters 4 and 5, and John Harris, "Organ procurement: dead interests, living needs," *Journal of Medical Ethics* 29 (2003), 130–134.

14. Such as, for example, Mark J. Cherry (in personal correspondence).

15. Gill, "Presumed Consent," 39.

16. C. Cohen, "The case for presumed consent to transplant human organs after death," *Transplantation Proceedings* 24 (1992), 2169. This datum is from The Gallup Organization, Inc., The American Public's Attitudes Toward Organ Donation, conducted for The Partnership for Organ Donation, Boston, MA. Feb 1993. Similarly, survey trends show that about 70% of persons in Britain are willing to have their kidneys removed postmortem for transplantation if they were suitable for this. See the British Kidney Patient Association, "Attitudes Towards Kidney Donating," (1–6 April), Surrey, Gallup Organisation, 1992; British Kidney Patient Association "Transplant Survey," (4–7 May), Surrey, Gallup Organisation, 1994; British Kidney Patient Association, "Organ Donor Scheme, Pre-Study Survey," (20–25 September), Gallup Organisation, 1995; British Kidney Patient Association, "Post-Study Survey," (1–6 November), Gallup Organisation; 1995; British Kidney Patient Association "Transplant Survey," (16–20 May), Surrey, Gallup Organisation, 1997; British Kidney Patient Association "Transplant Survey," (5–11 November), Surrey, Gallup Organisation, 1998. Cited by Gillian Haddow, "'Because

you're worth it?' The Taking and Selling of Transplantable Organs," *Journal of Medical Ethics* 32, no. 6 (2006), notes 2–7. Available at: http://www.ncbi. nlm.nih.gov/pmc/articles/PMC2563366/ . Accessed January 23rd, 2010. Gill notes that there are several problems associated with using such surveys as the basis for the debate over the ethical status of presumed consent policies. First, the data are old, and attitudes might have changed since they were taken. Second, persons might have said that they would be unlikely to donate their organs after their deaths might have answered this way not because they were opposed to their organs being transplanted, but because they believed that they would not be suitable for this. Third, the persons polled might have misinformed about organ retrieval procedures. Finally, such polls might not indicate how a person would actually behave in the hypothetical situation he is faced with. "Presumed Consent," 40.

17. Cohen, "The case for presumed consent," 2169.
18. At least in the United States and the United Kingdom, given the data cited above. Indeed, it is likely to be even more than this, since persons would have the option of registering their refusal to have their organs removed, and many persons who would so refuse would do this.
19. Veatch and Pitt, "The myth of presumed consent," 1888–1892.
20. At least within the American and British contexts.
21. Gill, "Presumed Consent," 41
22. Ibid., 41.
23. Ibid., 41.
24. Versions of this argument can be found in E.H. Kluge, "Improving organ retrieval rates: Various proposals and their ethical validity," *Health Care Analysis* 8 (2000), p. 286, and Veatch and Pitt, "The myth of presumed consent," 1890.
25. See, for example, J. Savulescu, "Death, us and our bodies: personal reflections," *Journal of Medical Ethics* 29 (2003), 129. It should be noted that the claims made here concerning autonomy will be claims that would be uncontroversial to contemporary autonomy theorists, for they do not rely on the acceptance of any particular model of autonomy for their truth. See James Stacey Taylor, "Introduction," *Personal Autonomy: New essays on personal autonomy and its role in contemporary moral philosophy* (Cambridge: Cambridge University Press, 2005), 1–32, for an outline of contemporary models of autonomy.
26. Gill, "Presumed Consent," 42
27. The view that mistaken uses of a person's body parts postmortem are worse than the equivalent mistaken failures to use is challenged by T. M. Wilkinson, "Consent and the Use of the Bodies of the Dead," *Journal of Medicine and Philosophy*, forthcoming.
28. Gill, "Presumed Consent," 43.
29. Ibid., 43.
30. Ibid., 44.
31. Ibid., 45.
32. Ibid., 44–45. Gill writes of the "non-interference model of autonomy" and the "respect-for-wishes model of autonomy". As he notes, however, these are not really "models of autonomy" at all, for they are not accounts of what it is for a person to be autonomous with respect to her actions or her desires. Rather, these are models of how one should *respect* the autonomy of persons.
33. Note that while all parties to the internecine debate over presumed consent (i.e., that between those who are concerned with respecting those desires that persons are autonomous with respect to concerning the disposal of their

postmortem remains) should accept this, this does not mean that persons with other ethical qualms about policies of presumed consent should do so too.

34. Before doing so, however, it is first necessary to rectify some conceptual unclarities in this argument. First, Gill's argument is not really concerned with respecting the autonomy of the brain-dead individuals whose organs are suitable for transplantation, as he writes. ("Presumed Consent," 45.) Such individuals have no autonomy to respect. They are, after all, brain-dead. Rather, Gill's argument is concerned with respecting the autonomy of such individuals as they were prior to their becoming brain-dead. Second, despite what Gill implies in naming the model of respect for autonomy that he endorses the "respect-for-wishes" model of autonomy, respecting an agent's wishes and respecting her autonomy are not the same. One might, for example, respect the wishes of a non-autonomous agent without thereby respecting her (non-existent) autonomy. Alternatively, one might respect a person's autonomy without respecting her wishes. For example, one might institute a prohibition against voluntary slavery on the grounds that the enslavement of persons, even if voluntary on the part of the enslaved, serves to compromise their autonomy to an extent that is incompatible with its value. If one institutes and enforces this prohibition without regard to the wishes of the population subject to it one will fail to respect their wishes where such a failure arises out of one's respect for their autonomy. Thus, with this final conceptual clarification in hand it is clear that rather than being concerned with respecting an agent's wishes *per se*, respect for a person's autonomy requires that those of her wishes that she is autonomous with respect to be respected, where such respect might *possibly* come with the caveat, "provided that the satisfaction of those wishes would not itself compromise her autonomy".

35. Ibid., 48

36. It should be acknowledged here that this answer to (iii) is be controversial, for one could readily argue that persons whose organs are taken for transplant are being used to provide benefits to others, rather than to prevent them from being harmed. This issue could only be resolved through a clear account of where to draw the appropriate baseline for the assessment of harms and benefits—and this will not be an easy matter. However, even with this acknowledgement in place, the answers to the other four questions to be asked in deciding how to respect a person's autonomy with respect to her wishes concerning the treatment of her postmortem body clearly support a proceduralist approach.

37. This situation might change were markets in organs to be legalized.

38. Note that giving due weight to a person's wishes does not commit one to abide by them. One might, for example, after giving due weight to a person's wishes decide that other considerations justify their being overridden. See Harris, "Organ procurement: dead interests, living needs," 131.

39. Gill mistakenly treats these as being coextensive. See, for example, "Presumed Consent," 43.

40. Although, as will be noted below, this is a necessary but not a sufficient condition for one person to respect the autonomy of another.

41. For this reason the malevolent conspirators in Feinberg's Case C fail to respect the autonomy of the woman whose trust they betray, with this failure occurring while she is still alive. Feinberg, "Harm to Others," 182–183. See, too, the discussion of Grover's views on posthumous harm and autonomy in Chapter 2.

42. This intent is defeasible.

43. It does not matter whether one believes that the reasons that a person gives for her desire to have her postmortem body treated in a certain way are mistaken,

or not. This is because respect for a person's autonomy requires that her desires be taken into account whether or not the person who is considering them as part of his deliberations believes them to be justifiable. An atheist, for example, would fail to respect the autonomy of a believer if he discounted her religiously-based desires on the grounds that they were mistaken.

44. There might also be other moral reasons as to why the wishes of persons who are now dead should be respected, in addition to the concern that this is required by the respect shown to their autonomy while they were alive. See the discussion at the end of Chapter 4, as well as, for example, Callahan "On Harming the Dead," 350–352, and Partridge, "Posthumous Interests and Posthumous Respect," 259–261.

45. Spital and Taylor, "Routine Recovery of Cadaveric Organs for Transplantation,"300–303.

46. While this argument is sound if the referent of "those" is taken to be the dead, it might well be unsound if it is taken to include the living, for they could be harmed by the knowledge that their organs would be subject to postmortem taking.

47. Such conscription is apparently endorsed by Fabre; see *Whose Body is it Anyway?* Chapter 5. However, although Fabre believes that her arguments support the conscription of live organs, they do not; see Taylor, "Liberalism, The Duty to Rescue, and Organ Procurement," 314–326.

48. Given Portmore's arguments, discussed in Chapter 1, this argument would not be one that a desire theorist of well-being could offer.

49. This latter assumption is especially forcefully accepted in France, where there is an "absolutist conception of all bodies belonging to the French state". See Donna Dickinson, *Property in the Body: Feminist Perspectives* (Cambridge; Cambridge University Press, 2007), 142.

50. Anthony M. Honore, "Ownership", in A.G. Guest, ed, *Oxford Essays in Jurisprudence: First Series* (Oxford: Clarendon Press, 1961), 107–147.

51. One might hold that (morally, even if not legally) a person's bodily remains would become the property of his heirs, and so any policy of organ conscription would be conscripting organs from them. However, that a person's remains should become the property of his heirs cannot merely be assumed, but must be argued for, and so this objection to a policy of organ taking will not be raised here.

52. Absent such a justification the classical liberals would be right: the taking of organs would simply amount to theft.

53. Three points must be noted here, however. First, this argument from subjective harm does not rest on the observation that the taking of organs from postmortem sources could involve conscripting them from living persons, for it could also be made with respect to the distress felt by the relatives of the organ source as the taking of her organs. Second, it must be recognized that not everyone believes that it is unethical to conscript organs from living sources—see, for example, Fabre's arguments in *Whose Body is it Anyway?* 98–125. Finally, it must be admitted that simply because the conscription of organs from living sources is generally held to be unethical this does not in itself make it so, and so this anti-conscription argument is weakened to the extent that this (albeit plausible) assumption on which it is based lacks theoretical support.

54. Tom L. Beauchamp and James F. Childress discuss this Principle in *Principles of Biomedical Ethics* (New York: Oxford University Press, sixth edition, 2008), Chapter 4.

55. Julia D. Mahoney, "Should We Adopt a Market Strategy to Increase the Supply of Transplantable Organs?" in Wayne Shelton and John Balint, eds., *The Ethics of Organ Transplantation* (Stamford, Conn.: Jai Press, 2001), 67–70.

56. This view is developed in James Stacey Taylor, "The Unjustified Assumptions of Organ Conscripters," *HEC Forum* 21, no. 2 (2009), 115–133.

57. Two points should be noted here. First, this claim could be endorsed by a consequentialist, for it is possible (indeed, likely) that a robust system of property rights of a sort that would require the provision of such compensation could be justified on consequentialist grounds. Second, it must be admitted that (unfortunately) the assumption that takings require compensation is not a *prima facie* obvious one to all. Cecile Fabre, for example, does not share it, believing instead that it can be legitimate for one group of individuals to take property from another, less powerful, group in order to advance the impositions of their own views on others. (See *Whose Body is it Anyway?* 11) Of course, when put this baldly it is hard to see why one would ever believe such violence-backed takings could ever be morally justified. Were one to make these same claims in terms of "states" and "citizens", however, a surprisingly (and worryingly) large number of people seem to believe this to be acceptable, even without arguments justifying this. (Fabre, for example, provides none, but simply assumes such forceful and uncompensated takings to be morally legitimate.) At least when it comes to the forcible taking of property, then, Shakespeare is mistaken to claim that a rose by any other name would smell as sweet—for it seems that for many persons the *prima facie* sweetness or otherwise of extorted takings depends on the names by which they extorter and extortee go by.

58. Note that such a belief need not be based on the belief that posthumous harm is possible; a person might believe that it is not, and yet still be concerned about what happens to her body after her death, perhaps for the sake of her relatives who she believes would be distressed by its dismemberment. Such a person might thus decide to buy out of having her organs taken to avoid the unpleasant feelings that she has when she contemplates the future distress of her relatives.

59. Arguments from autonomy that could be modified to support such sales can be found in Taylor, *Stakes and Kidneys*, although it should be noted that these arguments will only be offered by persons who hold autonomy to be of instrumental, rather than intrinsic, value. For further discussion of this latter point see Taylor, "Autonomy and Organ Sales, Revisited," 632–648.

60. Although note that in itself the moral requirement to pay compensation for a taken organ does not entail that organs are market alienable goods.

61. Note that this argument is not only of practical relevance to this bioethical debate, but also of theoretical interest insofar as it further supports the full-blooded Epicurean's rejection of Grover's "Knowledge and Autonomy" argument for the possibility of posthumous harm that was first discussed in Chapter 2.

62. Of course, persons might be harmed by the *belief* that their bodies would be mistreated after their deaths. But to accept this is not to accept that the cause of such harm would be the mistreatment itself.

63. Although the proponents of policies of presumed consent will still need to address other ethical worries that such policies give rise to. For example, they will have to address the worry that such policies evince an illegitimate relationship between the State and the individual. For such a worry, see Amitai Etzioni, "Organ Donation: A Communitarian Approach," *Kennedy Institute of Ethics Journal* 13 (2003), 2. For a response to such worries see D.R. McNeil, "Constitutionality of 'presumed consent' for organ donation," *Hamline Journal of Public Law and Policy* 9 (1989), 343–372.

64. One might wonder whether this debate was necessary, since, as T. M. Wilkinson notes, "Is it not obvious that we should follow the wishes of the dead

about organ retrieval, just as we respect wills for property?" However—and quite apart from arguing that in matters of life and death such as this it behooves us to have a thorough understanding of the issue at hand, even if the arguments canvassed do not lead us to any radical conclusions—as Wilkinson goes on to note there are significant disanalogies between "bequests and bodies". See *Ethics and the Acquisition of Organs*, 51–52.

NOTES TO CHAPTER 9

1. For a technical account of how such reproduction is possible, see James J. Finnerty, Ted S. Thomas, Robert J. Boyle, Stuart S. Howards, and Logan B. Karns, "Gamete retrieval in terminal conditions," *American Journal of Obstetrics and Gynecology* 185, no.2 (2001), 300—307.
2. In Western Australia, for example, posthumous reproduction is permitted when the deceased person has given written consent to this. See Human Reproductive Technology Act 1991 (WA), s 22(8)(a). Cited by Rebecca Collins, "Posthumous Reproduction and the Presumption against Consent in Cases of Death Caused by Sudden Trauma," *Journal of Medicine and Philosophy* 30 (2005), 411, n. 5; see also 433. This is also the case in England; see David T. Price, "Giving Blood: Posthumous Fertility Treatment and a Good Old British Compromise?" *International Review of Law, Computers and Technology* 11, no. 2 (1997), 302 ff.
3. B. Bennett, "Posthumous reproduction and the meanings of autonomy," *Melbourne University Law Review* 23, no. 2 (1999), 302.
4. Anne Reichman Schiff, "Posthumous conception and the need for consent," *Medical Journal of Australia* 170 (1999), 53.
5. Ibid., 53. Similar arguments have been offered against presumed consent with respect to organ procurement.
6. Schiff, "Arising from the Dead," 946. This concern is related to those discussed in the Conclusion to Chapter 4.
7. Schiff, "Posthumous conception and the need for consent," 54.
8. Collins, "Posthumous Reproduction and the Presumption against Consent," 437.
9. Ibid., 437.
10. A real example of this can be found in the case of Andrew Clough, whose fiancée Simone Baker desired to be impregnated with his sperm after his death from a fall in Queensland. It was clear from Clough's antemortem actions (including the expressed desire to have children with Baker, and his implicit willingness to have children in whose future he took no part, as shown by his prior donations to sperm banks) that he would have acceded to this desire. See M. Spriggs, "Woman wants dead fiancé's baby: who owns a dead man sperm," *Journal of Medical Ethics* 30 (2004), 384. For a response to Spriggs see M.J. Parker, "'Til Death Us Do Part: the ethics of postmortem gamete donation," *Journal of Medical Ethics* 30 (2004), 387–388.
11. Given full-blooded Epicureans' hedonism it is clear that there is at least one other thing that is of value besides autonomy—especially since a good case can be made for the claim that the value of autonomy is *derivative* from that of well-being. See here Taylor, *Practical Autonomy and Bioethics*, Chapter 10.
12. Although it is possible that he could be harmed by *thinking* that such harvesting would occur.
13. Recall that the presence or absence of a desire to continue living would be orthogonal to whether one was an Epicurean or not.

14. This does not, of course, *justify* taking numbers of persons to be normative in this way. Certain libertarians, for example, might simply deny that overriding a person's autonomously-formed decision for the benefit of a greater number of persons is ever legitimate. However, since such a person would be committed to denying the legitimacy of any such public policy her criticism here is external to this discussion, which is based on the (possibly mistaken) assumption that such a policy could be legitimate.

15. Harvesting organs from a single cadaver could benefit several people; the harvesting of gametes will only benefit the persons who request this—and typically only one person will do so. (Atypical cases in which there are multiple requests for harvested gametes might occur when they are harvested from persons whose reproductive capacities would be in higher demand than usual, such as, for example, film stars, persons in polygamous relationships, or analytic philosophers working on the metaphysics of death.)

16. The harm that such persons will be saved from will be the harm of having a life that is worse that that which they could have had; it is not the putative harm of death.

17. R. D. Orr and M. Siegler, "Is posthumous semen retrieval ethically permissible?" *Journal of Medical Ethics* 28 (2002), 301

18. The lack of evidence of harm caused to children by being brought up by a single parent is documented in A. Douglass and K. Daniels, "Posthumous reproduction: A consideration of the medical, ethical, cultural, psychosocial and legal perspectives in the New Zealand context," *Medical Law International* 4, no. 4 (2002), 268. For a weaker claim that supports the same conclusion concerning the possible harm to a future child, see ESHRE Task Force on Ethics and Law, "Posthumous assisted reproduction," *Human Reproduction* 21, no. 12 (2006), 3051–3052.

19. Or, at least, no objection can be leveled against this practice from the point of the view of the child so conceived in *typical* cases. One might, however, object to assisted posthumous reproduction in cases where it would produce a child who could charge that his life was a wrongful one.

20. See Tamar Lewin, "Taking After Father, a Frozen Sperm Riddle," *New York Times*, January 13th, 2002, A3.

21. Jamie Roswell, "Stayin' Alive: Postmortem Reproduction and Inheritance Rights," 41 *Family Court Review* 400 (2003), 411.

22. Indeed, this would have to be the case, for, as Steiner argues, it seems that there are no natural rights to inheritance, and so the discussion of this issue must be couched in terms of what legal policies should be adopted here. Steiner, *An Essay on Rights*, 249–261.

23. See, for example, Scarre, "Can archaeology harm the dead?" 181–198; Tarlow, "Archeological ethics and the people of the past," 199—216.

24. See Carolyn Abraham, *Possessing Genius: The Bizarre Odyssey of Einstein's Brain* (London: Icon Books Ltd., 2005).

25. Puzzlingly, even though Mark R. Wicclair and Michael DeVita recognize that it is at least an open question as to whether or not the dead can be harmed, they still claim that "deceased patients" "warrant protection in relation to postmortem research" for they need to be protected from being the subjects of research that is incompatible with their "premortem preferences and values". (Wicclair and DeVita, "Oversight of Research Involving the Dead," 144.) But since such protection could only be justified were one to believe that persons could be subjects of posthumous harm, and since Wicclair and DeVita do not seem to wish to endorse the possibility of such harm, it is unclear why they believe that such preferences and values need to be protected. Perhaps, though, since they have left open the possibility of

posthumous harm they wish to tailor their discussion so that their recommendations would be acceptable were it to be shown to be possible.

26. Wilkinson, "Last Rights," 37.

27. Ibid., 31.

28. Violating a person's privacy after her death would not itself affect her ability to direct her actions in accordance with her own values and desires. However, if while she was alive one intended to do this and kept this fact from her, then one could be said to be usurping her autonomy through this deceptive omission, insofar as it would then be the would-be deceiver, and not the agent herself, who was directing which type of actions she should perform (i.e., those that she would perform were she aware of this future violation, or those that she would perform were she to be unaware of it). For a more complete account of the relationship between autonomy and privacy, see James Stacey Taylor, "Privacy and autonomy: A reappraisal," *The Southern Journal of Philosophy* 40 (2002), 587–604.

29. Wilkinson, "Last Rights," 32.

30. The same claim would be justified, of course, if P's act benefitted someone other than T.

31. For a discussion of this incident, see Michael Redfern, Jean Keeling, Elizabeth Powell, *The Report of the Royal Liverpool Children's Inquiry*; available at: http://www.rlcinquiry.org.uk/index.htm. Accessed February 2, 2010. See also David Hall, "Reflecting on Redfern: What can we learn from the Alder Hey story?"*Archives of Disease in Childhood* 84 (2001), 455–456.

32. This point is made by James L. Werth, Jr., Caroline Burke, Rebekah J. Bardash, "Confidentiality in End-of-Life and After-Death Situations," *Ethics and Behavior* 12, no. 3 (2002), 215. More generally, see Partridge, "Posthumous Interests and Posthumous Respect," 259–264, and the Conclusion of Chapter 4.

33. This does not mean that medical confidentiality could never be breached, either antemortem or posthumously. A therapist, for example, could be legitimately required to breach her client's confidentiality if he makes threats to harm others. See *Tarasoff v. Regents of the University of California*, 17 Cal. 3d 425, 551 P.2d 334, 131 Cal. Rptr. 14 (Cal. 1976). Similarly, it could be ethically legitimate for a therapist to violate her client's confidentiality if she believes that he is in danger of causing harm to himself.

NOTES TO THE CONCLUSION

1. The fictitious "Plotinus" is based on Berkeley, California; the fictitious "Rummidge" is based on Birmingham, England.

2. David Lodge, *Changing Places* (New York: Penguin, 1978), 87–88.

3. Epicurus, *Gnomologium Vaticanum Epicureum* 31, in Graziano Arrighetti, ed., *Opere* (Torino: Giulio Einaudi, 1973), 147.

4. Homer, *Iliad*, 24.526 ff. Available at: http://www.perseus.tufts.edu/hopper/text?doc=Hom.+Il.+24+526&fromdoc=Perseus:text:1999.01.0133; accessed August 2nd, 2010. Alas, this recognition will not raise mortals to the status of the gods, for while mortals can be free from care about their deaths qua deaths and what comes after them, they might still be bowed down by other cares, including that pertaining to the manner of their deaths, whereas (at least according to Achilles) the gods will be free from cares *simpliciter*.

5. Belshaw, for example, holds that it "seems wrong on various counts". See *Annihilation*, 27.

6. Draper, "Epicurean Equanimity towards Death," 96.

7. Ibid., 96. See Brian Lombard, *Events* (Boston: Routledge, 1986), 131–144
8. Draper, "Epicurean Equanimity towards Death," 96.
9. See, respectively, Fred Feldman, *Pleasure and the Good Life,* Chapters 3, 4 and 5; Bradley *Well-Being & Death*, Chapter 1.
10. Some of these were outlined in the Introduction.

Bibliography

Abraham, Carolyn, *Possessing Genius: The Bizarre Odyssey of Einstein's Brain*. London: Icon Books Ltd., 2005.

Aeschines, trans. C. D. Adams, *Against Ctesiphon*. London: William Heinemann, 1919.

Annas, Julia, *The Morality of Happiness*. New York: Oxford University Press, 1993.

Aristotle, *Nicomachean Ethics*. In *The Basic Works of Aristotle*, translated and edited by Richard McKeon. New York: Random House, 1941.

———, *Nicomachean Ethics*, trans. H. Rackham. Cambridge, MA: Harvard University Press, 1934.

Armstrong, David, "All Things to All Men: Philodemus' Model of Therapy and the Audience of *De Morte*." In *Philodemus and the New Testament World*. Edited by John Fitzgerald, Dirk Obbink, and Glenn S. Holland, 15–54. Leiden: Brill, 2004.

Avramescu, Catalin, trans. Alistair Ian Blyth, *An Intellectual History of Cannibalism*, Princeton: Princeton University Press, 2009.

Baglow, John Sutton, "The Rights of the Corpse," *Mortality* 12, 3 (2007): 223–239.

Bahn, Paul, "Do Not Disturb? Archaeology and the Rights of the Dead." *Journal of Applied Philosophy* 1, no. 2 (1984): 213–225.

Baier, Annette C., *Death and Character: Further Reflections on Hume*. Cambridge, MA: Harvard University Press, 2008.

———, "The Rights of Past and Future Persons." In *Responsibilities to Future Generations: Environmental Ethics*, edited by Ernest Partridge, 171–183. Buffalo, NY: Prometheus Books, 1981.

Barber, H. E., "Ex Ante Desire and Post Hoc Satisfaction." In *Time and Identity: Topics in Contemporary Philosophy*, edited by Keim J. Campbell, M. O'Rourke, and H. Silverstein, 249–267. Cambridge, MA: MIT Press, 2010.

Barrington, Mary Rose, "Apologia for Suicide." In *Suicide: The Philosophical Issues*, edited by M. Pabst Battin and David J. Majo, 90–103. New York: St. Martin's Press, 1980.

Basset, Samuel Elliot, "Achilles' Treatment of Hector's Body." *Transactions and Proceedings of the American Philological Association* 64 (1933): 41–65.

Battin, Margaret P., *Ending Life: Ethics and the Way We Die*. New York: Oxford, 2005.

———, "Can Suicide Be Rational? Yes, Sometimes." In *Contemporary Perspectives on Rational Suicide*, edited by James L. Werth, Jr., 13–22. Philadelphia: Brunner/Mazel, 1999.

———, *The Least Worst Death: Essays in Bioethics on the End of Life*. New York: Oxford University Press, 1994.

——, "Age Rationing and the Just Distribution of Healthcare: Is There a Duty to Die?" *Ethics* 97, no. 2 (1987): 317–340.

——, "Suicide: A Fundamental Human Right?" In *Suicide: The Philosophical Issues*, edited by M. Pabst Battin and David J. Majo, 267–285. New York: St. Martin's Press, 1980.

Beauchamp, Tom L., and Childress, James F., *Principles of Biomedical Ethics*. New York: Oxford University Press, 6th edition, 2008.

Behrendt, Kathy, "A Special Way of Being Afraid." *Philosophical Psychology* 23, no. 5 (2010): 669–682.

Bellioti, Raymond A., "Do Dead Human Beings Have Rights?" *The Personalist* 60 (1979): 201–210.

Belshaw, Christopher, "Harm, Change, and Time." *Journal of Medicine and Philosophy*, forthcoming.

——, *Annihilation: The Sense and Significance of Death*. Stocksfield, UK: Acumen, 2009.

——, *10 Good Questions about Life and Death*. Oxford: Blackwell, 2005.

——, "Death, Pain, and Time." *Philosophical Studies* 97, no. 3 (2000): 317–341.

Benatar, David, "Suicide: A Qualified Defense." In *The Metaphysics and Ethics of Death*, edited by James Stacey Taylor. New York: Oxford University Press, forthcoming.

——, *Better Never to Have Been: The Harm of Coming Into Existence*. Oxford: Clarendon Press, 2006.

Bennett, B., "Posthumous Reproduction and the Meanings of Autonomy," *Melbourne University Law Review* 23, no. 2 (1999): 286–207.

Bentham, Jeremy, *Offences against One's Self*, available at: http://www.columbia.edu/cu/lweb/eresources/exhibitions/sw25/bentham/index.html. Accessed January 7, 2010.

Berg, Jessica, "Grave Secrets: Legal and Ethical Analysis of Postmortem Confidentiality." *Connecticut Law Review* 34, no. 1 (2001): 81–122.

Bering, Jesse M., and McLeod, Katrina, "Reasoning about Dead Agents Reveals Possible Adaptive Trends." *Human Nature* 16, no. 4 (2005): 360–381.

Bernstein, Mark H., *On Moral Considerability*. Oxford: Oxford University Press, 1998.

Bigelow, John, Campbell, John, and Pargetter, Robert, "Death and Well-Being." *Pacific Philosophical Quarterly* 71 (1990): 119–140.

Biggs, Hazel, "Speaking for the Dead—Life in Perpetuity." *Res Publica* 8 (2002): 93–104.

Blatti, Stephan, "Death's Distinctive Harm." *American Philosophical Quarterly*, forthcoming.

Blustein, Jeffrey, *The Moral Demands of Memory*. Cambridge: Cambridge University Press, 2008. .

Booth, W. James, *Communities of Memory: On Witness, Identity, and Justice*. Ithaca, NY: Cornell University Press, 2006.

Bortolotti, Lisa, "Agency, Life Extension, and the Meaning of Life," unpublished mss.

Bortolotti, Lisa, and Nagasawa, Y., "Immortality without Boredom." *Ratio* 22 (2009): 261–277.

Bourne, Craig, *A Future for Presentism*. New York: Oxford University Press, 2007.

Braddock, Glann, "Epicureanism, Death, and the Good Life." *Philosophical Inquiry* 22 (2000): 47–66.

Bradley, Ben *Well-Being & Death*. Oxford: Oxford University Press, 2009.

Bradley, Ben, and Kris McDaniel, "Death and Desires. " In *The Metaphysics and Ethics of Death*, edited by James Stacey Taylor. New York: Oxford University Press, forthcoming.

Brandt, Richard B. *Morality, Utilitarianism, and Rights*. Cambridge: Cambridge University Press, 1992.

Braun, S. Stewart, "Historical Entitlement and the Practice of Bequest: Is There a Moral Right of Bequest?" *Law and Philosophy* 29, no. 6 (2010): 695–715.

Brecher, Bob, "Our Obligation to the Dead." *Journal of Applied Philosophy* 19, no. 2 (2002): 109–119.

Brennan, Samantha, "The Badness of Death, the Wrongness of Killing, and the Moral Importance of Autonomy." *Dialogue* XL (2001): 723–737.

Brock, Edwin, "Five Ways to Kill a Man," available at: http://www.davidpbrown. co.uk/poetry/edwin-brock.html. Accessed January 18, 2010.

Broome, John, *Weighing Lives*. Oxford: Oxford University Press, 2004.

———, *Ethics out of Economics*. Cambridge: Cambridge University Press, 1999.

Brueckner, Anthony, and Fischer, John Martin, "Being Born Earlier." *Australasian Journal of Philosophy* 76, no. 1 (1998): 110–114.

———, "Why Is Death Bad?" *Philosophical Studies* 50 (1986): 213–221.

Burley, Mikel, "Anticipating Annihilation." *Inquiry* 49, no. 2 (2006): 170–185.

Callahan, Joan C., "On Harming the Dead." *Ethics* 97 (1987): 341–352.

Campbell, Alastair V., *The Body in Bioethics*. London: Routledge, 2009.

Cantor, Norman L., *After We Die: The Life and Times of the Human Cadaver*. Washington, DC: Georgetown University Press, 2010.

Carruthers, Peter, *The Animals Issue: Moral Theory in Practice*. Cambridge: Cambridge University Press, 1992.

Chan, David K., "Reasoning without Comparing." *American Philosophical Quarterly* 47, no. 2 (2010): 149–160.

Chappell, Timothy, "Infinity Goes Up on Trial: Must Immortality Be Meaningless?" *European Journal of Philosophy* 17, no. 1 (2007): 30–44.

Cherry, Mark J., "Why Should We Compensate Organ Donors When We Can Continue to Take Organs for Free? A Response to Some of My Critics." *Journal of Medicine and Philosophy* 34 (2009): 649–673.

———, *Kidney for Sale by Owner: Human Organs, Transplantation, and the Market*. Washington, DC: Georgetown University Press, 2005.

Chisholm, Roderick, *Person and Object: A Metaphysical Study*. LaSalle, IL: Open Court Publishing Co., 1976.

Christman, John "Defending Historical Autonomy: A Reply to Professor Mele," *Canadian Journal of Philosophy* 23, 2 (1993): 281–290.

Cicero, Marcus Tullius, *Tusculan Disputations*, trans. J. E. King. Cambridge, MA: Harvard University Press, 1960.

———, *De Finibus Bonorum et Malorum*, available at http://www.thelatinlibrary. com/cicero/fin1.shtml#49. Accessed July 17, 2010.

Cigman, Ruth, "Death, Misfortune, and Species Inequality." *Philosophy and Public Affairs* 10, no. 1 (1981): 47–64.

Cockburn, David, *Other Times: Philosophical Perspectives on Past, Present and Future*. Cambridge: Cambridge University Press, 1997.

Cohen, C., "The Case for Presumed Consent to Transplant Human Organs after Death." *Transplantation Proceedings* 24 (1992): 2168–2172.

Cohen, Esther, *The Crossroads of Justice: Law and Culture in Late Medieval France*. Leiden: E. J. Brill, 1993.

Collins, John M., "Feldman's Account of Death's Badness, and Life-Death Comparatives." *Southwest Philosophy Review* 21, no. 2 (2005): 83–99.

Collins, Rebecca, "Posthumous Reproduction and the Presumption against Consent in Cases of Death Caused by Sudden Trauma." *Journal of Medicine and Philosophy* 30 (2005): 431–442.

Conee, Earl, "Dispositions towards Counterfactuals in Ethics." In *The Good, the Right, Life and Death*, edited by Kris McDaniel, Jason R. Raibley, Richard

Feldman, and Michael J. Zimmerman, 173–187. Aldershot, UK: Ashgate, 2006.

Cooper, John M., *Reason and Emotion: Essays on Ancient Moral Psychology and Ethical Theory*. Princeton: Princeton University Press, 1999.

Cummins, R., "Reflection on Reflective Equilibrium." In *Rethinking Intuition: The Psychology of Intuition and Its Role in Philosophical Inquiry*, edited by M. DePaul and W. Ramsey, 113–128. Lanham, MD: Rowman & Littlefield, 1998.

Dalton, Peter C., "Death and Evil." *The Philosophical Forum* XI, no. 2 (1979–1980): 193–211.

Darwall, Stephen, *Welfare and Rational Care*. Princeton: Princeton University Press, 2002.

———, "Self-Interest and Self-Concern." In *Self-Interest*, edited by Ellen Frankel Paul, Fred D. Miller, Jr., and Jeffrey Paul, 158–178. New York: Cambridge University Press, 1997.

Davis, John K., "Surviving Interests and Living Wills." *Public Affairs Quarterly* 20, no. 1 (2006): 17–30.

Dennis, J. Michael, Hanson, Patricia, Hodge, Ernest E., Krom, Ridd A. F., and Veatch, Robert M., "An Evaluation of the Ethics of Presumed Consent and a Policy Based on Required Response." *UNOS Update* 1, no. 2 (1994): 16–21.

Devine, Philip E., *The Ethics of Homicide*. Ithaca, NY: Cornell University Press, 1978.

Devitt, Michael, "The Methodology of Naturalistic Semantics." *Journal of Philosophy* 91 (1994): 545–572.

Dickinson, Donna, *Property in the Body: Feminist Perspectives*. Cambridge: Cambridge University Press, 2007.

Digeser, P. E., *Political Forgiveness*. Ithaca, NY: Cornell University Press, 2001.

DiSilvestro, Russell, "The Ghost in the Machine Is the Elephant in the Room." *Journal of Medicine and Philosophy*, forthcoming.

Dodds, E. R., *The Greeks and the Irrational*. Berkeley: University of California Press, 1951.

Donnelly, John, "Suicide and Rationality." In *Language, Metaphysics, and Death*, edited by John Donnelly, 87–105. New York: Fordham University Press, 1978.

Douglass, A., and Daniels, K., "Posthumous Reproduction: A Consideration of the Medical, Ethical, Cultural, Psychosocial and Legal Perspectives in the New Zealand Context." *Medical Law International* 4, no. 4 (2002): 259–279.

Downie, R. S., "Research on Dead Infants." *Theoretical Medicine* 24 (2003): 161–175.

Draper, Kai, "Epicurus and the Anticipation of Death." In *The Metaphysics and Ethics of Death*, edited by James Stacey Taylor. New York: Oxford University Press, forthcoming.

———, "Epicurean Equanimity towards Death." *Philosophy and Phenomenological Research* 69, no. 1 (2004): 92–114.

———, "Disappointment, Sadness, and Death." *The Philosophical Review* 108, no. 3 (1999): 387–414.

Dresser, Rebecca, "Autonomy Revisited: The Limits of Anticipatory Choices." In *Dementia and Aging: Ethics, Values, and Policy Choices*, edited by Robert H. Binstock, Stephen G. Post, and Peter J. Whitehouse, 71–85. Baltimore; Johns Hopkins University Press, 1992.

Dworkin, Gerald, Frey, R. G., and Bok, Sissela, *Euthanasia and Physician-Assisted Suicide: For and Against*. Cambridge: Cambridge University Press, 1998.

Earle, William James, "Epicurus: 'Live Hidden!' " *Philosophy* 63, no. 243 (1988): 93–104.

Eberl, Jason T., "Do Human Persons Exist between Death and Resurrection?" In *Metaphysics and God: Essays in Honor of Eleonore Stump*, edited by Kevin Tempe, 188–205. New York: Routledge, 2009.

Englert, Walter, "Stoics and Epicureans on the Nature of Suicide." In *Proceedings of the Boston Area Colloquium in Ancient Philosophy: Volume X 1994*, edited by John J. Cleary and William Wians, 86–95. Lanham, MD: University Press of America, 1994.

Epicurus, *Kyriai Doxai*. In *Opere*, edited by Graziano Arrighetti, 121–137. Turin: Einaudi, 2nd edition, 1973.

———, *Gnomologium Vaticanum Epicureum*. In *Opere*, edited by Graziano Arrighetti, 139–157. Turin: Einaudi, 2nd edition, 1973.

———, "Letter to Menoeceus." In R. D. Hicks, *Stoic and Epicurean*, 169. New York, Russell & Russell, 1962.

ESHRE Task Force on Ethics and Law, "Posthumous Assisted Reproduction," *Human Reproduction* 21, no. 12 (2006): 3051–3052.

Etzioni, Amitai, "Organ Donation: A Communitarian Approach." *Kennedy Institute of Ethics Journal* 13 (2003): 1–18.

Ewin, R. E., *Reasons and the Fear of Death*. Boulder, CO: Rowman & Littlefield, Inc., 2002.

Fabre, Cecile, *Whose Body Is It Anyway?* New York: Oxford University Press, 2006.

Farsides, B., "Respecting Wishes and Avoiding Conflict: Understanding the Ethical Basis for Organ Donation and Retrieval." *British Journal of Anaesthesia* 108 (2012): 73–79.

Feinberg, Joel, "Harm to Others." In *The Metaphysics of Death*, edited by John Martin Fischer, 171–190. Stanford, CA: Stanford University Press, 1993.

———, *Harm to Others*. Oxford: Oxford University Press, 1984.

———, "The Rights of Animals and Unborn Generations." In *Responsibilities to Future Generations: Environmental Ethics*, edited by Ernest Partridge, 139–150. Buffalo, NY: Prometheus Books, 1981.

Feldman, Fred, *Pleasure and the Good Life: Concerning the Nature, Varieties, and Plausibility of Hedonism*. New York: Oxford University Press, 2004.

———, "Some Puzzles about the Evil of Death." In *The Metaphysics of Death*, edited by John Martin Fischer, 305–326. Stanford, CA: Stanford University Press, 1993.

———, *Confrontations with the Reaper*. New York: Oxford University Press, 1992.

———, "F.M. Kamm and the Mirror of Time." *Pacific Philosophical Quarterly* 71 (1990): 23–27.

Finnerty, James J., Thomas, Ted S., Boyle, Robert J., Howards, Stuart S., and Karns, Logan B., "Gamete Retrieval in Terminal Conditions." *American Journal of Obstetrics and Gynecology* 185, no. 2 (2001): 300–307.

Fischer, John Martin, "Epicureanism about Death and Immortality." *The Journal of Ethics* 10 (2006): 355–381.

———, "Earlier Birth and Later Death: Symmetry through Thick and Thin." In *The Good, the Right, Life and Death*, edited by Kris McDaniel, Jason R. Raibley, Richard Feldman, and Michael J. Zimmerman, 189–201. Aldershot, UK: Ashgate, 2006.

———, "Contribution to Symposium on Nussbaum's *The Therapy of Desire*." *Philosophy and Phenomenological Research* 59 (1999): 787–792.

———, "Why Immortality Is Not So Bad." *International Journal of Philosophical Studies* 2, no. 2 (1994): 257–270.

Fischer, John Martin, and Carl, Ruth, "Appendix: Philosophical Models of Immortality in Science Fiction." In *Our Stories: Essays on Life, Death, and Free Will*, edited by John Martin Fischer, 93–101. New York: Oxford University Press, 2009.

Fischer, John Martin, and Speak, Daniel, "Death and the Psychological Conception of Personal Identity." In *Our Stories: Essays on Life, Death, and Free Will*, edited by John Martin Fischer, 51–62. New York: Oxford University Press, 2009.

Fisher, Josie, "Harming and Benefiting the Dead." *Death Studies* 25 (2001): 557–568.

Frankfurt, Harry G., "On the Usefulness of Final Ends." In *Necessity, Volition, and Love*, edited by Harry G. Frankfurt, 82–94. Cambridge: Cambridge University Press, 1999.

———, "Freedom of the Will and the Concept of a Person." In *The Importance of What We Care About*, edited by Harry G. Frankfurt, 11–25. New York: Cambridge University Press, 1988.

Frey, R. G., "Autonomy, Diminished Life, and the Threshold for Use." In *Personal Autonomy: New Essays on Personal Autonomy and Its Role in Contemporary Moral Philosophy*, edited by James Stacey Taylor, 330–346. Cambridge: Cambridge University Press, 2005.

Friedman, Alan Warren, *Fictional Death and the Modernist Enterprise*. Cambridge: Cambridge University Press, 1995.

Friedman, David D. *Law's Order: What Economics Has to Do with Law and Why It Matters*. Princeton: Princeton University Press, 2000.

Fuchs, Alan E., "Posthumous Satisfactions and the Concept of Individual Welfare." In *Rationality, Morality, and Self-Interest: Essays Honoring Carl Overvold*, edited by John Heil, 215–220. Lanham, MD: Rowman & Littlefield Publishers, 1993.

Furley, David J., "Lucretius the Epicurean: On the History of Man." In *Lucretius: Oxford Readings in Classical Studies*, edited by Monica R. Gale, 157–181. Oxford: Oxford University Press, 2007.

———, "Nothing to Us?" In *The Norms of Nature: Studies in Hellenistic Ethics*, edited by Malcolm Schofield and Gisela Striker, 75–91. Cambridge: Cambridge University Press, 1986.

Gaita, Raimond, *The Philosopher's Dog: Friendships with Animals*. New York: Random House, 2002.

———, "Better One Than Ten," *Philosophical Investigations* 5, no. 2 (1982): 87–105.

Garrison, Elise P., *Groaning Tears: Ethical & Dramatic Aspects of Suicide in Greek Tragedy*. Leiden: Brill Academic Publishers, 1995.

Gasser, Georg, ed., *Personal Identity and Resurrection: How Do We Survive Our Death?* Aldershot, UK: Ashgate, 2010.

Geach, Peter, *God and the Soul*. New York: Schocken Books, 1969.

Gill, Michael B., "Presumed Consent, Autonomy, and Organ Donation," *Journal of Medicine and Philosophy* 29, no. 1 (2004): 37–59.

Glannon, Walter, "Brain Injury and Survival." In *The Metaphysics and Ethics of Death*, edited by James Stacey Taylor. New York: Oxford University Press, forthcoming.

———, "Do the Sick Have a Right to Cadaveric Organs?" *Journal of Medical Ethics*, 29 (2003): 153–156.

———, "Persons, Lives, and Posthumous Harms." *Journal of Social Philosophy* 32 (2001): 127–142.

———, "Temporal Asymmetry, Life, and Death," *American Philosophical Quarterly* 31, no. 3 (1994): 235–244.

———, "Epicureanism and Death," *Monist* 76 (1993): 222–234.

Glover, Jonathan, *Causing Death and Saving Lives*. Harmondsworth, UK: Penguin Books, 1977.

Goldman, Alvin, "Philosophical Intuitions: Their Target, Their Source, and Their Epistemic Status." *Grazer Philosophische Studien* 74 (2007): 1–26.

Goldstick, D., "The Welfare of the Dead," *Philosophy* 63 (1988): 111–113.

Gooch, Paul W., "Aristotle and the Happy Dead." *Classical Philology* 78, no. 2 (1983): 112–116.

Gordon, Robert M., *The Structure of Emotions: Investigations in Cognitive Philosophy*. Cambridge: Cambridge University Press, 1987.

Gosseries, Axel, "Intergenerational Justice." In *The Oxford Handbook of Practical Ethics*, edited by Hugh LaFollette, 459–484. New York: Oxford University Press, 2003.

Graver, Margaret, "Managing Mental Pain: Epicurus vs. Aristippus on the Pre-Rehearsal of Future Ills." *Proceedings of the Boston Area Colloquium in Ancient Philosophy* 17 (2002): 155–177.

Gray, John Chipman, *The Nature and Sources of the Law*. New York: Columbia University Press, 1916.

Green, O. H., "Fear of Death." *Philosophy and Phenomenological Research* XLIII, no. 1 (1982): 99–105.

Grey, William, "Epicurus and the Harm of Death." *Australasian Journal of Philosophy* 77 (1999): 358–364.

Griffin, James, *Well-Being*. Oxford: Clarendon Press, 1986.

Griseri, Paul, "Can a Dead Man Be Harmed?" *Philosophical Investigations* 10 (1987): 317–329.

Griswold, Charles L., *Forgiveness: A Philosophical Exploration*. New York: Cambridge University Press, 2007.

Grotius, Hugo, *The Rights of War and Peace, Including the Law of Nature and of Nations*, trans. A. C. Campbell. New York: M. Walter Dunne, 1901.

Grover, Dorothy, "Posthumous Harm." *The Philosophical Quarterly* 39 (1989): 334–353.

———, "Death, and Life." *Canadian Journal of Philosophy* 17, no. 4 (1987): 711–732.

Haddow, Gillian, "'Because You're Worth It?' The Taking and Selling of Transplantable Organs," *Journal of Medical Ethics* 32, no. 6 (2006). Available at: http://www.ncbi.nlm.nih.gov/pmc/articles/PMC2563366/. Accessed January 23, 2010.

Haji, Ishtiyaque, "Pre-vital and Post-vital Times." *Pacific Philosophical Quarterly* 72 (1991): 171–180.

Hall, David, "Reflecting on Redfern: What Can We Learn from the Alder Hey Story?" *Archives of Disease in Childhood* 84 (2001): 455–456.

Hamer, C. L., and Rivlin, M. M., "A Stronger Policy of Organ Retrieval from Cadaveric Donors: Some Ethical Considerations." *Journal of Medical Ethics*, 29 (2003): 196–200.

Hanser, Matthew, "The Metaphysics of Harm." *Philosophy and Phenomenological Research* 77, no. 2 (2008): 421–450.

Harman, Elizabeth, "Harming as Causing Harm." In *Harming Future Persons: Ethics, Genetics, and the Nonidentity Problem*, edited by Melinda A. Roberts and David T. Wasserstrom, 137–154. Dordrecht, Netherlands: Springer, 2009.

Harris, John, "Doing Posthumous Harm." In *The Metaphysics and Ethics of Death*, edited by James Stacey Taylor. New York: Oxford University Press, forthcoming.

———, "Mark Anthony or Macbeth: Some Problems Concerning the Dead and the Incompetent When It Comes to Consent." In *First Do No Harm: Law, Ethics, and Healthcare*, edited by Sheila A. M. Maclean, 287–302. Aldershot, UK: Ashgate, 2006.

———, "Organ Procurement: Dead Interests, Living Needs." *Journal of Medical Ethics* 29 (2003): 130–134.

———, "Four Legs Good, Personhood Better!" *Res Publica* 4, no. 1 (1998): 51–59.

Harrison, Robert Pogue, *The Dominion of the Dead*. Chicago: University of Chicago Press, 2003.

Hartley, James, *Suffering Witness*. Albany, NY: State University of New York, 2000.

Haslett, D. W., "Is Inheritance Justified?" *Philosophy and Public Affairs* 15, no. 2 (1986): 122–155.

Hershenov, David, "Do Dead Bodies Pose a Problem for Biological Approaches to Personal Identity?" *Mind* 114, no. 453 (2005): 31–59.

Hetherington, Stephen, "Lucretian Death: Asymmetries and Agency." *American Philosophical Quarterly* 42, no. 3 (2005): 211–219.

Hill, Thomas E., Jr., *Autonomy and Self-respect*. Cambridge: Cambridge University Press 1991.

Hinchliff, Mark, "The Puzzle of Change." *Nous* 30, Supplement: *Philosophical Perspectives* 10, Metaphysics (1996): 119–136.

Hinkley, Charles C., *Moral Conflicts of Organ Retrieval: A Case for Constructive Pluralism*. Amsterdam: Editions Rodophi, BV, 2005.

Hippen, Benjamin E., "In Defense of a Regulated Market in Kidneys from Living Vendors." *Journal of Medicine and Philosophy* 30, no. 6 (2005): 593–626.

Hobbes, Thomas, *Leviathan*. Indianapolis: Hackett Publishing Co., Inc., 1994.

Holland, Stephen, "On the Ordinary Concept of Death." *Journal of Applied Philosophy* 27, no. 2 (2010): 109–122.

Homer, *Iliad*. Available at: http://www.perseus.tufts.edu/hopper/text?doc=Hom.+Il.+24+526&fromdoc=Perseus:text:1999.01.0133, accessed August 2, 2010.

Honore, Anthony M., "Ownership." In *Oxford Essays in Jurisprudence: First Series*, edited by A. G. Guest, 107–147. Oxford: Clarendon Press, 1961.

Hooker, Brad, "A Breakthrough in the Desire Theory of Welfare." In *Rationality, Morality and Self-Interest: Essays Honoring Mark Carl Overold*, edited by J. Heil, 205–213. Lanham, MD: Rowan & Littlefield, 1993.

Hossenfelder, Malte, "Epicurus—hedonist malgre lui." In *The Norms of Nature: Studies in Hellenistic Ethics*, edited by Malcolm Schofield and Gisela Striker, 245–263. Cambridge: Cambridge University Press, 1986.

House of Commons, *Journal of the House of Commons, Vol. 8, 1660–1667*. London: House of Commons, 1802.

Howes, Craig, "Afterword." In *The Ethics of Life Writing*, edited by John Paul Eakin, 244–264. Ithaca, NY: Cornell University Press, 2004.

Iltis, Ana S., and Cherry, Mark J., eds., *Revisiting Death: Organ Donation and the Dead Donor Rule; The Journal of Medicine and Philosophy* 35, 3 (2010).

James, L., "Shape and the Meaningfulness of Life." In *Philosophy and Happiness*, edited by L. Bortolotti, 54–67. Basingstoke, UK: Palgrave, 2009.

Johansson, Jens, "The Time of Death's Badness." *Journal of Medicine and Philosophy*, forthcoming.

———, *Mortal Beings: On the Metaphysics and Value of Death*. Stockholm: Almquist & Wiksell International, 2005.

Johnston, Mark, *Surviving Death*. Princeton: Princeton University Press, 2010.

Kamm, F. M., *Morality, Mortality Volume I: Death and Whom to Save from It*. New York: Oxford University Press, 1993.

———, "Why Is Death Bad and Worse Than Pre-natal Non-existence?" *Pacific Philosophical Quarterly* 69 (1988): 161–164.

Kant, Immanuel, *The Metaphysics of Morals*, ed. Mary Gregor. Cambridge: Cambridge University Press, 1996.

Kaufman, Frederik, "Thick and Thin Selves: A Reply to Fischer and Speak." In *Midwest Studies in Philosophy Volume XXIV Life and Death: Metaphysics and Ethics*, edited by Peter A. French and Howard Wettstein, 94–97. Boston: Wiley-Blackwell, 2000.

———, "Pre-Vital and Post-Mortem Non-Existence." *American Philosophical Quarterly* 36, no. 1 (1999): 1–19.

———, "An Answer to Lucretius' Symmetry Argument against the Fear of Death." *Journal of Value Inquiry* 29, no. 1 (1995): 57–64.

———, "Death and Deprivation; Or, Why Lucretius' Symmetry Argument Fails." *Australasian Journal of Philosophy* 74, no. 2 (1996): 305–312.

Kavka, G., *Hobbesian Moral and Political Theory*. Princeton: Princeton University Press, 1986.

Kierkegaard, Søren, *Works of Love*, edited and translated by Howard V. Hong and Edna H. Hong. Princeton: Princeton University Press, 1995.

———, "At a Graveside." In Søren Kierkegaard, *Three Discourses on Imagined Occasions*, edited and translated by Howard V. Hong and Edna H. Hong, 71–102. Princeton: Princeton University Press, 1993.

Kivy, Peter, *The Fine Art of Repetition: Essays in the Philosophy of Music*. Cambridge: Cambridge University Press, 1993.

Kluge, E. H., "Improving Organ Retrieval Rates: Various Proposals and Their Ethical Validity." *Health Care Analysis* 8 (2000): 279–295.

Konstan, David, *Some Aspects of Epicurean Psychology*. Leiden: E.J. Brill, 1973.

Korsgaard, Christine M., *The Sources of Normativity*. Cambridge: Cambridge University Press, 1996.

Kripke, S., "Naming and Necessity." In *Semantics of Natural Language*, edited by D. Davidson and G. Harman, 253–355. Dordrecht, Netherlands: Reidel, 1972.

Laertius, Diogenes, "Life of Epicurus." In *Epicurus: The Extant Remains with Short Critical Apparatus*, translated and edited by Cyril Bailey, 140–171. New York: Georg Olms Verlag, 1970.

Lamont, Julian, "A Solution to the Puzzle of When Death Harms Its Victims." *Australasian Journal of Philosophy*, 76 (1998): 198–212.

Lande, Nelson P., "Posthumous Rehabilitation and the Dust-Bin of History." *Public Affairs Quarterly* 4, no. 3 (1990): 267–286.

Lenman, James, "On Becoming Extinct." *Pacific Philosophical Quarterly* 83 (2002): 253–269.

———, "Immortality: A Letter." *Cogito* 9 (1995): 164–169.

Leslie, John, "Why Not Let Life Become Extinct?" *Philosophy* 58 (1983): 329–338.

Levenbook, Barbara Baum, "Welfare and Harm after Death." In *The Metaphysics and Ethics of Death*, edited by James Stacey Taylor. New York: Oxford University Press, forthcoming.

———, "The Retroactivity Problem." In *Time and Identity*, edited by Joseph Keim Campbell, Michael O'Rourke, and Harry S. Silverstein, 287–308. Cambridge, MA: MIT Press, 2010.

———, "Harming the Dead, Once Again." *Ethics* 96 (1985): 162–164.

———, "Harming Someone after His Death." *Ethics* 94 (1984): 407–419.

Lewin, Tamar, "Taking after Father, a Frozen Sperm Riddle." *New York Times*, January 13, 2002, A3.

Lewis, David, *On the Plurality of Worlds*. New York: Blackwell, 1986.

———, *Counterfactuals*. New York: Blackwell, 1973.

Li, Jack, *Can Death Be a Harm to the Person Who Dies?* Dordrecht, Netherlands: Kluwer Academic Publishers, 2002.

Lindemann, James Nelson, "Death's Gender." In *Mother Time: Women, Aging, and Ethics*, edited by Margaret Urban Walker, 113–129. Lanham, MD: Rowman & Littlefield Publishers, Inc., 1999.

Lodge, David, *Changing Places*. New York: Penguin, 1978.

Lomasky, Loren, *Persons, Rights, and the Moral Community*. New York: Oxford University Press, 1987.

Lombard, Brian *Events*. Boston: Routledge, 1986.

Lucretius, *De Rerum Natura* , translated by W. H. D. Rouse and revised by Martin Ferguson Smith. Cambridge, MA: Harvard University Press, 2006.

Luper, Stephen, "Adaptation." In *The Metaphysics and Ethics of Death*, edited by James Stacey Taylor. New York: Oxford University Press, forthcoming.

———, *The Philosophy of Death*. Cambridge: Cambridge University Press, 2009.

———, "Mortal Harm." *The Philosophical Quarterly* 57, no. 227 (2007): 239–251.

———, "Past Desires and the Dead." *Philosophical Studies* 126 (2005): 331–345.

———, "Posthumous Harm." *American Philosophical Quarterly* 41 (2004): 63–72.

———, *Invulnerability: On Securing Happiness*. Chicago: Open Court Publishing Co., 1996.

Luper-Foy, Stephen, "Annihilation." In *The Metaphysics of Death*, edited by John Martin Fischer, 221–229. Stanford, CA: Stanford University Press, 1993.

Madoff, Ray D., *Immortality and the Law: The Rising Power of the American Dead*. New Haven: Yale University Press, 2010.

Mahoney, Julia D., "Should We Adopt a Market Strategy to Increase the Supply of Transplantable Organs?" In *The Ethics of Organ Transplantation*, edited by Wayne Shelton and John Balint, 65–88. Stamford, CT: Jai Press, 2001.

Markosian, Ned, "A Defense of Presentism." In *Oxford Studies in Metaphysics, Volume 1*, edited by Dean W. Zimmerman, 47–82. Oxford: Clarendon Press, 2004.

Marquis, Don, "Harming the Dead." *Ethics* 96 (1985): 159–161.

Masterton, Malin, Hansson, Matts G., Hoglund, Anna T., "In search of the missing subject: narrative identity and posthumous wrongdoing." *Studies in the History and Philosophy of Biological and Biomedical Sciences* 41 (2010): 340–346.

Masterton, M., Hansson, M. G., Hoglund, A. T., and Helgesson, G., "Can the Dead Be Brought into Disrepute?" *Theoretical Medicine and Bioethics* 28, no. 2 (2007): 137–149.

———, "Queen Christina's Moral Claim on the Living: Justification of a Tenacious Moral Intuition." *Medicine, Health Care, and Philosophy* 10, no. 3 (2007): 321–327.

Matson, Wallace I., "Hegesias the Death-Persuader: Or, the Gloominess of Hedonism." *Philosophy* 73 (1998): 553–557.

May, Larry, "Metaphysical Guilt and Moral Taint." In *Collective Responsibility: Five Decades of Debate in Theoretical and Applied Ethics*, edited by Larry May and Stacey Hoffman, 239–254. Savage, MD: Rowman & Littlefield, 1991.

May, Todd, *Death*. Stocksfield, UK: Acumen, 2009.

McGonagall, William, "Railway Bridge of the Silvery Tay." In *The Penguin Book of Scottish Verse*, edited by Robert Crawford and Mick Imlah, 349–350. London: Penguin, 2006.

McMahan, Jeff, "The Lucretian Argument." In *The Good, the Right, Life and Death: Essays in Honor of Fred Feldman*, edited by Kris McDaniel, Jason R. Raibley, Richard Feldman, and Michael J. Zimmerman, 213–226. Aldershot, UK: Ashgate Publishing Co., 2006.

———, "Death and the Value of Life." In *The Metaphysics of Death*, edited by John Martin Fischer, 231–266. Stanford, CA: Stanford University Press, 1993.

McNeil, D. R., "Constitutionality of 'Presumed Consent' for Organ Donation," *Hamline Journal of Public Law and Policy* 9 (1989): 343–372.

Mellor, D. H., *Real Time*. Cambridge: Cambridge University Press, 1981.

Mendola, Joseph, "Intuitive Hedonism." *Philosophical Studies* 128 (2006): 441–477.

Meyer, Lukas H., "Reparations and Symbolic Restitution." *Journal of Social Philosophy* 37, no. 3 (2006): 406–422.

Mill, J. S., *Utilitarianism*. Indianapolis: Hackett Publishing Company, 1979.

Miller, Fred D., Jr., "Epicurus on the Art of Dying." *The Southern Journal of Philosophy* 14, no. 2 (1976): 169–177.

Mitchell, Gregory, "Libertarian Paternalism Is an Oxymoron." *Northwest University Law Review* 99 (2005): 1245–1277.

Mitsis, Philip, "Epicurus on Death and the Duration of Life," in *Proceedings of the Boston Area Colloquium in Ancient Philosophy* 4 (1989): 303–322.

———, *Epicurus' Ethical Theory: The Pleasures of Invulnerability*. Ithaca, NY: Cornell University Press, 1988.

Momeyer, Richard W., *Confronting Death*. Bloomington: Indiana University Press, 1988.

Mothersill, Mary, "Death." In *Life and Meaning: A Reader*, edited by Oswald Hanfling, 83–92. Oxford: Basil Blackwell, 1987.

Mulgan, Tim, "The Place of the Dead in Liberal Political Philosophy." *The Journal of Political Philosophy* 7, no. 1 (1999): 52–70.

Murphy, Jeffrie, "Rationality and the Fear of Death." *The Monist* 59 (1976): 187–203.

Mustakallio, Katariina, *Death and Disgrace: Capital Penalties with Post Mortem Sanctions in Early Roman Historiography*. Helsinki: Suomalainen Tiedeakatemia, 1994.

Nabokov, Vladimir, *Speak, Memory*. New York: Everyman's Library, 1999.

Nagel, Thomas, "Death." In *The Metaphysics of Death*, edited by John Martin Fischer, 61–69. Stanford, CA: Stanford University Press, 1993.

———, *The View from Nowhere*. New York: Oxford University Press, 1986.

Nelkin, Dorothy, and Andrews, Lori, "Do the Dead Have Interests? Policy Issues for Research After Life." *American Journal of Law and Medicine* XXIV, nos. 2&3 (1998): 261–291.

Nikolsky, Boris, "Epicurus on Pleasure." *Phronesis* XLVI, no. 4 (2001): 440–465.

Noggle, Robert, "Autonomy, Value, and Conditioned Desire." *American Philosophical Quarterly* 32, no. 1 (1995): 57–69.

Nozick, Robert, *Anarchy, State, and Utopia*. Oxford: Blackwell, 1974.

Nussbaum, Martha, "The Damage of Death: Incomplete Arguments and False Consolations." In *The Metaphysics and Ethics of Death*, edited by James Stacey Taylor. New York: Oxford University Press, forthcoming.

———, "Reply to Papers in Symposium on Nussbaum, *The Therapy of Desire*." *Philosophy and Phenomenological Research* 59 (1999): 811–819.

———, *The Therapy of Desire: Theory and Practice in Hellenistic Ethics*. Princeton: Princeton University Press, 1994.

———, "Therapeutic Arguments: Epicurus and Aristotle." In *The Norms of Natures: Studies in Hellenistic Ethics*, edited by Malcolm Schofield and Gisela Striker, 31–74. Cambridge: Cambridge University Press, 1986.

O'Callaghan, E., Sham, P., Takei, N., Glover, G., and Murray, R. M., "Schizophrenia after Prenatal Exposure to 1957 A2 Influenza Epidemic." *The Lancet* 337 (1991): 1248–1250.

Ochs, Carol, *Women and Spirituality*. Lanham, MD: Rowman & Littlefield, Inc., 2nd edition, 1997.

O'Keefe, Tim, "Lucretius on the Cycle of Life and the Fear of Death." *Apeiron* 36, no. 1 (2003): 43–65.

Olick, Robert S., *Taking Advance Directives Seriously: Prospective Autonomy and Decisions Near the End of Life*. Washington, DC: Georgetown University Press, 2001.

Orr, R. D., and Siegler, M., "Is Posthumous Semen Retrieval Ethically Permissible?" *Journal of Medical Ethics* 28 (2002): 299–302.

Oshana, Marina A. L., "Moral Taint." *Metaphilosophy* 37, nos. 3–4 (2006): 353–375.

Overall, Christine, *Aging, Death, and Human Longevity: A Philosophical Inquiry*. Berkeley: University of California Press, 2003.

Overvold, Mark, "Self-Interest and Getting What You Want." In *The Limits of Utilitarianism*, edited by H. B. Miller and W. H. Williams, 186–194. Minneapolis: University of Minnesota Press, 1982.

Page, Edward A., *Climate Change, Justice and Future Generations*. Cheltenham, UK: Edward Elgar, 2006.

Paine, Thomas, *Rights of Man*. Harmondsworth, UK: Penguin, 1969.

Parfit, Derek, *Reasons and Persons*. Oxford: Oxford University Press, 1984.

Parker, M. J., " 'Til Death Us Do Part: The Ethics of Postmortem Gamete Donation." *Journal of Medical Ethics* 30 (2004): 387–388.

Parker, R., *Miasma: Pollution and Purification in Early Greek Religion*. Oxford: Clarendon Press, 1983.

Partridge, Ernest, "Posthumous Interests and Posthumous Respect." *Ethics* 91 (1981): 259–264.

Philodemus, *On Death*, translated by W. Benjamin Henry. Atlanta: Society of Biblical Literature, 2009.

Pitcher, George, "The Misfortunes of the Dead." In *The Metaphysics of Death*, edited by John Martin Fischer, 157–168. Stanford, CA: Stanford University Press, 1993.

Porphyry, *Porphyry the Philosopher to Marcella*, 31. Available at http://www.tertullian.org/fathers/porphyry_marcella_03_revised_text.htm. Accessed June 16, 2010.

Portmore, Douglas, "Desire Fulfillment and Posthumous Harm." *American Philosophical Quarterly* 44, 1 (2007): 27–38.

———, "Welfare, Achievement, and Self-Sacrifice." *Journal of Ethics & Social Philosophy* 2, no. 2 (2007). Available at: http://www.jesp.org/PDF/Douglas-Portmore.pdf. Accessed January 8, 2010.

Prado, C. G., *Coping with Choices to Die*. Cambridge: Cambridge University Press, 2010.

———, *Choosing to Die: Elective Death and Multiculturalism*. Cambridge: Cambridge University Press, 2008.

Price, David T., *Legal and Ethical Aspects of Organ Transplantation*. Cambridge: Cambridge University Press, 2000.

———, "Giving Blood: Posthumous Fertility Treatment and a Good Old British Compromise?" *International Review of Law, Computers and Technology* 11, no. 2 (1997): 299–311.

Prior, A. N., "Now." In *Papers on Time and Tense*, edited by A. N. Prior, 171–193. Oxford: Clarendon Press, 2003.

Pritzl, Kurt, "Aristotle and Happiness after Death: *Nicomachean Ethics* 1. 10–11," *Classical Philology* 78, no. 2 (1983): 101–111.

Rabieh, Linda R., *Plato and the Virtue of Courage*. Baltimore, MD: Johns Hopkins University Press, 2006.

Raz, Joseph, *Value, Respect, and Attachment*. Cambridge: Cambridge University Press, 2001.

Redfern, Michael, Keeling, Jean, and Powell, Elizabeth, *The Report of the Royal Liverpool Children's Inquiry*. Available at: http://www.rlcinquiry.org.uk/index.htm. Accessed February 2, 2010.

Renteln, Alison Dundes, *The Cultural Defense*. Oxford: Oxford University Press, 2004.

Ridge, Michael, "Giving the Dead Their Due." *Ethics* 114 (2003): 38–59.

Rivera-Lopez, Eduardo, "Are Mental State Welfarism and Our Concern for Non-experiential Goals Incompatible?" *Pacific Philosophical Quarterly* 88 (2007): 74–91.

Robertson, John A., "Second Thoughts on Living Wills." *The Hastings Center Report* 21, no. 6 (1991): 6–10.

Rosenbaum, Stephen E., "Concepts of Value and Our Thinking about Death." In *The Metaphysics and Ethics of Death*, edited by James Stacey Taylor. New York: Oxford University Press, forthcoming.

———, "Death as a Punishment: A Consequence of Epicurean Thanatology." In *Epicurus: His Continuing Influence and Contemporary Relevance*, edited by Dane R. Gordon and David B. Suits, 195–207. Rochester, NY: RIT Cary Graphic Arts Press, 2003.

———, "How to Be Dead and Not Care: A Defense of Epicurus." In *The Metaphysics of Death*, edited by John Martin Fischer, 117–134. Stanford, CA: Stanford University Press, 1993.

———, "Epicurus and Annihilation." In *The Metaphysics of Death*, edited by John Martin Fischer, 293–304. Stanford, CA: Stanford University Press, 1993.

———, "Epicurus on Pleasure and the Complete Life." *Monist* 73, no. 1 (1990): 21–41.

———, "The Symmetry Argument: Lucretius against the Fear of Death." *Philosophy and Phenomenological Research* 50, no. 2 (1989): 353–373.

———, "The Harm of Killing: An Epicurean Perspective." In *Contemporary Essays on Greek Ideas: The Kilgore Festschrift*, edited by Robert M. Baird, William F. Cooper, Elmer H. Duncan, and Stuart E. Rosenbaum, 207–226. Waco, TX: Baylor University Press, 1987.

Ross, W. D., *Foundations of Ethics*. Oxford: Oxford University Press, 1939.

Roswell, Jamie, "Stayin' Alive: Postmortem Reproduction and Inheritance Rights." *41 Family Court Review* 400 (2003): 400–415.

Ruben, David-Hillel, *Action and Its Explanation*. Oxford: Clarendon Press, 2003.

———, "A Puzzle about Posthumous Predication." *The Philosophical Review* 98 (1988): 211–236.

Russell, Bertrand, "Lectures of the Philosophy of Logical Atomism." In Bertrand Russell, *Logic and Knowledge. (Essays 1901–1950)*, edited by R. C. Marsh, 175–281. London: Routledge, 1956.

———, "Knowledge by Acquaintance and Knowledge by Description." *Proceedings of the Aristotelian Society* 11 (1911): 108–128.

Savulescu, J., "Death, Us and Our Bodies: Personal Reflections." *Journal of Medical Ethics* 29 (2003): 127–130.

Sayers, Brian, "Death as a Loss." *Faith and Philosophy* 4, no. 2 (1987): 149–159.

Scarre, Geoffrey, "The Invulnerability of the Dead." In *The Metaphysics and Ethics of Death*, edited by James Stacey Taylor. New York: Oxford University Press, forthcoming.

———, *Death*. Montreal: McGill-Queen's University Press, 2007.

———, "Can Archaeology Harm the Dead?" In *The Ethics of Archeology: Philosophical Perspectives on Archaeological Practice*, edited by Chris Scarre and Geoffrey Scarre, 181–198. Cambridge: Cambridge University Press, 2006.

———, "Archeology and Respect for the Dead." *Journal of Applied Philosophy* 20, no. 3 (2003): 237–249.

———, "On Caring about One's Posthumous Reputation." *American Philosophical Quarterly* 38, no. 2 (2001): 209–219.

———, "Should We Fear Death?" *European Journal of Philosophy* 5, no. 3 (1997): 269–282.

Schaller, Barry R., *Understanding Bioethics and the Law: The Promises and Perils of the Brave New World of Biotechnology.* Westport, CT: Praeger, 2008.

Schiff, A. R., "Posthumous Conception and the Need for Consent." *Medical Journal of Australia* 170 (1999): 53–54.

———, "Arising from the Dead: Challenges of Posthumous Procreation." *North Carolina Law Review* 75, 3 (1997): 901–965.

Scott, Dominic, "Aristotle on Posthumous Fortune." *Oxford Studies in Ancient Philosophy* XVIII (2000): 211–229.

Sedley. D. N., "Chrysippus on Psychophysical Causality." In *Passions and Perceptions: Studies in Hellenistic Philosophy of Mind,* edited by J. Brunschwig and M. Nussbaum, 313–331. Cambridge: Cambridge University Press, 1993.

Segal, Charles, *Lucretius on Death and Anxiety: Poetry and Philosophy in "De Rerum Natura."* Princeton: Princeton University Press, 1990.

Seneca, Lucius Annaeus, *Epistulae Morales,* 77.12. Trans. R. M. Gummere. Available at: http://www.molloy.edu/sophia/seneca/epistles/ep77.htm. Accessed July 20, 2010.

Serafini, Anthony, "Callahan on Harming the Dead." *Journal of Philosophical Research* XV (1989–1990): 329–339.

Sewell-Rutter, N. J., *Guilt by Descent: Moral Inheritance and Decision Making in Greek Tragedy.* Oxford: Oxford University Press, 2007.

Shakespeare, William, *Macbeth.* New York: Longman's, Green, & Co., 1896.

———, *Hamlet.* In *The Complete Works of William Shakespeare.* New York: Avenel Books, 1975.

Silverstein, Harry S., "The Evil of Death One More Time: Parallels between Time and Space." In *The Metaphysics and Ethics of Death,* edited by James Stacey Taylor. New York: Oxford University Press, forthcoming.

———, "The Time of the Evil of Death." In *Time and Identity,* edited by Joseph Keim Campbell, Michael O'Rourke, and Harry S. Silverstein, 283–295. Cambridge, MA: MIT Press, 2010.

———, "The Evil of Death Revisited." In *Midwest Studies in Philosophy Volume XXIV, Life and Death: Metaphysics and Ethics,* edited by Peter A. French and Howard K. Wettstein, 116–134. Boston: Wiley-Blackwell, 2000.

———, "The Evil of Death." *Journal of Philosophy* 77 (1980): 401–424.

Singer, Peter, *Animal Liberation.* New York: New York Review, 1975.

Sinnott-Armstrong, Walter, "You Can't Lose What You Ain't Never Had: A Reply to Marquis on Abortion." *Philosophical Studies* 96 (1997): 59–72.

Smith, Alexander McCall, *Friends, Lovers, Chocolate.* New York: Pantheon Books, 2005.

Smith, Nick. *I Was Wrong: The Meanings of Apologies.* New York: Cambridge University Press, 2008.

Soll, Ivan, "On the Purported Insignificance of Death: Whistling before the Dark?" In *Death and Philosophy,* edited by Jeff Malpas and Robert C. Solomon, 20–34. London: Routledge, 1998.

Solomon, Robert C., "Is There Happiness after Death?" *Philosophy,* 51 (1976): 189–193.

Sorabji, Richard, *Self: Ancient and Modern Insights about Individuality, Life, and Death.* Chicago: University of Chicago Press, 2006.

———, *Time, Creation, and the Continuum: Theories in Antiquity and the Early Middle Ages.* Ithaca, NY: Cornell University Press, 1983.

Spawn, Clay, "Updating Epicurus's Concept of *Katastematic* Pleasure." *The Journal of Value Inquiry* 36 (2002): 473–482.

Sperling, Daniel, *Posthumous Interests: Legal and Ethical Perspectives*. Cambridge: Cambridge University Press, 2008.

———, *Management of Post-Mortem Pregnancy: Legal and Philosophical Aspects*. Aldershot, UK: Ashgate, 2006.

Spital, Aaron, "Conscription of Cadaveric Organs for Transplantation: Neglected Again." *Kennedy Institute of Ethics Journal* 13, no. 2 (2003): 169–174.

Spital, Aaron, and Taylor, James Stacey, "In Defense of Routine Recovery of Cadaveric Organs: A Response to Walter Glannon." *Cambridge Quarterly of Healthcare Ethics* 17, no. 3 (2008): 337–343.

———, "Routine Recovery of Cadaveric Organs for Transplantation: Consistent, Fair, and Life Saving." *Clinical Journal of the American Society of Nephrology* 2 (2007): 300–303.

Spriggs, M., "Woman Wants Dead Fiancé's Baby: Who Owns a Dead Man's Sperm." *Journal of Medical Ethics* 30 (2004): 384–385.

Stalnaker, Robert, *Inquiry*. Cambridge, MA: MIT Press, 1984.

Steiner, Hillel, *An Essay on Rights*. Oxford: Blackwell, 1994.

Striker, Gisela, "Epicurean Hedonism." In *Passions and Perceptions: Studies in Hellenistic Philosophy of Mind Proceedings of the Fifth Symposium Hellenisticum*, edited by Jacques Brunschwig and Martha C. Nussbaum, 1–17. Cambridge: Cambridge University Press, 1993.

Suits, David B., "Why Death Is Not Bad for the One Who Dies." *American Philosophical Quarterly* 38, no. 1 (2001): 69–84.

Sumner, L. W., "A Matter of Life and Death." *Nous* 10 (1976): 145–171.

Tarlow, Sarah, "Archeological Ethics and the People of the Past." In *The Ethics of Archeology: Philosophical Perspectives on Archaeological Practice*, edited by Chris Scarre and Geoffrey Scarre, 199–216. Cambridge: Cambridge University Press, 2006.

Taylor, C. C. W., *Pleasure, Mind, and Soul: Selected Papers in Ancient Philosophy*. Oxford: Clarendon Press, 2008.

Taylor, James Stacey, *Practical Autonomy and Bioethics*. New York: Routledge, 2009.

———, "Autonomy and Organ Sales, Revisited." *Journal of Medicine and Philosophy* 34 (2009): 632–648.

———, "Nothing in the Dark: Deprivation, Death, and the Good Life." In *Philosophy in the Twilight Zone*, edited by Noel Carroll and Lester H. Hunt, 171–186. Oxford: Blackwell, 2009.

———, "The Unjustified Assumptions of Organ Conscripters." *HEC Forum* 21, no. 2 (2009): 115–133.

———, "Harming the Dead." *Journal of Philosophical Research* 33 (2008): 185–202.

———, "Liberalism, the Duty to Rescue, and Organ Procurement." *Political Studies Review* 6, no. 3 (2008): 314–326.

———, "The Myth of Posthumous Harm." *American Philosophical Quarterly* 42, no. 4 (2005): 311–322.

———, *Stakes and Kidneys: Why Markets in Human Body Parts Are Morally Imperative*. Aldershot, UK: Ashgate Publishing, 2005.

———, "Introduction." In *Personal Autonomy: New Essays on Personal Autonomy and Its Role in Contemporary Moral Philosophy*, edited by James Stacey Taylor, 1–32. Cambridge: Cambridge University Press, 2005.

———, "Privacy and Autonomy: A Reappraisal." *The Southern Journal of Philosophy* 40 (2002): 587–604.

Taylor, James Stacey, and Spital, Aaron "Corpses Do Not Have Rights: A Response to Baglow." *Mortality* 13, 3 (2008): 282–286.

Thaler, Richard H., and Sunstein, Cass R., *Nudge: Improving Decisions about Health, Wealth, and Happiness*. New Haven, CT: Yale University Press, 2008.

Thompson, Janna, "Intergenerational Responsibilities and the Interests of the Dead." In *Time and Ethics: Essays at the Intersection*, edited by H. Dyke, 71–83. Dordrecht, Netherlands: Kluwer Academic Publishers, 2003.

———, "Inherited Obligations and Generational Continuity." *Canadian Journal of Philosophy* 29, no. 4 (1999): 493–516.

Tooley, Michael, *Time, Tense, and Causation*. Oxford: Clarendon Press, 1997.

Trapp, Michael, *Philosophy in the Roman Empire: Ethics, Politics, and Society*. Aldershot, UK: Ashgate, 2007.

Tsouna, Voula, *The Ethics of Philodemus*. Oxford: Oxford University Press, 2007.

Varner, Eric R., "Punishment after Death: Mutilation of Images and Corpse Abuse in Ancient Rome." *Mortality* 6, no. 1 (2010): 46–64.

Veatch, R. M., and Pitt, J. B., "The Myth of Presumed Consent: Ethical Problems in Organ Procurement Strategies." *Transplantation Proceedings* 27 (1995): 1888–1892.

von Dehsen, Christian D., *Philosophers and Religious Leaders: An Encyclopedia of People Who Changed the World*. Phoenix, AZ: Oryx Press, 1999.

Wallach, Barbara Price, *Lucretius and the Diatribe against the Fear of Death: "De Rerum Natura III,"* 830–1094. Leiden: E. J. Brill, 1976.

Walton, Kendall L., "Fearing Fictions." *The Journal of Philosophy* 75, no. 1 (1978): 5–27.

Waluchow, W. J., "Feinberg's Theory of 'Preposthumous' Harm." *Dialogue* 25 (1986): 727–734.

Warren, James, "The Harm of Death in Cicero's First Tusculan Disputation." In *The Metaphysics and Ethics of Death*, edited by James Stacey Taylor. New York: Oxford University Press, forthcoming.

———, *Facing Death: Epicurus and His Critics*. Oxford: Clarendon Press, 2004.

———, *Epicurus and Democritean Ethics: An Archaeology of Ataraxia*. Cambridge: Cambridge University Press, 2002.

———"Epicurus and the Pleasures of the Future." In *Oxford Studies in Ancient Philosophy XXI*, edited by David Sedley, 135–179. Oxford: Clarendon Press, 2001.

———, "Lucretius, Symmetry Arguments, and Fearing Death." *Phronesis* LXVI, no. 4 (2001): 466–480.

Watkins, Joe, "Archaeological Ethics and American Indians." In *Ethical Issues in Archeology*, edited by Larry J. Zimmerman, Karen D. Vitelli, and Julie Hollowell-Zimmer, 129–141. Lanham, MD: AltaMira Press, 2003.

Waugh, Evelyn, *Brideshead Revisited*. New York: Alfred A. Knopf, 1993.

Weinberg, J., Nichols, S., and Stich, S., "Normativity and Epistemic Intuitions." *Philosophical Topics* 29, nos. 1–2 (2001): 429–460.

Weis, Charles McC., and Pottle, Frederick A., eds., *Boswell in Extremes 1776–1778*. New York: McGraw-Hill Book Company, Inc., 1970.

Werth, James L., Jr., Burke, Caroline, and Bardash, Rebekah J., "Confidentiality in End-of-Life and After-Death Situations." *Ethics and Behavior* 12, no. 3 (2002): 205–222.

Wicclair, Mark R., and deVita, Michael, "Oversight of Research Involving the Dead." *Kennedy Institute of Ethics Journal* 14, no. 2 (2004): 143–164.

Wilkinson, T. M., "Consent and the Use of the Bodies of the Dead." *Journal of Medicine and Philosophy*, forthcoming.

———, *Ethics and the Acquisition of Organs*. New York: Oxford University Press, 2011.

——, "Last Rights: The Ethics of Research on the Dead." *Journal of Applied Philosophy*, 19 (2002): 31–41.

——, "Parental Consent and the Use of Dead Children's Bodies." *Kennedy Institute for Ethics Journal* 11, no. 4 (2001): 337–358.

Williams, Bernard, "The Makropulos Case: Reflections on the Tedium of Immortality." In *The Metaphysics of Death*, edited by John Martin Fischer, 71–92. Stanford, CA: Stanford University Press, 1993.

Willis, Connie, *Doomsday Book*. New York: Spectra, 1993.

Winter, Stephen, "Against Posthumous Rights." *Journal of Applied Philosophy* 27, no. 2 (2010): 186–199.

Wisnewski, J. Jeremy, "What We Owe the Dead." *Journal of Applied Philosophy* 27, no. 1 (2009): 54–70.

——, "Is the Immortal Life Worth Living?" *International Journal for the Philosophy of Religion* 58 (2005): 27–36.

Woolf, Raphael, "Pleasure and Desire." In *The Cambridge Companion to Epicureanism*, edited by James Warren, 158–178. New York: Cambridge University Press, 2009.

——, "What Kind of Hedonist Was Epicurus?" *Phronesis* X:IX, no. 4 (2004): 303–322.

Wright, Ronald, *A Scientific Romance: A Novel*. New York: Picador, 1999.

Wyndham, John, *Trouble with Lichen*. New York: Walker and Company, 1960.

Yost, Benjamin S., "The Irrevocability of Capital Punishment." *Journal of Social Philosophy* 42, no. 3 (2011): 321–340.

Young, Robert, *Medically Assisted Death*. Cambridge: Cambridge University Press, 2007.

Younger, Stuart J., Arnold, Robert M., and Schapiro, Renie, eds., *The Definition of Death: Contemporary Controversies*. Baltimore: Johns Hopkins University Press, 1999.

Yourgrau, Palle, "Kripke's Moses." In *The Metaphysics and Ethics of Death*, edited by James Stacey Taylor. New York: Oxford University Press, forthcoming.

Index